# Pharmacology

## Examination & Board Review

a LANGE medical book

# Pharmacology

## Examination & Board Review

**third edition**

**Bertram G. Katzung, MD, PhD**
Professor of Pharmacology
Department of Pharmacology
University of California, San Francisco

**Anthony J. Trevor, PhD**
Professor of Pharmacology and Toxicology
Department of Pharmacology
University of California, San Francisco

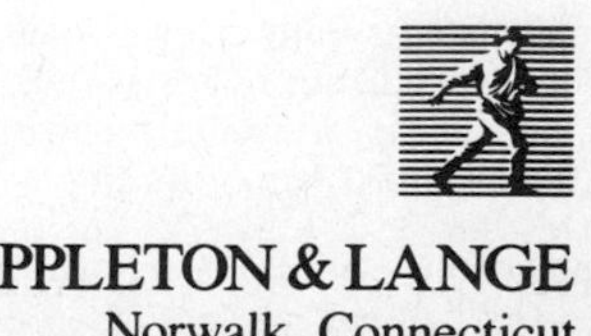

APPLETON & LANGE
Norwalk, Connecticut

0-8385-7807-1

Notice: The authors and the publisher of this volume have taken care to make certain that the doses of drugs and schedules of treatment are correct and compatible with the standards generally accepted at the time of publication. Nevertheless, as new information becomes available, changes in treatment and in the use of drugs become necessary. The reader is advised to carefully consult the instruction and information material included in the package insert of each drug or therapeutic agent before administration. This advise is especially important when using new or infrequently used drugs. The publisher and authors disclaim any liability, loss, injury, or damage incurred as a consequence, directly or indirectly, of the use and application of any of the contents of this volume.

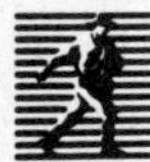



94 95 96 97 / 10 9 8 7 6 5 4 3

Prentice Hall International (UK) Limited, *London*
Prentice Hall of Australia Pty. Limited, *Sydney*
Prentice Hall Canada, Inc., *Toronto*
Prentice Hall Hispanoamericana, S.A., *Mexico*
Prentice Hall of India Private Limited, *New Delhi*
Prentice Hall of Japan, Inc., *Tokyo*
Simon & Schuster Asia Pte. Ltd., *Singapore*
Editora Prentice Hall do Brasil Ltda., *Rio de Janeiro*
Prentice Hall, *Englewood Cliffs, New Jersey*

**ISBN: 0-8385-7807-1**
**ISSN: 1063-8636**

Acquisitions Editor: John Dolan
Production Editor: Charles F. Evans
Cover Designer: Janice Bielawa
Copy Editor: Yvonne Strong

PRINTED IN THE UNITED STATES OF AMERICA

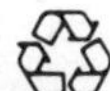

Printed on recycled paper.

# Contents

## . DRUGS WITH IMPORTANT ACTIONS ON SMOOTH MUSCLE



## V. DRUGS THAT ACT IN THE CENTRAL NERVOUS SYSTEM



## VI. DRUGS WITH IMPORTANT ACTIONS ON BLOOD, INFLAMMATION, & GOUT



## VII. ENDOCRINE DRUGS

## X. SPECIAL TOPICS

# Preface

This review book is designed to help students prepare for both regular course exams and "board" exams. Preparing for a large pharmacology examination is a difficult task. It is with good reason, then, that students seek a review or study guide that can make the process more efficient. This book takes a unique approach to the challenge, an approach that has been well tested by successful students over a 10-year period.

First, the book breaks the subject down into the topics used in most courses and textbooks, rather than combining them into larger, unwieldy groups. Major introductory sections (eg, autonomic pharmacology and central nervous system pharmacology) are included, so that students can integrate their review of pharmacology with a review of physiology and biochemistry. This chapter-based approach also encourages students to use the *Review* in conjunction with their course notes or with a larger text.

Second, it explicitly lists the objectives in each unit, providing students with a checklist against which they can challenge themselves as they progress through the book.

Third, each chapter provides a concise and highly organized review of the material that is considered core subject matter by experts in the field. The determination of what is core is based on a careful analysis of the content of actual board examinations over the past several years as well as the content of major medical school courses.

Fourth, a table of important drug names is provided in every chapter dealing with a specific drug group. Recognition of drug names is an important part of board exams. We make the process more efficient by distinguishing between drugs important as prototypes, drugs recognized as major variants of the prototypes, and drugs that should simply be recognized as belonging to a particular drug group.

Finally, each chapter ends with a generous sampling of questions followed by a list of answers and explanations. Because each area of pharmacology is represented by a separate chapter, students are assured of having practice questions in every important area. Questions that require analysis of graphic data or short case descriptions are included. Appendixes I and II comprise long examinations that, together, cover the entire field. According to a 1990 announcement of the National Board of Medical Examiners, the United States Medical Licensure Examination (USMLE) Step 1 will no longer include "K-type" (multiple true/false) and "C-type" (A/B/Both/Neither) questions, starting with the June 1991 exam. "A-type" (best answer) and "B-type" (matching) questions will be retained. However, many faculty members have been using all four of these question types in course exams and will probably continue to do so. We have addressed the needs of students preparing for both board and course examinations by using A-type and B-type questions in individual chapters and Appendix II, but retaining a sampling of K-type questions in the long examination in Appendix I.

The book provides several additional sections of value to the student preparing for a board exam: (1) a set of 18 case histories, with questions and answers, providing additional review and testing of the student's preparation for questions about clinical pharmacology; and (2) a short chapter on test strategies, which summarizes time-saving devices for approaching specific types of questions used on most "objective" exams.

It is recommended that this book be used with a regular text. The reader will find that *Basic & Clinical Pharmacology,* by Katzung (Appleton & Lange, 1992), follows the chapter sequence used here. However, the *Review* is designed to complement any standard medical pharmacology text.

Because it was developed in parallel with the textbook *Basic & Clinical Pharmacology*, the Review represents the authors' interpretations of chapters written by contributors to that text. We are very grateful to these authors, to our other faculty colleagues, and to our students—who have taught us most of what we know about teaching.

Suggestions and criticisms regarding this study guide should be mailed to us at the following address:

Pharmacology Department, Box 0450
University of California
San Francisco, CA 94143-0450, USA

Bertram G. Katzung, MD, PhD
Anthony J. Trevor, PhD
San Francisco
September 1991

# Part I. Basic Principles

# Introduction 1

## OBJECTIVES

**Define the following terms:**

- Absorption
- Biodisposition
- Distribution
- Drug
- Elimination
- Excretion
- Metabolism
- Permeation
- Pharmacodynamics
- Pharmacokinetics
- Pharmacology
- $pK_a$
- Special carrier
- Termination of action
- Toxicology
- Weak acid, weak base
- Zero-order, first-order elimination

**You should be able to:**

- Predict the relative ease of permeation of a weak acid or base if you are given its $pK_a$ and the pH of the medium.
- List and discuss the common routes of drug administration and excretion.
- Draw graphs of the blood level versus time for drugs subject to zero-order elimination and for drugs subject to first-order elimination.

## GENERAL DEFINITIONS

**A. Pharmacology:** Pharmacology is the study of the interaction of chemicals with living systems.

**B. Drugs:** Drugs are substances that act on living systems at the chemical (molecular) level.

**C. Medical Pharmacology:** Medical pharmacology is the study of drugs used for the diagnosis, prevention, and treatment of disease.

**D. Toxicology:** Toxicology is the study of the untoward effects of chemical agents on living systems. It is usually considered an area of pharmacology.

**E. Pharmacodynamics:** Pharmacodynamics refers to the action of a drug on the body, including receptor interactions, dose-response phenomena, and mechanisms of therapeutic and toxic action.

**F. Pharmacokinetics:** Pharmacokinetics refers to the action of the body on the drug, including absorption, distribution, metabolism, and excretion. A drug may be eliminated by metabolism or by excretion. **Biodisposition** is a term sometimes used to describe the processes of metabolism and excretion.

## CONCEPTS

**A. Permeation:** Permeation is the movement of drug molecules within the biologic environment. Permeation involves several processes. The 4 most important are the following:

1. **Aqueous diffusion.** Aqueous diffusion is the simple diffusion of molecules through the watery extracellular and intracellular spaces. Membranes of most capillaries have small aqueous pores that permit the aqueous diffusion of molecules up to the size of small proteins.
2. **Lipid diffusion.** Lipid diffusion of molecules refers to solution in and diffusion through membranes and other lipid structures.
3. **Transport by special carriers.** Transport of drugs across barriers sometimes occurs by carrier mechanisms developed for related endogenous substances, eg, the secretory and reabsorptive carriers for weak acids located in the renal tubule.
4. **Endocytosis, pinocytosis.** Endocytosis refers to binding of a molecule to specialized components of the membrane with subsequent internalization by infolding of that area of the membrane. Some drugs, especially peptides, enter cells by this mechanism. Exocytosis is the reverse process, ie, the expulsion of membrane-encapsulated material from cells.

## B. Water & Lipid Solubility of Drugs:

1. The aqueous solubility of a drug is often a function of the electrostatic charge (degree of ionization, polarity) of the molecule, because water molecules behave as dipoles and are attracted to charged drug molecules, forming an aqueous shell around them. Conversely, the lipid solubility is inversely proportionate to the charge.
2. A large number of drugs are weak bases or weak acids. The pH of the medium determines the fraction of molecules charged (ionized) if the molecule is a weak acid or base. If the $pK_a$ of the drug and the pH of the medium are known, this fraction can be predicted by means of the Henderson-Hasselbalch equation:

$$\log\left(\frac{\text{Protonated form}}{\text{Unprotonated form}}\right) = pK_a - pH$$

"Protonated" means *associated with a proton* (a hydrogen ion); this form of the equation is applicable to both acids and bases.

3. Weak bases are ionized—and therefore more polar and more water soluble—when they are protonated; weak acids are less ionized—and so less water soluble—when they are protonated. The following equations summarize these points:

| $RNH_3^+$ | $\rightleftharpoons$ | $RNH_2$ | + | $H^+$ |
|---|---|---|---|---|
| **protonated weak base (charged, more water-soluble)** | | **unprotonated weak base (uncharged, more lipid-soluble)** | | **proton** |

| RCOOH | $\rightleftharpoons$ | $RCOO^-$ | + | $H^+$ |
|---|---|---|---|---|
| **protonated weak acid (uncharged, more lipid-soluble)** | | **unprotonated weak acid (charged, more water-soluble)** | | **proton** |

## C. Absorption of Drugs:

1. Drugs usually enter the body at sites remote from the target tissue or organ and must be carried by the circulation to the intended site of action. Before a drug can enter the bloodstream, it must be absorbed; the rate and efficiency of absorption differ depending on the route of administration. Common routes of administration of drugs and some of their features include the following:
   a. **Oral (swallowed):** Offers maximum convenience but may be slower and less complete than parenteral routes. Is subject to the first-pass effect (metabolism of a significant amount of the agent in the gut wall and the liver before it reaches the systemic circulation).
   b. **Buccal (in the pouch between gums and cheek):** Permits direct absorption into the systemic venous circulation, bypassing the hepatic portal circuit and first-pass metabolism. May be fast or slow depending on the physical formulation of the product.
   c. **Sublingual (under the tongue):** Offers the same features as the buccal route.
   d. **Rectal (suppository):** Offers partial escape from the first-pass effect (though not as complete as the sublingual route). Larger amounts of drug may be administered than by the buccal or sublingual route. Some drugs may cause significant irritation.

e. **Intramuscular:** Absorption is sometimes (not always) faster and more complete than with oral administration. Large volumes (eg, 5–10 mL) may be given.

f. **Subcutaneous:** Offers slower absorption than intramuscular. Large volumes are not feasible.

g. **Inhalation:** For respiratory diseases, offers delivery closest to the target tissue; often provides rapid absorption because of the large alveolar surface area available.

h. **Topical:** Application to the skin or mucous membrane of the eye, nose, throat, airway, or vagina for *local* effect. The rate of absorption varies with the area of application and the drug formulation, but is usually lower than for any of the routes listed above.

i. **Transdermal:** Application to the skin for *systemic* effect. Absorption is usually very slow, but the first-pass effect is avoided.

j. **Intravenous:** Offers instantaneous and complete absorption (by definition, 100%); potentially more dangerous than less direct routes.

## D. Distribution of Drugs:

1. The distribution of drugs to the various tissues depends upon the following:

   a. **Size** of the organ. For example, skeletal muscle is a very large organ and can take up a large amount of drug. In contrast, the brain is smaller, and therefore the same drug concentration is achieved with a much smaller dose of drug if other factors are equal.

   b. **Blood flow** to the tissue (important in the *rate* of uptake).

   c. **Solubility** of the drug in the tissue. For example, some organs (eg, the brain) have a high lipid content and thus dissolve a higher concentration of lipid-soluble agents than organs with a low lipid content (eg, skeletal muscle).

   d. **Binding** of the drug to macromolecules in the blood or tissue.

2. The **apparent volume of distribution (Vd)** is an important pharmacokinetic parameter, which relates the amount of drug in the body to its concentration in the plasma. See Chapter 3.

## E. Metabolism of Drugs:

1. The action of many drugs (eg, local anesthetics, phenothiazines) is terminated before they are excreted because they are metabolized (chemically converted) to biologically inactive derivatives.

2. Some drugs (**pro-drugs,** eg, levodopa) are inactive as administered and must be metabolized in the body to become active.

3. Other drugs (eg, lithium) are not modified by the body and continue to act until they are excreted.

## F. Elimination of Drugs:

1. The rate of elimination (disappearance of the active molecule from the bloodstream or body) is usually related to termination of effect. A knowledge of the time course of a drug's concentration in plasma is therefore important in predicting the intensity and duration of its effect. ***Note:*** *Elimination* is not the same as *excretion;* a drug may be eliminated by metabolism long before the molecules are excreted from the body. Conversely, for drugs with active metabolites (eg, diazepam), elimination by metabolism is *not* synonymous with termination of action. For drugs (such as penicillin G) that are not metabolized, excretion is the mode of elimination.

   a. **First-order elimination:** First order implies that the rate of elimination is proportionate to the concentration; the result is that the concentration of the drug in plasma decreases exponentially with time. Drugs with first-order elimination have a characteristic **half-life of elimination** that is constant regardless of the amount in the body. The concentration of such a drug in the blood will decrease by 50% for every half-life. Most of the drugs in clinical use demonstrate first-order kinetics.

   b. **Zero-order elimination:** Zero order implies that the rate of elimination is constant regardless of concentration. A few drugs saturate their elimination mechanisms even at low concentrations. As a result, the concentration of the drug in plasma decreases in a linear fashion over time. This is typical of ethanol (over most of its concentration range in plasma) and of phenytoin and aspirin at high therapeutic or toxic concentrations.

## G. Pharmacokinetic Models:

1. Many drugs undergo an early distribution phase, followed by a slower elimination phase, after intravenous administration. Mathematically, this behavior can be modeled by means of a

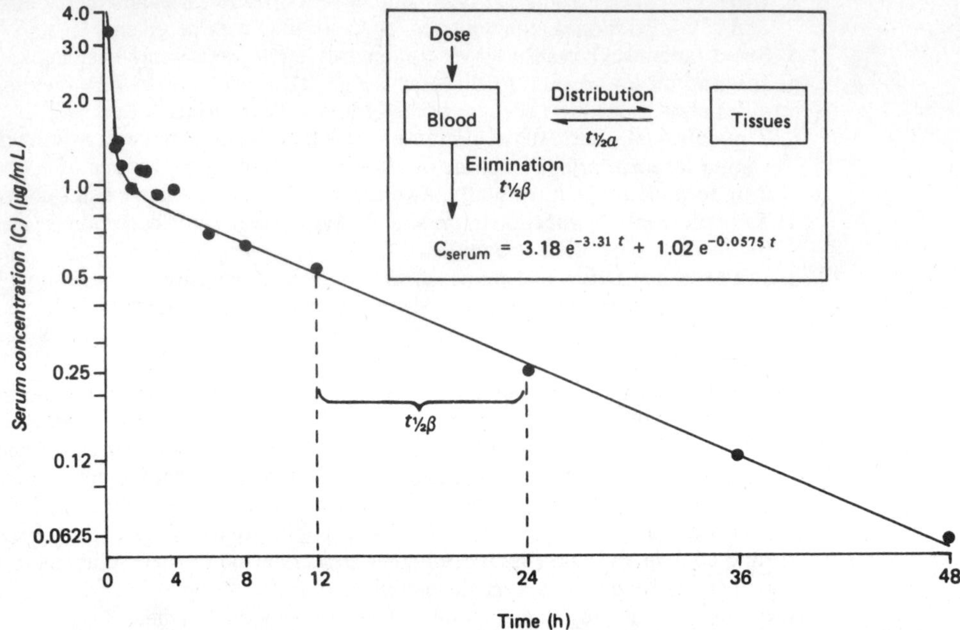


**Figure 1–1.** Serum concentration-time curve after administration of 25 mg of chlordiazepoxide as an intravenous bolus to a 75-kg man. The experimental data are plotted on a semilogarithmic scale as filled circles. If the drug is assumed to follow 2-compartment kinetics (inset), the initial curvilinear portion of the data represents the distribution phase, with drug moving into the tissues. The linear portion of the curve represents drug elimination. The equation shown in the inset was fitted to the data and generated the smooth curve passing through the data points. The elimination half-life ($t_{½β}$) can be extracted in 2 ways: graphically, by measuring the time between any 2 points that differ by 2-fold plasma concentration; and numerically, from the exponent of the second term of the equation, ie, $t_{½β} = 0.693 \div 0.0575 = 12$ hours ($t$ = time). See Chapter 3 for additional details. (Modified and reproduced, with permission, from Greenblatt DJ, Koch-Weser J: Drug therapy: Clinical pharmacokinetics. *N Engl J Med* 1975;293:702.)

"2-compartment model" as shown in Fig 1–1. (Note that each phase is associated with a characteristic half-life: $t_{½α}$ for the first phase, $t_{½β}$ for the second, etc.)

2. A few drugs may behave as though they are distributed to only one compartment (eg, if they are restricted to the vascular compartment). Others have more complex distributions that require 2 or more compartments for accurate modeling.

## QUESTIONS

**DIRECTIONS (items 1–8):** Each numbered item or incomplete statement in this section is followed by answers or by completions of the statement. Select the ONE lettered answer or completion that is BEST in each case.

**1.** All of the following are mechanisms of drug permeation EXCEPT:
- **(A)** aqueous diffusion
- **(B)** aqueous hydrolysis
- **(C)** lipid diffusion
- **(D)** pinocytosis or endocytosis
- **(E)** special carrier transport

2. Promethazine is an antihistaminic drug. It is a weak base with a $pK_a$ of 9.1. In the treatment of an overdose of the drug,
   (A) urinary excretion would be accelerated by administration of $NH_4Cl$
   (B) urinary excretion would be accelerated by giving $NaHCO_3$
   (C) more of the drug would be ionized at blood pH than at stomach pH
   (D) the drug would be absorbed faster from the stomach than from the small intestine
   (E) hemodialysis is the only effective therapy for overdose.

3. All of the following statements about routes of drug administration are correct EXCEPT:
   (A) Concentrations in blood often rise faster after intramuscular injection than after oral dosing
   (B) The "first-pass" effect is the result of metabolism of a drug after administration and before it enters the systemic circulation
   (C) Administration of antiasthmatic drugs by aerosol is usually associated with more adverse effects than is giving the drug systemically
   (D) Bioavailability of most drugs is lower with rectal (suppository) administration than with the intravenous route
   (E) Administration of a drug by transdermal patch is often slow, but is associated with less first-pass metabolism than oral administration

4. Aspirin is a weak organic acid with a $pK_a$ of 3.5. What percentage of a given dose will be in the lipid-soluble form at a stomach pH of 2.5?
   (A) 1%
   (B) 10%
   (C) 50%
   (D) 90%
   (E) 99%

5. If the plasma concentration of a drug is said to decline with first-order kinetics, it means that
   (A) there is only one metabolic path for drug disposition
   (B) the half-life is the same regardless of the plasma concentration
   (C) the drug is largely metabolized in the liver after oral administration and has low bioavailability
   (D) the rate of elimination is proportionate to the rate of administration
   (E) the drug is not distributed outside the vascular system

6. Regarding the termination of action of drugs that have no endogenous counterparts,
   (A) drugs must be excreted from the body to terminate their action
   (B) metabolism of drugs always increases their water solubility
   (C) metabolism of drugs always abolishes their pharmacologic activity
   (D) hepatic metabolism and renal excretion are the 2 most important mechanisms
   (E) distribution of drug out of the bloodstream terminates its effects

7. Distribution of drugs to tissues
   (A) is independent of blood flow to the organ
   (B) is independent of the solubility of the drug in a given tissue
   (C) depends on the concentration gradient between blood and tissue
   (D) is increased for drugs that are strongly bound to plasma proteins
   (E) has no effect on the half-life of the drug

8. Physiologic blood flows and volumes are important in drug distribution because
   (A) skeletal muscle receives the largest fraction of the cardiac output at rest
   (B) drugs that are restricted to the plasma vascular space have a volume of distribution of about 12% of body weight
   (C) in pregnancy, the placenta and uterus receive the largest fraction of the cardiac output
   (D) drugs that are strongly bound to proteins outside the vascular space may have a volume of distribution greater than the body volume
   (E) the larger the blood flow to the major organs, the larger the volume of distribution will be

**DIRECTIONS (items 9–12):** Each group of items in this section consists of lettered headings followed by a numbered phrase or statement. For each numbered phrase or statement, select the ONE lettered heading that is most closely associated with it. Each lettered heading may be selected once, more than once, or not at all.

Item 9

**(A)** Weak acid with $pK_a$ of 2.5
**(B)** Weak base with $pK_a$ of 2.5
**(C)** Weak acid with $pK_a$ of 7.5
**(D)** Weak base with $pK_a$ of 7.5

**9.** Excretion will be most significantly accelerated by acidification of the urine.

Items 10–12

**(A)** Distribution
**(B)** Pharmacodynamics
**(C)** First-pass effect
**(D)** Pharmacokinetics
**(E)** Elimination

**10.** Word that refers to the effects of a drug on the body

**11.** Word that refers to the effects of the body on a drug

**12.** Word that refers to the process by which the amount of active drug in the body is reduced

## ANSWERS

**1.** Hydrolysis has nothing to do with the mechanisms of permeation; rather, it is one mechanism of drug metabolism. The answer is **(B).**

**2.** Questions that deal with acid-base (Henderson-Hasselbalch) manipulations are found on almost every board exam. This is one form. Since absorption involves permeation across lipid membranes, we can treat an overdose by decreasing reabsorption from the tubular urine by making the drug *less lipid soluble.* We know that ionization attracts water molecules and decreases lipid solubility. The drug is a weak base, which means that it will be more ionized (protonated) at acid pH than at a basic pH. All of the choices are variations on the theme of lipid permeation. Choice **(C)** puts it directly: it suggests that the drug would be more ionized at pH 7.4 than at pH 2. So **(C)** is wrong. **(D)** says (in effect) that the more ionized form will be absorbed faster and that is wrong. **(A)** and **(B)** are opposites, since $NH_4Cl$ is an acidifying salt and sodium bicarbonate an alkalizing one. From a purely test strategy point of view, opposites always deserve careful attention and, in this case, permit us to exclude **(E)**, a distractor. If we consider the fact that lipid solubility favors reabsorption from the renal tubule back into the body, it should be clear that ionizing the molecule would reduce reabsorption. Since an acidic environment favors ionization, we should give $NH_4Cl$. The answer is **(A).**

**3.** **(A), (B), (D),** and **(E)** are correct statements. **(C)** is wrong: delivering the drug directly to the target organ usually reduces adverse effects, because the total dose is lower and the concentration reaching other organs is lower.

**4.** Henderson-Hasselbalch principles again. The drug is an acid, so it will be more ionized at a basic pH. The equation says the ratio will change from 50/50 at the pH equal to the $pK_a$ to 10/1 (protonated/unprotonated) at 1 pH unit more acid than the $pK_a$. For acids, the protonated form is the nonionized, more lipid-soluble form. The answer is **(D).**

**5.** Definitions, see the first page of this unit. First-order means that the elimination is proportionate to the concentration perfusing the organ of elimination. The result is that a plot of the logarithm of the plasma concentration on the vertical axis versus time on the horizontal axis is a straight line. The half-life is a constant. (Zero-order elimination means that a constant number of moles or grams are eliminated per unit of time, regardless of plasma concentration. The half-life will then be concentration-dependent and is not a useful variable. Ethanol is the most common drug with zero-order elimination.) The rate of elimination is equal to the rate of administration when the amount of drug in the body is at steady-state; it is independent of whether elimination is zero or first order. Most drugs, regardless of order of elimination, are distributed outside the vascular compartment. The answer is **(B)**.

**6.** Note the "trigger" words (must, always) in choices **(A)**, **(B)**, and **(C)**. All drugs that affect tissues other than circulating blood act outside of the "bloodstream." The answer is **(D)**.

**7.** Fairly straightforward. There are no trigger words to give the answer away, but it can be reasoned out without much trouble. Given the above list of determinants of drug distribution (Concepts, item D), choice **(C)** is correct.

**8.** Choice **(A)** is wrong because resting muscle is specified. At rest, skeletal muscle receives about 16% of the cardiac output while the liver receives 28% and the kidneys 23%. During maximal exercise, muscle would indeed receive the largest fraction of cardiac output. The plasma volume is normally about 3–4% of the body weight. Uterine and placental blood flow is only about 9% of cardiac output, even at term. High total blood flow (cardiac output) may affect the *rate* of distribution to the tissues, but has no effect on the *volume* of distribution. The answer is **(D)**.

**9.** Since acceleration of excretion requires an increase in the ionized fraction in the urine, the basic drugs are the ones to be considered here. How much would their excretion be affected by the degree of urinary acidification achievable (ie, within the physiologic range of pH 5.5 to 8)? Clearly, a basic drug with a $pK_a$ much lower than this range will not be significantly ionized: The drug of $pK_a$ 2.5 will go from 1 part in 300,000 ionized at pH 8 to 1 part in 1000 ionized at pH 5.5—ie, less than 0.1% change in the total nonionized fraction. In contrast, the basic drug of $pK_a$ 7.5 is about 32% ionized, 68% nonionized at pH 8 but changes to 1% nonionized, 99% ionized at pH 5.5. The answer is **(D)**.

**10.** More definitions. Pharmacodynamics—choice **(B)**— is the term given to the processes of drug action on the body.

**11.** Pharmacokinetics is the general term that describes all the actions of the body on the drug. The answer is **(D)**.

**12.** The amount of active drug is reduced by excretion and metabolism, processes that are included in the term "elimination." The answer is **(E)**.

# 2 Pharmacodynamics

## OBJECTIVES

**Define the following terms:**

- Chemical antagonist
- Competitive antagonist
- Coupling protein
- Drug efficacy
- Drug potency
- ED50, TD50, LD50
- Effector
- Effector mechanism
- Graded dose-response curve
- Irreversible antagonist
- Partial agonist
- Physiologic antagonist
- Quantal dose-response curve
- Receptor
- Receptor agonist
- Spare receptor

**You should be able to:**

- Specify whether an antagonist is competitive or irreversible on the basis of its effect on the dose-response curve of the agonist.
- Compare the efficacy and potency of drugs on the basis of their dose-response curves.
- Predict the effect of a partial agonist on a system in the presence and in the absence of a full agonist.
- Name an important inert binding-site protein in blood.
- Predict the effect of adding drug ***B*** when a barely subtoxic dose of drug ***A*** is present if drug ***A*** and drug ***B*** both bind to the same inert binding site.
- Give examples of partial agonists, competitive and irreversible antagonists, and physiologic and chemical antagonists.
- Name the coupling and effector proteins that are activated by the beta adrenoceptor.
- Name 4 methods by which drug-receptor signals bring about effects.

## DEFINITIONS & CONCEPTS

**A. Receptors:** Receptors are the specific molecular components of a biologic system with which drugs interact to produce changes in the function of the system. Receptors must be selective in their ligand-binding characteristics (so as to respond to the proper chemical signal and not to meaningless ones) and must be modifiable as a result of binding (to bring about the functional change). Many receptors have been identified, purified, and chemically characterized. The receptors characterized to date are proteins and other macromolecules such as DNA. The receptor site for a drug is a specific area of the macromolecule that has a high and selective affinity for the drug molecule. The interaction of a drug with its receptor is the fundamental event that initiates the action of the drug.

**B. Effectors:** Molecules that translate the drug-receptor interaction into a change in cellular activity. The best examples of effectors are enzymes such as adenylyl (formerly called adenylate) cyclase. Some receptors are also effectors.

**C. Spare Receptors:** Spare receptors are said to exist when the maximum drug response is obtained at less than saturation (complete occupation) of the receptors. This might result from one of several mechanisms. First, the effect of the drug-receptor interaction may persist much longer than the interaction itself. Second, the actual number of receptors may exceed the number of effector molecules available. The effect of having spare receptors in a system is to increase its sensitivity to the agonist.

**D. Inert Binding Sites:** Inert binding sites are sites on endogenous molecules that bind a drug without initiating events leading to the drug's effects. In many compartments of the body (eg, the plasma), they play an important role in buffering the concentration of a drug. The 2 most important plasma proteins with significant binding capacity are albumin and orosomucoid ($\alpha_1$-acid glycoprotein).

E. **Agonist, Partial Agonist:** An agonist is a drug capable of fully activating the effector system when it binds to the receptor. A partial agonist produces less than the full effect, even when it has saturated the receptors (Fig 2–1). In the presence of a full agonist, a partial agonist acts like a competitive inhibitor.

F. **Competitive & Irreversible Antagonists:** Competitive antagonists are drugs that bind to the receptor in a reversible way without activating the effector system for that receptor. The effects of competitive antagonists can be overcome by adding more agonist. However, the effects of irreversible antagonists cannot be overcome by adding more agonist. The graded dose-response curves generated in the presence of these 2 types of inhibitors differ (Fig 2–2).

G. **Physiologic Antagonist:** A physiologic antagonist is a drug that binds to some other receptor, producing an effect opposite to that produced by the drug it is antagonizing.

H. **Chemical Antagonist:** A chemical antagonist is a chelator or similar agent that interacts directly with the drug being antagonized to remove it or to prevent it from reaching its target. A chemical antagonist does not depend on interaction with the agonist's receptor (although such interaction may occur).

I. **Efficacy:** Efficacy refers to the effect that a drug can produce, regardless of dose. Thus, *maximal efficacy* is the maximum effect an agonist can produce if the maximum dose is taken. Efficacy, which is determined by the nature of the receptor and its associated effector system, can be measured only by using a graded dose-response curve (Fig 2–1).

J. **Potency:** Potency denotes the amount of a drug needed to produce a given effect. In graded dose-response measurements, the effect usually chosen is 50% of the maximum effect (the EC50). Potency is determined mainly by the affinity of the receptor for the drug. In quantal dose-response measurements, ED50, TD50, and LD50 are typical potency measurements (effective, toxic, and lethal doses, respectively, in 50% of a population). Thus, potency can be determined from either graded or quantal dose-response curves (eg, Figs 2–1 and 2–3), but the numbers obtained are not identical.

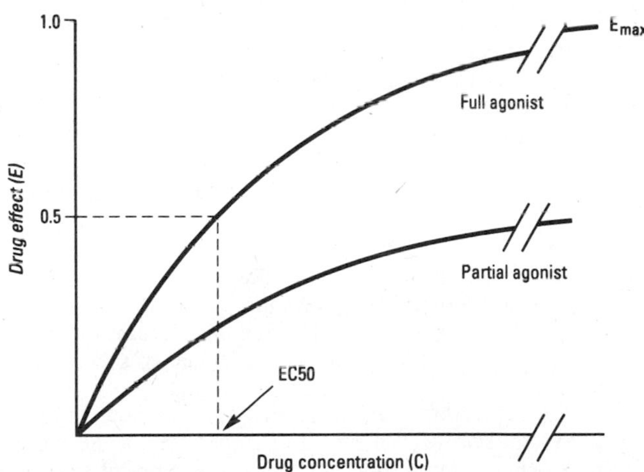


**Figure 2–1.** Relation between drug concentration and drug effect. The concentration at which the effect is half-maximal is denoted EC50. If receptor-bound drug is plotted against drug concentration, a similar curve is obtained, and the concentration at which 50% of the receptors are associated with drug is denoted $K_D$. (Modified and reproduced, with permission, from Katzung BG [editor]: *Basic & Clinical Pharmacology,* 5th ed. Appleton & Lange, 1992.)

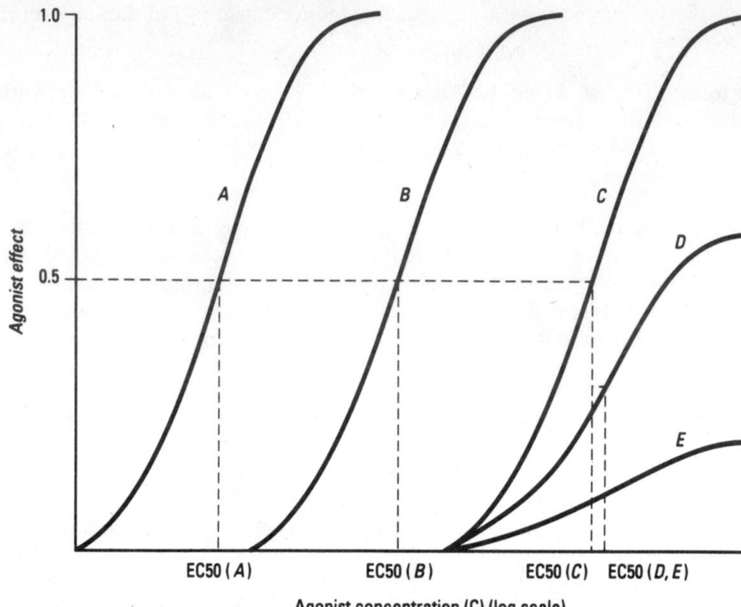


**Figure 2–2.** Agonist dose-response curves in the presence of competitive and noncompetitive antagonists. Note the use of a logarithmic scale for drug concentration. A competitive antagonist has an effect illustrated by curves *A*, *B*, and *C*. A noncompetitive antagonist shifts the curves downward (curves *D* and *E* ). (Modified and reproduced, with permission, from Katzung BG [editor]: *Basic & Clinical Pharmacology,* 5th ed. Appleton & Lange, 1992.)

**K. Graded Dose-Response Relationships:** When the response of a particular system (isolated tissue, animal, or patient) is measured against increasing concentrations of a drug, the graph of the response versus the drug concentration or dose is called a graded dose-response curve (Fig 2–1). In the presence of a competitive antagonist, the log dose versus response curve is shifted to higher doses (ie, horizontally on the dose axis) but still reaches the same maximum effect. In contrast, an irreversible antagonist causes a downward shift of the maximum, with no shift of the curve on the dose axis unless spare receptors are present (Fig 2–2).

**L. Quantal Dose-Response Relationships:** When the dose required to produce a specified response is determined in each member of a large population, the quantal dose-response relationship is defined (Fig 2–3). When plotted as the fraction of the population that responds at each dose level versus the log of the dose administered, a cumulative quantal dose-response curve, which is usually sigmoid, is obtained. The median effective (ED50), median toxic (TD50), and median lethal (LD50) doses are determined from experiments carried out in this manner.

**M. Therapeutic Index:** The therapeutic index is the ratio of the TD50 (or LD50) to the ED50. It represents an estimate of the safety of a drug, since a very safe drug might be expected to have a very large toxic dose and a small effective dose. Unfortunately, several factors make this estimate a poor safety index (see textbook discussions of this variable).

**N. Signaling Mechanisms:** Once an agonist drug has bound to its receptor, some effector mechanism is activated. For many useful drugs, the effector mechanism is located inside the cell or modifies some intracellular process. Four major types of transmembrane signaling mechanisms for drugs have been defined:

1. Some drugs, especially more lipid-soluble agents (eg, steroid hormones) may cross the membrane and combine with an intracellular receptor.
2. Ion channel-regulating drugs (eg, acetylcholine at the nicotinic receptor) may directly regulate the opening of an ion channel.

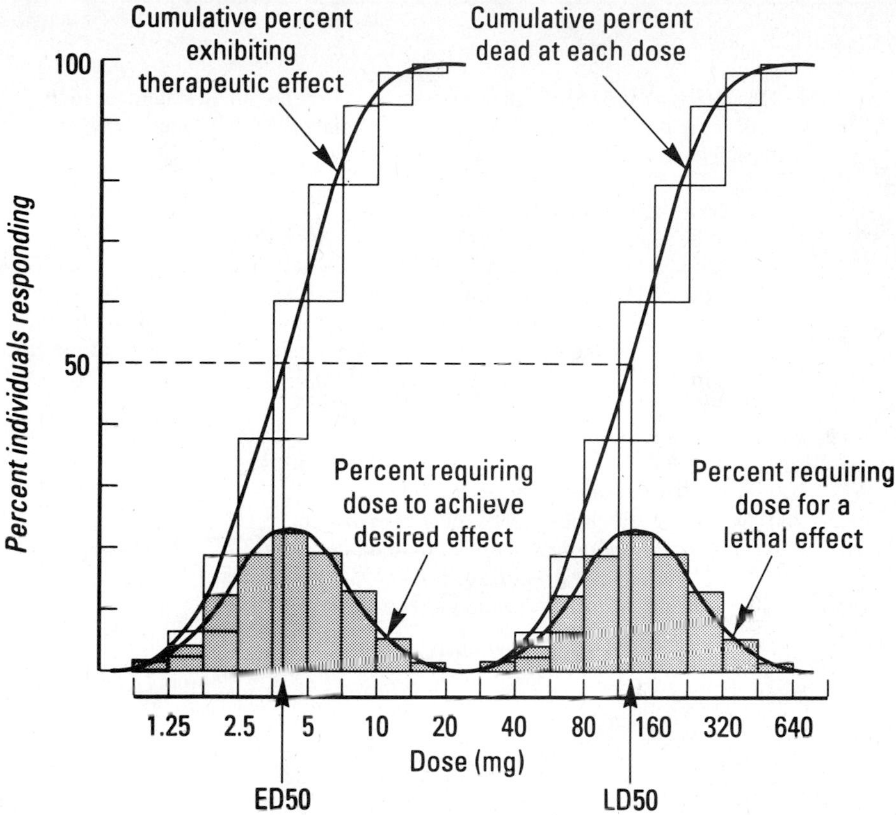


**Figure 2–3.** Quantal dose-effect plots. Shaded boxes (and the accompanying curves) indicate the frequency distribution of doses of drug required to produce a specified effect, ie, the percentage of animals that required a particular dose to exhibit the effect. Open boxes (and corresponding curves) indicate the cumulative frequency distribution of responses, which are lognormally distributed. (Reproduced, with permission, from Katzung BG [editor]: *Basic & Clinical Pharmacology,* 5th ed. Appleton & Lange, 1992.)

3. Enzyme-regulating drugs (eg, insulin) may combine with the extracellular portion of membrane-spanning enzymes and modify their intracellular activity.
4. Drugs may bind to receptors that are linked by coupling proteins to intracellular effectors. The best defined examples are the sympathomimetic drugs, which activate or inhibit adenylyl cyclase by activating "G" proteins that have either stimulant or inhibitory effects on the cyclase.
   a. Activation is brought about by drugs that bind to beta adrenoceptors; the drug-receptor interaction is coupled to the effector (adenylyl cyclase) by a stimulatory coupling protein, $G_s$.
   b. Inhibition is accomplished by binding of drug to alpha adrenoceptors; this interaction is coupled to adenylyl cyclase by another G protein, $G_i$.

## QUESTIONS

**DIRECTIONS (items 1–5):** Each numbered item or incomplete statement in this section is followed by answers or by completions of the statement. Select the ONE lettered answer or completion that is BEST in each case.

**1.** Quantal dose-response curves are
(A) used in determining the therapeutic index for a drug
(B) used for determining the maximal efficacy of a drug
(C) invalid in the presence of inhibitors of the drug being studied
(D) obtainable from the study of intact subjects but not from isolated tissue
(E) used to determine the statistical variation (standard deviation) of the maximal response to the drug

**2.** Two drugs, ***A*** and ***B***, have the same mechanism of action. Drug ***A*** in a dose of 5 mg produces the same magnitude of effect as drug ***B*** in a dose of 500 mg.
(A) Drug ***B*** is less efficacious than drug ***A***
(B) Drug ***A*** is 100 times more potent than drug ***B***
(C) The toxicity of drug ***A*** is lower than that of drug ***B***
(D) Drug ***A*** is a better drug if maximal efficacy is needed
(E) Drug ***A*** has a shorter duration of action

**3.** The results shown in Graph 2–1 were obtained in a comparison of positive inotropic agents.

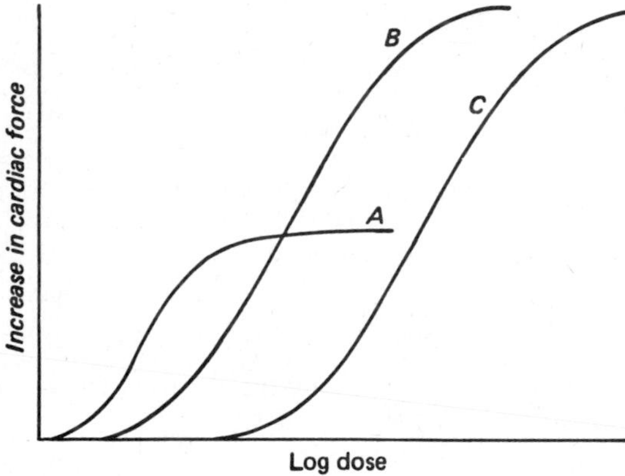


**Graph 2–1.**

(A) Drug ***A*** is the most effective
(B) Drug ***B*** is the least potent
(C) Drug ***C*** is the most potent
(D) Drug ***B*** is more potent than drug ***C*** and more effective than drug ***A***
(E) Drug ***A*** is more potent than drug ***B*** and more effective than drug ***C***

**4.** In the absence of other drugs, pindolol causes an increase in heart rate by activating beta receptors. However, in the presence of highly effective beta stimulants, pindolol causes a dose-dependent, reversible decrease in heart rate. Therefore, pindolol is probably a
(A) noncompetitive antagonist
(B) physiologic antagonist
(C) chemical antagonist
(D) partial agonist
(E) spare receptor agonist

**5.** All of the following statements about spare receptors are correct EXCEPT:
- **(A)** Spare receptors are identical, in the absence of drug, to nonspare receptors
- **(B)** Spare receptors do not bind drug when the maximal drug effect first occurs
- **(C)** Spare receptors influence the sensitivity of the receptor system to the drug
- **(D)** Spare receptors activate the effector machinery of the cell without the need for a drug
- **(E)** Spare receptors may be detected by the finding that the EC50 is less than the $K_D$ for the agonist

**DIRECTIONS (items 6–11):** Each group of items in this section consists of lettered headings followed by a set of numbered statements or phrases. For each numbered statement or phrase, select the ONE lettered heading that is most closely associated with it. Each lettered heading may be selected once, more than once, or not at all.

Items 6–8

- **(A)** Pharmacologic antagonist
- **(B)** Partial agonist
- **(C)** Physiologic antagonist
- **(D)** Chemical antagonist
- **(E)** Noncompetitive antagonist

**6.** A drug that mediates the reversal of histamine bronchoconstriction (mediated at histamine receptors), eg, epinephrine (acting at adrenoceptors)

**7.** A drug that interacts directly with the agonist and not at all, or only incidentally, with the receptor

**8.** A drug that blocks the action of epinephrine at its receptors by occupying those receptors without activating them

Items 9–11

- **(A)** Maximum efficacy
- **(B)** Therapeutic index
- **(C)** Inert binding site
- **(D)** Graded dose-response curve
- **(E)** Quantal dose-response curve

**9.** Provides information about the standard deviation of sensitivity to the drug in the population studied

**10.** Binds drug molecules but causes no biologic response

**11.** The largest effect a drug can produce, regardless of dose

## ANSWERS

**1.** Graded dose-response curves must be used for determining maximal efficacy (maximal response). Quantal dose-response curves show only the frequency of occurrence of a specified response. This specified response may be either therapeutic (ED) or toxic (TD). Dividing the TD50 by the ED50 gives the therapeutic index. The answer is **(A)**.

**2.** No information is given regarding the magnitude of the maximum response to either drug. Similarly, no information about toxicity is available, since the "response" mentioned is not defined as either therapeutic or toxic. The answer is **(B)**.

**3.** These are straightforward graded dose-response curves. Drug ***A*** is the most potent, drug ***C*** the least. Drug ***A*** is less effective than drugs ***B*** and ***C***. The answer is **(D)**.

4. (B) and (C) are clearly incorrect, since pindolol is said to act at beta receptors and to block beta stimulants. The drug is not noncompetitive, since its effect is reversible. "Spare receptor agonist" is a nonsense distracter. The answer is **(D)**.

5. There is no difference between "spare" and other receptors. Spare receptors may be defined as receptors that do not bind drug when the maximal effect is achieved. Spare receptors do influence the sensitivity of the system to an agonist since the statistical probability of a drug-receptor interaction increases with the total number of receptors. Spare receptors do not activate the effector molecule without agonist binding. The answer is **(D)**.

6. Because epinephrine interacts with adrenoceptors and histamine with histamine receptors, epinephrine cannot be a pharmacologic antagonist of histamine. Because the results of adrenoceptor activation oppose the effects of histamine receptor activation, epinephrine must be a physiologic antagonist of histamine. The answer is **(C)**.

7. A chemical antagonist is one that interacts directly (chemically) with the agonist drug and not with a receptor. The answer is **(D)**.

8. See definitions and concepts. The answer is **(A)**.

9. Quantal dose-response curves provide information about the statistical distribution of sensitivity to a drug. The answer is **(E)**.

10. Inert binding sites bind drug molecules (both agonists and antagonists) but cause no biologic response, even when fully saturated. The answer is **(C)**.

11. The largest response a drug can produce represents its maximum efficacy. The answer is **(A)**.

# 3 Pharmacokinetics

## OBJECTIVES

**Define the following terms:**

- Area under the curve (AUC)
- Bioavailability
- Clearance
- Extraction
- First-pass effect
- Half-life
- Hepatic blood flow-limited elimination
- Minimum therapeutic concentration
- Peak and trough concentrations
- Volume of distribution

**You should be able to:**

- Compute the half-life of a drug from its clearance and volume of distribution.
- Calculate loading and maintenance dosage regimens for oral or intravenous administration of a drug when the minimum therapeutic concentration, clearance, and volume of distribution are known.

## DEFINITIONS

**A. Volume of Distribution (Apparent):** The ratio of the amount of a drug in the body to its concentration in the plasma or blood.

**B. Clearance:** The ratio of the rate of elimination of a drug to its concentration in plasma or blood.

**C. Half-Life:** The time it takes for the amount or concentration of a drug to fall to 50% of an earlier measurement. This number is a constant, regardless of concentration, for drugs eliminated by first-order kinetics. It is not a constant—and therefore not particularly useful—for drugs eliminated by zero-order kinetics (eg, ethanol).

**D. Bioavailability:** The fraction (or percentage) of the administered dose of a drug that reaches the systemic circulation.

**E. Area Under the Curve (AUC):** The graphic area under a plot of drug concentration in plasma versus time after a single dose of the drug. AUC is important for calculating the bioavailability of a drug given by any route other than intravenous.

**F. Peak & Trough Concentrations:** The maximum and minimum drug concentrations—in plasma or blood—measured during cycles of repeated dosing.

**G. Minimum Therapeutic Concentration:** The plasma concentration below which a patient's response is too weak for therapeutic benefit.

**H. First-Pass Effect:** The elimination of drug that occurs after administration but before it reaches the systemic circulation, ie, during passage through the gut wall, portal blood, and liver for an orally administered drug.

**I. Extraction:** The fraction of drug in the plasma that is removed by an organ as it passes through that organ.

## CONCEPTS

**A. Effective Drug Concentration:** Effective drug concentration is the concentration of a drug at the receptor site. Except for topically active agents, this concentration is often a function of the concentration of the drug in plasma. This, in turn, is a function of the rate of **input** of the drug (by absorption) into the plasma, the rate of **distribution** to the peripheral tissues (including the target organ), and the rate of **elimination** from the body. These are all functions of time, but if the rate of input is known the remaining processes are reasonably approximated by 2 primary variables: volume of distribution and clearance.

**B. Volume of Distribution (Vd):**

$$\mathbf{Vd} = \frac{\textbf{amount of drug in the body}}{\textbf{plasma drug concentration}}$$

The calculated parameter for the apparent volume of distribution has no direct physical equivalent. If a drug is avidly bound in peripheral tissues, its concentration in plasma may drop to very low levels even though the total amount in the body is large. As a result, the volume of distribution may greatly exceed the total volume of the body (eg, 50,000 L is the Vd for the drug quinacrine in a person whose physical body volume is 70 L). On the other hand, a drug that is completely retained in the plasma compartment will have a volume of distribution equal to the plasma volume (about 4% of body weight). The volume of distribution of drugs that are normally bound to plasma protein, especially albumin, can be altered by liver disease (through reduced protein synthesis) and kidney disease (through urinary protein loss).

**C. Clearance (CL):**

$$\mathbf{CL} = \frac{\textbf{rate of elimination of the drug}}{\textbf{plasma drug concentration}}$$

The magnitude of this computed parameter may range from a minimum of a few milliliters per minute to a maximum of the total blood flow to the organ of elimination. Clearance depends upon the drug and the perfusion and condition of the organs of elimination in the patient. The clearance by an individual organ is equivalent to the extraction by that organ multiplied by the rate of delivery of drug to the organ. Thus the clearance of a drug that is very effectively extracted by an organ is often flow-limited (ie, the blood is completely cleared of the drug as it passes through the organ) and total clearance from the body is simply a function of blood flow through that organ (ie, it is limited by the blood flow to the organ). In this situation, other conditions—disease, or other drugs that change blood flow—may have more dramatic effects on clearance than disease of the organ of elimination.

**D. Half-Life:** Half-life is a secondary variable, completely determined by volume of distribution and clearance. It can be determined graphically from a plot of the blood level versus time, or from the following relationship:

$$t_{1/2} = \frac{\mathbf{0.693 \times Vd}}{\mathbf{CL}}$$

One must know both primary variables (Vd and CL) to predict changes in half-life. In practice, clearance changes with disease, age, and other variables much more than does volume of distribution. However, the half-life of a drug may not change despite a decreased rate of clearance if the volume of distribution decreases at the same time (as occurs, for example, in the case of lidocaine administration to patients with congestive heart failure).

**E. Bioavailability:** The bioavailability of a drug is the fraction of the administered dose that reaches the systemic circulation. It is defined as unity (or 100%) in the case of intravenous administration. After administration by other routes, bioavailability is generally reduced by incomplete absorption, first-pass metabolism, and any distribution into other tissues (eg, gut wall or liver) that occurs before the drug enters the systemic circulation. To account for differing rates of absorption into the blood, the concentration appearing in the plasma must be integrated over time to obtain an integrated total from the area under the plasma concentration-time curve (AUC).

**F. Extraction:** Removal of a drug by an organ can be specified as the **extraction ratio,** or the fraction of the drug removed from the perfusing blood during its passage through the organ. After steady-state concentration in plasma has been achieved, the extraction ratio is one measure of the elimination of the drug by that organ. Drugs that have a high hepatic extraction ratio have a large first-pass effect, and their bioavailability after oral administration will be low.

**G. Dosage Regimens:** A dosage regimen is a plan for drug administration over a given period. An appropriate dosage regimen will result in therapeutic levels of the drug in the blood without exceeding the minimum toxic concentration. Ideally, the plan is based on knowledge of both the minimum therapeutic and minimum toxic concentrations for a given drug as well as its clearance and volume of distribution.

1. **Maintenance dosage.** This is a function of clearance:

$$\textbf{Dosing rate} = \textbf{clearance} \times \textbf{desired plasma concentration}$$

Note that the volume of distribution is not involved in the above calculation. The dosing rate computed for a maintenance dosage is the average dose per unit time. If clearance is given in milliliters per minute, the resulting dosing rate is a per-minute rate. For chronic therapy, oral administration is desirable and doses should be given only once or a few times per day. The size of the daily dose (dose per minute × 60 minutes per hour × 24 hours per day) is a simple extension of the above information. The number of doses to be given per day is usually determined by the half-life of the drug and the difference between the minimum therapeutic and toxic concentrations. Thus, for a drug with a short half-life (eg, 1 hour), the plasma concentration will decrease to 50% of its peak after 1 hour, to 25% of its peak after 2 hours, etc. If it is important to maintain a concentration above the minimum therapeutic level at all times, either a large dose must be given at long intervals or smaller doses at frequent intervals. If the difference between the toxic and therapeutic concentrations is small, then small doses must be administered frequently to avoid toxicity.

2. **Loading dose:** If the therapeutic concentration must be achieved rapidly, a large loading dose may be needed at the onset of therapy. This is calculated from the following equation:

$$\textbf{Loading dose} = \textbf{volume of distribution} \times \textbf{desired plasma concentration}$$

Note that clearance does not enter into this computation. If the loading dose is very large (Vd much larger than body size), the dose should be given slowly to avoid excessively high peak plasma levels during the distribution phase.

## QUESTIONS

**DIRECTIONS (items 1–10):** Each numbered item or incomplete statement in this section is followed by answers or by completions of the statement. Select the ONE lettered answer or completion that is BEST in each case.

1. Mr Jones is admitted to General Hospital with pneumonia due to gram-negative bacteria. The antibiotic tobramycin is ordered. The CL and Vd of tobramycin in Mr Jones are 80 mL/min and 40 L, respectively. What maintenance dosage must be administered intravenously every 6 hours to eventually obtain average steady-state plasma concentrations of 4 mg/L?
   (A) 0.32 mg
   (B) 115 mg
   (C) 160 mg
   (D) 230 mg
   (E) None of the above

2. If you wish to give Mr Jones (of question 1) a loading dose to achieve the therapeutic plasma concentration of 4 mg/L immediately, how much should you give?
   (A) 0.1 mg
   (B) 10 mg
   (C) 115.2 mg
   (D) 160 mg
   (E) None of the above

3. Despite your careful adherence to basic pharmacokinetic principles, your patient on digoxin therapy has developed digitalis toxicity. The plasma digoxin level is 4 ng/mL. Renal function is normal, and the plasma $t_{1/2}$ of digoxin is 1.6 days. How long should you withhold digoxin to reach a safer yet probably therapeutic level of 1 ng/mL?
   (A) 1.6 days
   (B) 2.4 days
   (C) 3.2 days
   (D) 4.8 days
   (E) 6.4 days

4. Verapamil and phenytoin are both eliminated from the body by metabolism in the liver. Verapamil has a clearance of 1.5 L/min, approximately equal to liver blood flow, whereas phenytoin has a clearance of 0.1 L/min. When these compounds are administered along with a drug that is a hepatic enzyme inducer, which of the following is most likely?
   (A) The clearance of both compounds will be increased
   (B) The clearance of both compounds will be decreased
   (C) The clearance of verapamil will be unchanged, whereas the clearance of phenytoin will be increased
   (D) The clearance of phenytoin will be unchanged, whereas the clearance of verapamil will be increased

5. Drug *X* has a narrow therapeutic index: the minimum toxic plasma concentration is 150 mg/L while the minimum therapeutic plasma concentration is 100 mg/L. The half-life is 6 hours. It is essential to maintain the plasma concentration above the minimum therapeutic level. The most appropriate dosing regimen would be
   (A) once a day
   (B) twice a day
   (C) 3 times a day
   (D) 4 times a day
   (E) none of the above

6. With regard to design of a dosing regimen,
   (A) when a drug is given at an interval equal to twice its half-life or longer, it will not cumulate
   (B) a drug with a very short half-life will be ineffective unless given at intervals less than the half-life
   (C) the steady-state concentration of a drug in the plasma will be equal to the dose multiplied by 0.693 times the volume of distribution divided by the clearance
   (D) if an immediate therapeutic plasma level is desired, the appropriate loading dose is the target plasma concentration times the volume of distribution
   (E) the drug should not be given more than 4 times per day

7. The bioavailability of drugs is
   (A) established by FDA regulation at 100% for preparations for intramuscular injection
   (B) 100% for oral preparations that are not metabolized in the liver
   (C) equal to the amount of drug in the body at the time of peak concentration relative to the dose administered
   (D) important in that bioavailability determines what fraction of the administered dose reaches the systemic circulation
   (E) is less than unity (or 100%) only for orally administered drugs

8. The pharmacokinetics of theophylline include the following average parameters: Vd, 35 L; CL, 48 mL/min; half-life, 8 hours. If an intravenous infusion of theophylline is started, how long will it take to approach a steady-state plasma level, ie, 93.75% of final steady state?
   (A) Approximately 6 hours
   (B) Approximately 48 minutes
   (C) Approximately 8 hours
   (D) Approximately 5.8 hours
   (E) Approximately 32 hours

9. A patient with myocardial infarction has a severe cardiac arrhythmia. A continuous intravenous infusion of lidocaine, 1.92 mg/min, was started at 8 AM. The average pharmacokinetic parameters of lidocaine are as follows: Vd, 77 L; CL, 640 mL/min; half-life, 1.8 hours. The expected steady-state plasma concentration is approximately
   (A) 40 mg/L
   (B) 3.0 mg/L
   (C) 0.025 mg/L
   (D) 7.2 mg/L
   (E) 3.46 mg/L

**10.** Your patient with the lidocaine infusion (question 9) has been receiving the drug for 8 hours, and you decide to obtain a plasma concentration measurement. When the results come back, the plasma level is exactly half of what you expected. The most probable explanation is:
**(A)** The patient's lidocaine volume of distribution is twice the average value
**(B)** The patient's lidocaine clearance is twice the average
**(C)** The patient's lidocaine half-life is twice the average
**(D)** The patient's infusion rate was accidentally decreased by half
**(E)** The laboratory made a mistake in the assay for lidocaine

## ANSWERS

**1.** Maintenance dosage is a function of plasma level and clearance only:

**Rate in = Rate out at steady state**

**Dosage = Plasma level × clearance**
**= 4 mg/L × 0.08 L/min**
**= 0.32 mg/min**
**= 0.32 mg/min × 60 min/h × 6 h**
**= 115.2 mg/dose when given at 6 hour intervals**

The answer is **(B)**.

**2.** Loading dose is a function of volume of distribution and target plasma concentration:

**Loading dose = 40 L × 4 mg/L**

**= 160 mg**

The answer is **(D)**.

**3.** Since the blood level will drop by 50% during each half-life, the level will be 2 ng/mL after 1.6 days and 1 ng/mL after 3.2 days. The answer is **(C)**.

**4.** Apparently verapamil is already metabolized so rapidly that only the rate of delivery to the liver regulates its disappearance; ie, it is blood flow-limited. Further increases in liver enzyme levels could not increase its elimination. However, the rate of elimination of phenytoin is apparently limited by its rate of metabolism (clearance is much less than hepatic blood flow). Therefore, the clearance of phenytoin can rise if some agent causes an increase in liver enzyme levels. The answer is **(C)**.

**5.** The minimum therapeutic plasma concentration of hypothetic drug *X* is 100 units, the minimum toxic concentration is 150 units. If a dose is given that brings the plasma concentration to 150 units, it will fall to 75 units in one half-life, or 6 hours. Since 75 units is less than the minimum therapeutic concentration, even the shortest dosing interval proposed (4 times a day or 6 hours) is too long. The answer is **(E)**.

**6.** "Cumulation" is theoretically possible for any dosing interval; even after 4 half-lives, approximately 6% of the drug remains in the body. The efficacy of a particular drug depends on many variables; some drugs are actually more effective when given at long intervals. The steady-state concentration of a drug is not a function of volume of distribution. The answer is **(D)**.

**7.** Bioavailability is calculated from the ratio of the area under the curve (AUC) after oral administration to the AUC after intravenous administration of the same dose. Many drugs given orally are incompletely absorbed or metabolized in the lumen of the gut, and so they will have a bioavailability less than unity even if they are not metabolized in the liver. Some drugs have a bioavailability of less than unity even when given transdermally or intramuscularly. This parameter is the ratio of the amount found in the circulating blood to the amount administered. The answer is **(D)**.

8. The approach of the drug plasma concentration to steady-state concentration during continuous infusion follows a stereotypic curve that rises rapidly at first and gradually levels off. It reaches 50% of steady state at one half-life, 75% at 2 half-lives, 87.5% at 3, and 93.75% at 4, and progressively decreases the difference between its current level and 100% with each half-life. The answer is **(E)**.

9. The drug is being administered continuously; the steady-state concentration for a continuously administered drug is given by the equation given in question 1. Thus

$$\begin{aligned}
\textbf{Dosage} &= \textbf{Plasma level} \times \textbf{clearance} \\
\textbf{1.92 mg/min} &= \textbf{Plasma level} \times \textbf{clearance} \\
\textbf{Plasma level} &= \textbf{1.92 mg/min} \div \textbf{clearance} \\
\textbf{Plasma level} &= \textbf{1.92 mg/min} \div \textbf{640 mL/min} \\
\textbf{Plasma level} &= \textbf{0.003 mg/mL (3 mg/L)}
\end{aligned}$$

The answer is **(B)**.

10. If the half-life is 1.8 hours, the plasma concentration should be approaching steady state after 8 hours (more than 4 half-lives). As indicated by the equation, the steady-state concentration is a function of dosage and clearance, not volume of distribution. If the plasma level is lower than predicted, the clearance must be greater than average in this patient. (In a question of this type, do not assume errors of analysis or administration as answers unless all other possible answers can be positively ruled out.) The answer is **(B)**.

# 4 Drug Metabolism

## OBJECTIVES

**Define the following terms:**

- Phase I and phase II biotransformation
- Microsomal mixed-function oxidase system
- Enzyme induction
- Slow acetylators

**You should be able to:**

- List the major phase I and phase II metabolic reactions.
- Describe the mechanism of hepatic enzyme induction.
- List 3 drugs that inhibit the metabolism of other drugs.
- List 3 drugs for which there are well-defined genetically determined differences in metabolism.
- Discuss the effects of smoking, liver disease, and kidney disease on drug elimination.
- Describe the pathways by which acetaminophen is metabolized (1) to harmless products if taken in normal doses and (2) to hepatotoxic products if taken in excess.

## DEFINITIONS

**A. Phase I Reactions:** Reactions that convert the parent drug to a more polar (water-soluble) or more reactive product by unmasking or inserting a polar functional group such as OH, SH, or $NH_2$.

**B. Phase II Reactions:** Reactions that increase water solubility or decrease lipid solubility by conjugation of the drug molecule with a polar moiety such as glucuronate, acetate, or sulfate.

**C. Enzyme Induction:** Stimulation of drug-metabolizing capacity; usually manifested in the liver by increased synthesis of smooth endoplasmic reticulum (which contains a high concentration of phase I enzymes).

## CONCEPTS

**A. Need for Drug Metabolism:** Biotransformation of drugs is an important mechanism by which the body terminates the action of some drugs. Conversely, an inactive pro-drug may be converted to an active product by similar enzymatic action. In most cases, the drug as given is relatively lipid-soluble to ensure good absorption. The same property would result in very slow removal from the body because the molecule would also be readily reabsorbed from the urine in the renal tubule. The body hastens excretion by transforming the drug to a less lipid-soluble form.

**B. Types of Metabolic Reactions:**

1. **Phase I reactions** include oxidation (especially by the cytochrome P-450 group of enzymes, mixed-function oxidases), reduction, and hydrolysis. Examples are listed in Table 4–1.
2. **Phase II reactions** are synthetic reactions that involve addition (conjugation) of subgroups to OH, $NH_2$, and SH functions on the drug molecule. These subgroups include glucuronate (from UDP glucuronic acid), acetate (from acetyl coenzyme A), glutathione, glycine, sulfate, and methyl groups (from S-adenosylmethionine). Note that most of these groups are relatively polar. Examples of phase II reactions are listed in Table 4–2.

**C. Sites of Drug Metabolism:** The most important organ for drug metabolism is the liver. The kidneys play an important role in the metabolism of some drugs. A few drugs (eg, esters) are metabolized in many tissues because of the broad distribution of their metabolic enzymes.

**Table 4–1.** Phase I reactions.

| Reaction Type | Typical Drug Substrates |
|---|---|
| Oxidations, P-450-dependent | |
| Hydroxylations | Barbiturates, amphetamines, phenylbutazone, phenytoin |
| N-dealkylation | Morphine, caffeine, theophylline |
| O-dealkylation | Codeine |
| N-oxidation | Acetaminophen, nicotine, methaqualone, chlorphenteramine |
| S-oxidation | Thioridazine, cimetidine, chlorpromazine |
| Deamination | Amphetamine, diazepam |
| Oxidations, P-450-independent | |
| Amine oxidation | Epinephrine |
| Dehydrogenation | Ethanol, chloral hydrate |
| Reductions | Chloramphenicol, clorazepam, dantrolene, naloxone |
| Hydrolyses | |
| Esters | Procaine, succinylcholine, aspirin, clofibrate |
| Amides | Procainamide, lidocaine, indomethacin |

**Table 4–2.** Phase II reactions.[1]

| Reaction Type | Typical Drug Substrates |
|---|---|
| Glucuronidation | Nitrophenol, morphine, acetaminophen, diazepam, N-hydroxydapsone, sulfathiazole, meprobamate, digitoxin, digoxin. |
| Acetylation | Sulfonamides, isoniazid, clonazepam, dapsone, mescaline. |
| Glutathione conjugation | Ethacrynic acid, bromobenzene. |
| Glycine conjugation | Salicylic acid, benzoic acid, nicotinic acid, cinnamic acid, cholic acid, deoxycholic acid. |
| Sulfate conjugation | Estrone, aniline, phenol, 3-hydroxycoumarin, acetaminophen, methyldopa. |
| Methylation | Dopamine, epinephrine, pyridine, histamine, thiouracil. |

[1]Adapted, with permission, from Katzung BG (editor): *Basic & Clinical Pharmacology,* 5th ed. Appleton & Lange, 1992.

**D. Determinants of Biotransformation Rate:** The rate of biotransformation of a drug may vary markedly among different subjects. This variation may be due to age or to genetic, drug-induced, or disease-related differences in drug metabolism. Since the rate of biotransformation is often the primary determinant of clearance, variations in drug metabolism must be considered carefully when designing a dosage regimen. Smoking is a common cause of enzyme induction in the liver and may alter the metabolism of some drugs (eg, theophylline).

1. **Genetic factors.** Several drug-metabolizing systems have been shown to differ among families or populations in genetically determined ways.
   a. **Hydrolysis of esters.** Succinylcholine is an ester that is metabolized by plasma cholinesterase ("pseudocholinesterase" or butyrylcholinesterase). In most individuals, this process occurs very rapidly and the drug has a duration of action of about 5 minutes. Approximately one person in 2500 has abnormal variants of this enzyme that result in much slower metabolism of succinylcholine and similar esters. In such individuals, the neuromuscular paralysis produced by succinylcholine may last many hours.
   b. **Acetylation of amines.** Isoniazid and some other amines such as procainamide are inactivated by N-acetylation. Individuals deficient in acetylation capacity, termed **slow acetylators,** may have prolonged or toxic responses to normal doses of these drugs. Slow acetylators constitute about 50% of white and black persons in the USA and a much smaller fraction of Asian and Inuit (Eskimo) populations. The slow acetylation trait is inherited as an autosomal recessive gene.
   c. **Oxidation.** The rate of oxidation of debrisoquin, sparteine, phenformin, dextromethorphan, metoprolol, and some tricyclic antidepressants by certain P-450 isozymes has been shown to be genetically determined.
2. **Other drugs.** Coadministration of certain agents may stimulate or inhibit the metabolism of many drugs. Mechanisms include the following:
   a. **Enzyme induction.** As indicated above, induction usually results from increased synthesis of cytochrome P-450-dependent drug-oxidizing enzymes in the liver. Many isozymes of

**Table 4–3.** Partial list of drugs that enhance drug metabolism in humans.[1]

| Inducer | Drug Whose Metabolism Is Enhanced |
|---|---|
| Chlorcyclizine | Steroid hormones |
| Ethchlorvynol | Warfarin |
| Glutethimide | Antipyrine, glutethimide, warfarin |
| Griseofulvin | Warfarin |
| Phenobarbital and other barbiturates | Barbiturates, chloramphenicol, chlorpromazine, cortisol, coumarin, anticoagulants, desmethylimipramine, digitoxin, doxorubicin, estradiol, phenylbutazone, phenytoin, quinine, testosterone |
| Phenylbutazone | Aminopyrine, cortisol, digitoxin |
| Phenytoin | Cortisol, dexamethasone, digitoxin, theophylline |
| Rifampin | Coumarin anticoagulants, digitoxin, glucocorticoids, methadone, metoprolol, oral contraceptives, prednisone, propranolol, quinidine |

[1]Reproduced, with permission, from Katzung BG (editor): *Basic & Clinical Pharmacology,* 5th ed. Appleton & Lange, 1992.

**Table 4–4.** Partial list of drugs that inhibit drug metabolism in humans.

| Inhibitor | Drug Whose Metabolism Is Inhibited |
|---|---|
| Allopurinol, chloramphenicol, isoniazid | Antipyrine, dicumarol, probenicid, tolbutamide |
| Cimetidine | Chlordiazepoxide, diazepam, warfarin |
| Dicumarol | Phenytoin |
| Diethylpentenamide | Diethylpentenamide |
| Disulfiram | Antipyrine, ethanol, phenytoin, warfarin |
| Ethanol | Chlordiazepoxide (?), diazepam (?), methanol |
| Ketoconazole | Cyclosporine |
| Nortriptyline | Antipyrine |
| Oral contraceptives | Antipyrine |
| Phenylbutazone | Phenytoin, tolbutamide |
| Secobarbital | Secobarbital |
| Troleandomycin | Theophylline, methylprednisone |

this family exist, and inducers selectively increase subgroups of isozymes. Several days are usually required to reach maximum induction, and a similar period is required to regress after withdrawal of the inducer. Common inducers and drugs whose metabolism is increased are indicated in Table 4–3. In addition, some toxic chemicals, such as the carcinogens in cigarette smoke, are hepatic enzyme inducers.

**b. Metabolism inhibitors:** Common inhibitors and the drugs whose metabolism is diminished are indicated in Table 4–4. **Suicide inhibitors** are drugs that are metabolized to products which inhibit the metabolizing enzyme. Such agents include ethinyl estradiol, norethindrone, spironolactone, secobarbital, allobarbital, fluroxene, and propylthiouracil. Metabolism may also be decreased by pharmacodynamic factors, such as a reduction in blood flow to the metabolizing organ (eg, propranolol reduces hepatic blood flow).

**E. Toxic Metabolism:** Drug metabolism is not synonymous with drug inactivation. Some drugs are converted to active products by metabolism. If these products are toxic, severe injury may result. An important example is acetaminophen when it is taken in a large overdose. Acetaminophen is conjugated to harmless glucuronide and sulfate metabolites when it is taken in normal doses. If a large overdose is taken, however, the metabolic pathways are overwhelmed and a P-450-dependent system converts some of the drug to a reactive intermediate. The intermediate is conjugated with glutathione to a third harmless product if glutathione stores are adequate. However, if glutathione stores are exhausted, the reactive intermediate will combine with essential hepatic cell proteins, resulting in cell death. Prompt administration of other sulfhydryl donors (eg, acetylcysteine) may be life-saving in such a situation.

## QUESTIONS

**DIRECTIONS (items 1–5):** Each numbered item or incomplete statement in this section is followed by answers or by completions of the statement. Select the ONE lettered answer or completion that is BEST in each case.

**1.** Biotransformation (metabolism) usually results in a product that is
**(A)** more likely to distribute intracellularly
**(B)** less lipid-soluble than the original drug
**(C)** more likely to be reabsorbed by kidney tubules
**(D)** more lipid-soluble than the original drug
**(E)** more likely to produce side effects

2. "Induction" of drug metabolism
   (A) results in increased production of smooth endoplasmic reticulum
   (B) results in increased production of rough endoplasmic reticulum
   (C) results in decreased enzyme levels in the soluble cytoplasmic fraction
   (D) requires 3–4 months to reach completion
   (E) is irreversible

3. Factors that are likely to increase the duration of action of a drug that is partially metabolized in the liver and partially excreted as the unchanged drug by the kidneys include
   (A) chronic administration of phenobarbital prior to and during therapy with the drug in question
   (B) chronic renal disease
   (C) displacement from tissue-binding sites by another drug
   (D) increased cardiac output
   (E) chronic administration of rifampin

4. Which of the following is NOT a phase I drug-metabolizing reaction?
   (A) Oxidation
   (B) Reduction
   (C) Hydrolysis
   (D) Acetylation
   (E) Deamination

5. Which of the following statements about drug metabolism is NOT correct?
   (A) Succinylcholine metabolism is accelerated in individuals with abnormal cholinesterase
   (B) Metabolism of isoniazid varies in different ethnic groups
   (C) Incidence of lupuslike drug-induced toxicity is more common in patients who have an increased ability to oxidize drugs via the P-450 system
   (D) Metabolism of most drugs is not markedly affected by gender in humans

## ANSWERS

1. **(B)** is correct. Biotransformation usually results in a product that is less lipid-soluble.

2. **(A)** is correct. The smooth endoplasmic reticulum, containing the mixed function oxidase drug metabolizing enzymes, is selectively increased by "inducers."

3. The answer is **(B)**. Phenobarbital and rifampin induce drug-metabolizing enzymes and thereby reduce their duration of action. Displacement of drug from tissue will transiently increase the intensity of the effect, but it will decrease the volume of distribution and thereby reduce the half-life.

4. Acetylation is a phase II reaction. The answer is **(D)**.

5. Succinylcholine metabolism is slowed in persons with genetically determined "abnormal" cholinesterase. The speed of isoniazid acetylation varies among different genetically determined groups. The drug is not converted to toxic products as a result of this change in metabolic rate. Lupuslike toxicity is caused by hydralazine and procainamide, drugs that are metabolized by acetylation. Gender has significant effects on drug metabolism in rodents but not in humans. (A possible exception is the metabolism of ethanol, which appears to be significantly faster in men than in women.) The answer is **(A)**.

# Drug Evaluation 5

## OBJECTIVES

**Define the following terms:**

- Single-blind study
- Double-blind study
- IND
- NDA
- Placebo
- Positive control
- Phases I, II, III, and IV of clinical trials
- Crossover design
- Mutagenesis
- Teratogenesis
- Carcinogenesis
- Ames test
- Dominant lethal test
- Orphan drugs

## CONCEPTS

**A. Safety & Efficacy:** Because society expects prescription drugs to be safe and effective, governments have regulated the development and marketing of new drugs. Each country has its own regulatory body and its own set of more or less stringently enforced standards for drug safety and efficacy. The Food & Drug Administration (FDA) administers these regulations in the USA. Regulatory agencies require evidence of relative safety (from animal toxicity testing) and probable therapeutic action (from the pharmacologic profile in animals) before human testing is permitted. Often some information about the pharmacokinetics of a compound is also required before clinical evaluation is begun. Chronic toxicity test results are generally not required before human studies are started.

**B. Animal Testing:** The extent of animal testing that is required before human studies are begun is a function of the proposed use and the urgency of the application. Thus, a drug proposed for occasional nonsystemic use requires less extensive testing than one destined for chronic systemic administration. Anticancer drugs and drugs proposed for use in AIDS, because of the urgency of the need for new agents, require less testing than do drugs used in less threatening diseases.

1. **Acute toxicity** studies are required for all drugs. These involve single administrations of the agent up to the lethal level in several species.
2. Both **subacute** testing and **chronic toxicity** testing are required for most agents, especially those intended for chronic use. Tests are usually carried out for at least the period proposed for human application, eg, 2–4 weeks (subacute) or 6–24 months (chronic), in several species.

**C. Types of Animal Tests:** Tests done with animals often include general screening tests for pharmacologic effects, hepatic and renal function monitoring, blood and urine tests, gross and histopathologic examination of tissues, and tests of teratogenicity, mutagenicity, and carcinogenicity.

1. The **pharmacologic profile** is a description of all the pharmacologic effects of a drug (eg, effects on blood pressure, gastrointestinal activity, respiration, renal function, endocrine function, and the central nervous system).
2. **Teratogenesis** can be defined as induction of developmental defects, generally of a nonheritable type, in the fetus (by a drug or by exposure of the fetus to other harmful substances). It is studied by treating pregnant female animals at selected times during early pregnancy when organogenesis is known to take place and later examining the fetuses or neonates for abnormalities. Drugs known to have teratogenic effects include thalidomide, ethanol, valproic acid, isotretinoin, warfarin, lithium, and androgens.
3. **Mutagenesis** is defined as induction of changes in the genetic material of animals of any age and therefore induction of heritable abnormalities. The Ames test is the standard in vitro test for mutagenicity. The dominant lethal test is an in vivo mutagenicity test. Many carcinogens (eg, aflatoxin, cancer chemotherapeutic drugs, and other agents that bind to DNA) have mutagenic effects.
4. **Carcinogenesis** is defined as induction of malignant characteristics in cells. Because carcino-

genicity is difficult and expensive to study, the Ames test is often used to screen chemicals, since there is a moderately high degree of correlation between mutagenicity in the Ames test and carcinogenicity in some animal tests. Agents with known carcinogenic effects include coal tar, aflatoxin, dimethylnitrosamine and other nitrosamines, urethane, vinyl chloride, and the polycyclic aromatic hydrocarbons in tobacco smoke.

**D. Clinical Trials:** Human testing in the USA requires the approval of an **Investigational New Drug (IND)** application, submitted by the manufacturer to the FDA. The major testing period is formally divided into 3 phases before a **New Drug Application (NDA)** can be submitted. The NDA constitutes the request for approval of general marketing of the new agent for prescription use. A fourth phase of study follows NDA approval.

1. **Phase I** consists of careful evaluation of the dose-response relationship in a small number (20–30) of normal human volunteers, ie, the effects of an agent as a function of dosage. An exception is in phase I trials of cancer chemotherapeutic agents; these are carried out by administering the agents to patients with cancer.
2. **Phase II** involves evaluation of a drug in a small number (10–100) of patients with the target disease, often with a placebo or positive control drug included in a single-blind design.
3. **Phase III** consists of a larger design involving hundreds of patients (sometimes in many centers) and many clinicians. Such studies usually include placebo and positive controls in a double-blind crossover design.
4. **Phase IV** represents the postmarketing surveillance phase of evaluation, in which it is hoped that toxicities that occur infrequently will be detected and reported early enough to prevent major therapeutic disasters. Unlike the first 3 phases, phase IV is not rigorously monitored by the FDA.

**E. Drug Legislation:** In the USA, many laws regulating drugs have been passed during this century. Refer to Table 5–1 for a selective list of this legislation.

**F. Orphan Drugs:** An orphan drug is a drug for a rare disease (one affecting fewer than 200,000 people). The study of such agents has often been neglected in the past because the sales of an effective agent for an uncommon ailment might not even pay the costs of development. In the USA, legislation that provides regulatory incentives encouraging the development of orphan drugs is now in place.

**Table 5–1.** Selected legislation pertaining to drugs in the USA.[1]

| Law | Purpose and Effect |
|---|---|
| Pure Food & Drug Act of 1906 | Prohibited mislabeling and adulteration of drugs. |
| Harrison Narcotics Act of 1914 | Established regulations for the use of opium, opiates, and cocaine (marihuana added in 1937). |
| Food, Drug, & Cosmetic Act of 1938 | Required that new drugs be safe as well as pure (but did not require proof of efficacy). |
| Kefauver-Harris Amendment (1962) to the Food, Drug, & Cosmetic Act | Required proof of efficacy as well as safety for new drugs and for drugs released since 1938; established guidelines for reporting of information about adverse reactions, clinical testing, and advertising of new drugs. |
| Comprehensive Drug Abuse Prevention & Control Act (1970) | Outlined strict controls on the manufacture, distribution, and prescribing of habit-forming drugs; established programs to prevent and treat drug addiction. |
| Drug Price Competition & Patent Restoration Act of 1984 | Abbreviated new drug applications for generic drugs. Requires bioequivalence data. Patent life extended by amount of time drug was delayed by FDA review process. Cannot exceed 5 extra years or extend to more than 14 years post-NDA approval. |

[1]Modified and reproduced, with permission, from Katzung BG (editor): *Basic & Clinical Pharmacology,* 5th ed. Appleton & Lange, 1992.

## QUESTIONS

**DIRECTIONS (items 1–5):** Each numbered item or incomplete statement in this section is followed by answers or by completions of the statement. Select the ONE lettered answer or completion that is BEST in each case.

**1.** With regard to clinical trials of new drugs, all of the following are correct EXCEPT:
**(A)** Phase I involves the study of a small number of normal volunteers
**(B)** Phase II involves the use of the new drug in a small number of patients (10–100) with the disease to be treated
**(C)** Phase III involves the determination of the drug's therapeutic index by cautious induction of toxicity by highly trained clinical pharmacologists in a hospital setting
**(D)** Phase IV involves the recording of unusual events, especially toxic reactions, after the drug is approved for general prescription use
**(E)** Phase II does not require the use of a positive control (known effective drug) or placebo

**2.** Animal testing of potential new therapeutic agents
**(A)** extends over different periods depending on the projected human use
**(B)** requires the use of at least 2 primate species, eg, monkey and baboon
**(C)** requires the submission of a set of histopathologic slides and specimens to the FDA for government evaluation
**(D)** has good predictability for drug allergy-type reactions
**(E)** both **(B)** and **(C)** are correct

**3.** The "dominant lethal" test involves the treatment of a male adult animal with a chemical before mating; the pregnant female is later examined for fetal death and abnormalities. The dominant lethal test therefore is a test of
**(A)** teratogenicity
**(B)** mutagenicity
**(C)** carcinogenicity
**(D)** all of the above
**(E)** none of the above

**4.** An optimum clinical trial of a new analgesic drug would include all of the following EXCEPT:
**(A)** a negative control (placebo)
**(B)** a positive control (current standard therapy)
**(C)** double-blind protocol (neither patient nor immediate observers of the patient know which agent is which)
**(D)** prior submission of an IND (investigational new drug) application to the FDA
**(E)** prior submission of an NDA (new drug application) to the FDA

**5.** In the testing of new compounds (eg, antihypertensives) for potential therapeutic use,
**(A)** animal tests cannot be used to predict the types of toxicities that may occur because there is so little correlation with human toxicity
**(B)** human studies in normal individuals will be done before studies in diseased individuals
**(C)** the degree of risk must be assessed in at least 3 species of animals including one primate species
**(D)** the animal therapeutic index must be known before the agents are tested in humans

## ANSWERS

**1.** The induction of toxicity is not required in any phase of clinical testing, although some toxicity is usually seen. The answer is **(C)**.

**2.** For some drugs, no primates are used; for others, only one species is used. The answer is **(A)**.

**3.** The description of the test indicates that a chromosomal change (passed from father to fetus) is the toxicity detected. This is a mutation. The answer is **(B).**

**4.** The first 4 items **(A–D)** are correct. An NDA cannot be submitted until the first 3 phases of clinical trials have been completed. The answer is **(E).**

**5.** Animal tests in a single species do not always predict human toxicities, but when they are carried out in several species, most of the acute toxicities that occur in humans will also appear in at least one animal species. According to current FDA rules, the "degree of risk" must be determined in at least 2 species. Use of primates is rarely required. The therapeutic index is not required. Except for cancer chemotherapeutic agents and AIDS drugs, phase I clinical trials are always carried out in normal subjects. The answer is **(B).**

# Part II. Autonomic Drugs

# Pharmacology 6

## OBJECTIVES

**Define the following terms:**

- Adrenergic
- Adrenoceptor
- Autonomic effector cells
- Autonomic ganglion
- Baroreceptor reflex
- Cholinergic
- Cholinoceptor
- Dopaminergic
- Homeostatic reflexes
- Parasympathetic
- Postsynaptic receptor
- Presynaptic receptor
- Sympathetic

**You should be able to:**

- Describe the steps in the synthesis and the termination of action of the major autonomic transmitters.
- Name 2 cotransmitter substances.
- Describe the organ system effects of stimulation of the parasympathetic and sympathetic systems.
- Name examples of inhibitors of acetylcholine and norepinephrine synthesis, storage, and release.
- Predict the effects of these inhibitors on the function of the major organ systems.
- List the determinants of blood pressure and describe the baroreceptor reflex responses for the following perturbations: blood loss, administration of (1) a vasodilator, (2) a vasoconstrictor, (3) a cardiac stimulant, and (4) a cardiac depressant.
- Name the major types of receptors found on autonomic effector tissues.
- Describe the differences between the effects of surgical sympathetic ganglionectomy (interruption of ganglionic transmission by surgical removal of the sympathetic ganglia) and those of pharmacologic ganglion block.
- Describe the action of several toxins that affect nerve function: tetrodotoxin, saxitoxin, botulinum toxin, and latrotoxin.

## CONCEPTS

The autonomic nervous system (ANS) may be compared to and contrasted with the somatic (voluntary) nervous system. Its anatomy, neurotransmitter chemistry, receptor characteristics, and functional integration are discussed below.

A. **Anatomic Facts:** The motor (efferent) portion of the ANS may be thought of as a pathway for information transmission from the central nervous system (CNS) to the effector tissues (smooth muscle, vascular endothelium, cardiac muscle, and exocrine glands). There are also many sensory (afferent) fibers in autonomic nerves, but these are of importance for only a few drugs.
   1. **Spinal roots of origin.** The parasympathetic preganglionic motor fibers originate exclusively in the cranial nerve nuclei (III, VII, IX, and X) and the sacral segments (usually S2–S4) of the spinal cord. The sympathetic preganglionic fibers originate in the thoracic (T1–T12) and lumbar (L1–L5) segments of the cord.
   2. **Location of ganglia.** Most of the sympathetic ganglia are located in 2 paravertebral chains that lie along the spinal column. A few (the prevertebral ganglia) are located on the anterior aspect of the vertebral column. Most of the parasympathetic ganglia are located in the organs innervated, more distant from the spinal cord.

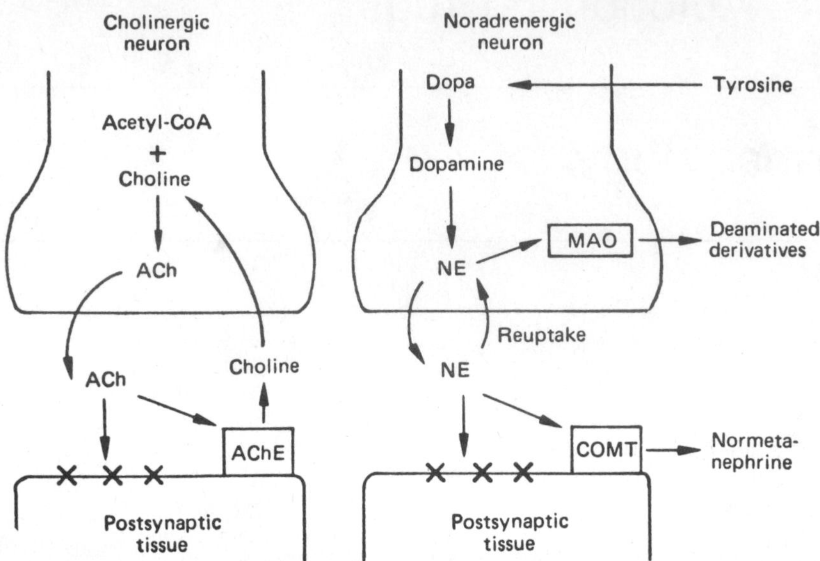


**Figure 6–1.** Comparison of the biochemical events at cholinergic endings with those at noradrenergic endings. ACh, acetylcholine; AChE, acetylcholinesterase; NE, norepinephrine; X, receptor. Note that monoamine oxidase (MAO) is intracellular, so that some norepinephrine is being constantly deaminated in noradrenergic endings. Catechol-O-methyltransferase (COMT) acts on norepinephrine after it is secreted. (Modified and reproduced, with permission, from Ganong WF: *Review of Medical Physiology,* 15th ed. Appleton & Lange, 1991.)

3. **Length of pre- and postganglionic fibers.** Because of the locations of the ganglia noted above, the preganglionic sympathetic fibers are short and the postganglionic fibers are long. The opposite is true for the parasympathetic system.

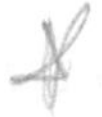

4. **Uninnervated receptors.** Some receptors that respond to autonomic transmitters receive no innervation. These include muscarinic receptors on the endothelium of blood vessels and, in some species, the adrenoceptors on apocrine sweat glands.

## B. Neurotransmitter Facts:

1. **Major transmitters (Fig 6–1).** Acetylcholine (ACh) is the major transmitter in all autonomic ganglia and at the parasympathetic postganglionic neuron-effector cell synapses. Norepinephrine (NE) is the primary transmitter at the sympathetic postganglionic neuron-effector cell synapses in most tissues. Important exceptions include vasodilator sympathetic fibers in skeletal muscle and thermoregulatory sweat glands, which release ACh. Dopamine (DA) is an important vasodilator transmitter in some splanchnic blood vessels, especially renal vessels.
2. **Cotransmitters.** Many (perhaps all) autonomic transmitter vesicles contain other transmitter molecules in addition to the major agents described above. These other molecules are often purine nucleotides or peptides. Such cotransmitters may include ATP, neuropeptide Y, neurotensin, somatostatin, substance P, vasoactive intestinal polypeptide (VIP), and others. Their role in autonomic function is not well understood.
3. **Synthesis of transmitters.** ACh is synthesized by the enzyme choline acetyltransferase from acetyl coenzyme A (acetyl-CoA) and choline. The rate-limiting step is probably the transport of choline into the nerve terminal. The synthesis of NE is more complex. Tyrosine is hydroxylated (the rate-limiting step) to dihydroxyphenylalanine (DOPA), decarboxylated to dopamine, and hydroxylated to norepinephrine. Drugs that block the synthesis of ACh (eg, hemicholinium) or the release of ACh (eg, botulinum toxin*) are not very useful in therapy, because their effects are not sufficiently selective (see section on **Major transmitters,** above). Drugs that block catecholamine synthesis (eg, metyrosine) or catecholamine storage (eg, reserpine), or catecholamine release (eg, guanethidine) are useful in several diseases (eg, hypertension) because their effects are sufficiently selective.

*Botulinum toxin (botulin) has been used by local injection to achieve a medically useful selective effect.

4. **Metabolism of transmitters:**
   a. **Acetylcholine.** The action of ACh is normally terminated by metabolism (by cholinesterase to acetate and choline). These products are not excreted but are recycled in the body. Inhibition of cholinesterase is an important therapeutic and toxicologic effect of several drugs.
   b. **Catecholamines.** Metabolism is not responsible for the termination of action of the catecholamine transmitters. Instead, diffusion and reuptake reduce the concentration of norepinephrine and dopamine in the synaptic cleft and stop their action. However, these substances are also metabolized—by monoamine oxidase (MAO) and catechol-O-methyltransferase (COMT)—and the products of these enzymatic reactions are excreted. Determination of the 24-hour excretion of metanephrine, normetanephrine, 3-methoxy-4-hydroxymandelic acid (VMA), and other metabolites provides a measure of the total body production of catecholamine transmitters, which is useful in diagnosing several clinical conditions. Blockade of MAO increases stores of catecholamines and has both therapeutic and toxic potential.

**C. Receptor Characteristics:** The major receptor systems include the following:

1. **Cholinoceptors or acetylcholine receptors.** Often referred to as "cholinergic receptors,"* these receptors respond to ACh and its analogs. Cholinoceptors are subdivided as follows:
   a. **Muscarinic receptors.** These receptors respond to muscarine, an ACh analog whose effects resemble those of postganglionic parasympathetic nerve stimulation. They are located primarily on autonomic effector cells (of the heart, vascular endothelium, smooth muscle, presynaptic nerve terminals, and exocrine glands). Evidence has been found for several subtypes.
   b. **Nicotinic receptors.** These receptors respond to nicotine, another ACh analog. The 2 major subtypes are those located in ganglia and those located in skeletal muscle endplates. They are the primary receptors for transmission at these sites.
2. **Adrenoceptors.** Often referred to as "adrenergic receptors," adrenoceptors are divided into the following subtypes:
   a. **Alpha-receptors.** Located on vascular smooth muscle, presynaptic nerve terminals, blood platelets, and fat cells (lipocytes) and in the brain, alpha receptors are further divided into 2 major types, $\alpha_1$ and $\alpha_2$.
   b. **Beta-receptors.** Located on most types of smooth muscle, cardiac muscle, some presynaptic nerve terminals, and lipocytes and in the brain, beta receptors are divided into 3 major subtypes, $\beta_1$, $\beta_2$, and $\beta_3$.
3. **Dopamine receptors.** A subclass of adrenoceptors, but with rather different distribution and function, dopamine receptors are especially important in the renal and splanchnic vessels and in the brain. Although at least 2 subtypes exist, the $D_1$ (or $DA_1$) subtype appears to be the most important peripheral effector cell dopamine receptor. $D_2$ (or $DA_2$) receptors are found on presynaptic nerve terminals; both $D_1$ and $D_2$ types occur in the CNS.

**D. Integration of Autonomic Function:** Functional integration is provided through the mechanism of negative feedback. This process utilizes presynaptic receptors at the local level and homeostatic reflexes at the systemic level.

1. **Local feedback** control has been found at the level of the nerve endings in some systems. The best documented of these is the negative feedback of norepinephrine upon its own release from the presynaptic adrenergic terminals. This effect is mediated by $\alpha_2$ receptors located on the presynaptic nerve membrane.

   Presynaptic receptors that regulate the release of their own transmitter substance have been called **autoreceptors.** Control of transmitter release is not limited to inhibition by the transmitter itself. Adrenergic nerve terminals also carry regulatory receptors **(heteroreceptors)** for ACh ($M_1$ receptors), prostaglandins, and polypeptides. Presynaptic regulation by a variety of endogenous chemicals probably occurs in all nerve fibers.
2. **Systemic reflexes** include very important mechanisms that regulate blood pressure, especially the baroreceptor neural reflex and the renin-angiotensin-aldosterone hormonal response (Fig 6–2).

---

*"Cholinergic" means acting through the release of ACh. The word should be reserved for denoting nerves that release ACh and the synapses at which such release takes place.

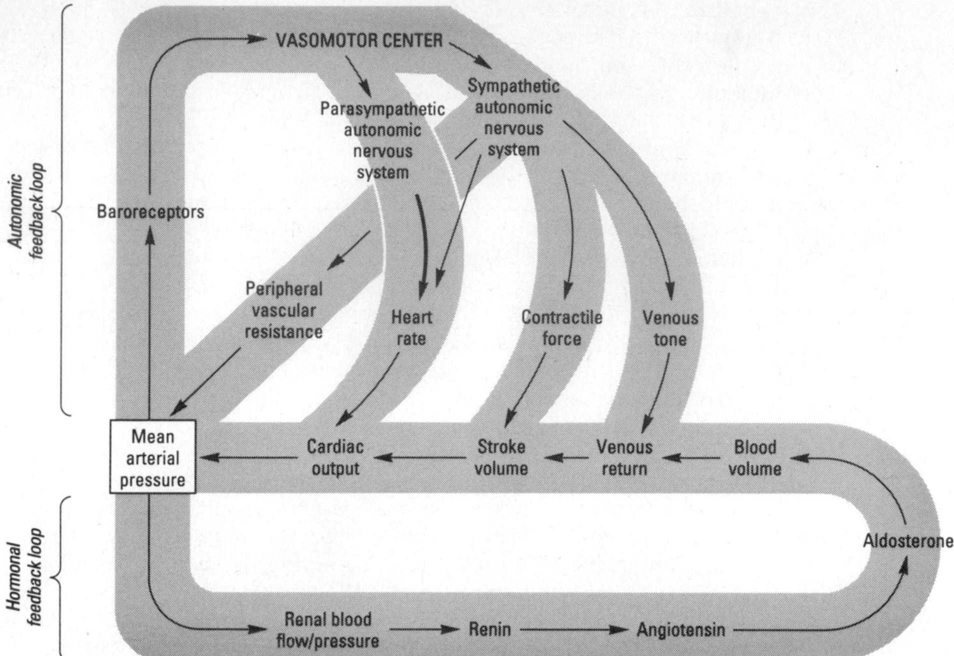


**Figure 6–2.** Autonomic and hormonal control of cardiovascular function. Note that at least 2 feedback loops are present, the autonomic nervous system loop and the hormonal loop. In addition, each major loop has several components. Thus, the sympathetic nervous system directly influences 4 major variables, peripheral vascular resistance, heart rate, force, and venous tone. The parasympathetic nervous system directly influences heart rate. Angiotensin II directly increases peripheral vascular resistance (not shown), and the sympathetic nervous system directly increases renin secretion (not shown). Because these control mechanisms are designed to maintain normal blood pressure, the net feedback effect of each loop is negative in that it tends to compensate for the change in arterial blood pressure that evoked the response. Thus, decreased blood pressure due to blood loss would be compensated for by increased sympathetic outflow and renin release. Conversely, elevated pressure due to the administration of a vasoconstrictor drug would cause reduced sympathetic outflow and renin release and increased parasympathetic (vagal) outflow.

**E. Effects of the Activation of Autonomic Nerves:** Each division of the ANS has specific effects on organ systems. These effects are summarized in Table 6–1. Dually innervated organs—such as the iris of the eye and the sinoatrial node of the heart—receive both sympathetic and parasympathetic innervation. Pharmacologic ganglionic blockade will result in the removal of both sympathetic and parasympathetic tone; how will the muscle respond if this occurs? The answer is predictable if one knows which system is dominant. For example, the pupil and, in young individuals, the sinoatrial node are dominated by the parasympathetic system. Therefore, blockade of both systems will result in an effect that resembles increased sympathetic activity (mydriasis and tachycardia).

**F. Sites of Autonomic Drug Action:** Because of the number of steps in the transmission of autonomic commands from the CNS to the effector, there are many sites at which autonomic drugs may act. These sites include the CNS centers, the ganglia, the postganglionic nerve terminals, the effector cell receptors, and the mechanisms responsible for termination of transmitter action. The most selective action is achieved by drugs acting at receptors that mediate very selective actions (Table 6–1). In addition, many natural and synthetic toxins have significant effects on autonomic and somatic nerve function. Some of these toxins are listed in Table 6–2.

**G. Nonadrenergic, Noncholinergic Transmission:** Autonomic effector tissues contain nerve fibers that do not show the histochemical characteristics of either cholinergic or adrenergic fibers. Some of these fibers appear to be motor fibers and cause the release of ATP and

**Table 6–1.** Direct effects of autonomic nerve activity on some organ systems.[1]

| Organ | Effect of Sympathetic Action[2] | Sympathetic Receptor[3] | Parasympathetic Action | Parasympathetic Receptor[3] |
|---|---|---|---|---|
| Eye | | | | |
| Iris | | | | |
| Radial muscle | Contracts | $\alpha_1$ | ... | ... |
| Circular muscle | ... | ... | Contracts | M |
| Ciliary muscle | [Relaxes] | $\beta$ | Contracts | M |
| Heart | | | | |
| Sinoatrial node | Accelerates | $\beta_1$ | Decelerates | M |
| Ectopic pacemakers | Accelerates | $\beta_1$ | ... | ... |
| Contractility | Increases | $\beta_1$ | Decreases (atria) | M |
| Vascular smooth muscle | | | | |
| Skin, splanchnic vessels | Contracts | $\alpha$ | ... | M[4] |
| Skeletal muscle vessels | Relaxes | $\beta_2$ | ... | ... |
| | [Contracts] | $\alpha$ | ... | ... |
| | Relaxes | M[5] | ... | M4 |
| Bronchiolar smooth muscle | Relaxes | $\beta_2$ | Contracts | M |
| Gastrointestinal tract | | | | |
| Smooth muscle | | | | |
| Walls | Relaxes | $\alpha_2$[6], $\beta_2$ | Contracts | M |
| Sphincters | Contracts | $\alpha_1$ | Relaxes | M |
| Secretion | ... | ... | Increases | M |
| Myenteric plexus | Inhibits | $\alpha$ | ... | ... |
| Genitourinary smooth muscle | | | | |
| Bladder wall | Relaxes | $\beta_2$ | Contracts | M |
| Sphincter | Contracts | $\alpha_1$ | Relaxes | M |
| Uterus, pregnant | Relaxes | $\beta_2$ | ... | ... |
| | Contracts | $\alpha$ | ... | ... |
| Penis, seminal vesicles | Ejaculation | $\alpha$ | Erection | M |
| Skin | | | | |
| Pilomotor smooth muscle | Contracts | $\alpha$ | ... | ... |
| Sweat glands | | | | |
| Thermoregulatory | Increases | M | ... | ... |
| Apocrine (stress) | Increases | $\alpha$ | ... | ... |
| Metabolic functions | | | | |
| Liver | Gluconeogenesis | $\alpha/\beta_2$[7] | ... | ... |
| Liver | Glycogenolysis | $\alpha/\beta_2$ | ... | ... |
| Fat cells | Lipolysis | $\alpha_2, \beta_1$[8] | ... | ... |
| Kidney | Renin release | $\beta_1$ | ... | ... |

[1]Reproduced, with permission, from Katzung BG (editor): *Basic & Clinical Pharmacology,* 5th ed. Appleton & Lange, 1992.
[2]Less important actions are in brackets.
[3]Specific receptor type: $\alpha$ = alpha, $\beta$ = beta, M = muscarinic.
[4]The endothelium of most blood vessels releases "endothelium-derived relaxing factor," which causes marked vasodilation in response to muscarinic stimuli. However, unlike the receptors innervated by sympathetic cholinergic fibers in skeletal muscle blood vessels, these muscarinic receptors are not innervated and respond only to *circulating* muscarinic agonists.
[5]Vascular smooth muscle in skeletal muscle has sympathetic cholinergic dilator fibers.
[6]Probably through presynaptic inhibition of parasympathetic activity.
[7]Depends on species.
[8]$\alpha_2$ inhibits; $\beta_1$ stimulates.

**Table 6-2.** Steps in autonomic transmission: Effects of drugs.[1]

| Process | Drug Example | Site | Action |
|---|---|---|---|
| Action potential propagation | Local anesthetics, tetrodotoxin,[2] saxitoxin[3] | Nerve axons. | Block sodium channels; block conduction. |
| Transmitter synthesis | Hemicholinium | Cholinergic nerve terminals: membrane. | Blocks uptake of choline and slows synthesis. |
| | α-Methyltyrosine (metyrosine) | Adrenergic nerve terminals and adrenal medulla: cytoplasm. | Blocks synthesis. |
| Transmitter storage | Vesamicol | Cholinergic terminals: vesicles. | Prevents uptake. |
| | Reserpine | Adrenergic terminals: vesicles | Prevents uptake. |
| Transmitter release | Many[4] | Nerve terminal membrane receptors. | Modulate release. |
| | Botulinum toxin | Cholinergic vesicles. | Prevents release. |
| | Latrotoxin[5] | Cholinergic and adrenergic vesicles. | Causes explosive release. |
| | Tyramine, amphetamine | Adrenergic nerve terminals. | Promote transmitter release. |
| Transmitter uptake after release | Cocaine, tricyclic antidepressants | Adrenergic nerve terminals. | Inhibit uptake: increase transmitter effect on postsynaptic receptors. |
| | 6-Hydroxydopamine | Adrenergic nerve terminals. | Destroys the terminals. |
| Receptor activation/blockade | Norepinephrine | Receptors at adrenergic junctions. | Binds α receptors; causes activation. |
| | Phentolamine | Receptors at adrenergic junctions. | Binds α receptors; prevents activation. |
| | Isoproterenol | Receptors at adrenergic junctions. | Binds β receptors; activates adenylate cyclase. |
| | Propranolol | Receptors at adrenergic junctions. | Binds β receptors; prevents activation. |
| | Nicotine | Receptors at nicotinic cholinergic junctions (autonomic ganglia, neuromuscular end-plates). | Binds nicotinic receptors; opens ion channel in postsynaptic membrane. |
| | Tubocurarine | Neuromuscular end-plates. | Prevents activation. |
| | Bethanechol | Receptors, parasympathetic effector cells (smooth muscle, cardiac muscle, glands). | Binds muscarinic receptors; releases inositol triphosphate and activates guanylate cyclase. |
| | Atropine | Receptors, parasympathetic effector cells. | Binds muscarinic receptors; prevents activation. |
| Enzymatic inactivation of transmitter | Neostigmine | Cholinergic synapses (acetylcholinesterase). | Inhibits enzyme; prolongs and intensifies transmitter action. |
| | Tranylcypromine | Adrenergic nerve terminals (monoamine oxidase). | Inhibits enzyme; increases stored transmitter pool. |

[1]Reproduced, with permission, from Katzung BG (editor): *Basic & Clinical Pharmacology,* 5th ed. Appleton & Lange, 1992.
[2]Toxin of puffer fish, California newt.
[3]Toxin of *Gonyaulax* (red tide organism).
[4]Norepinephrine, dopamine, acetylcholine, angiotensin II, various prostaglandins, etc.
[5]Black widow spider venom.

possibly other purines related to it. These fibers are therefore called **purinergic** fibers, and at least 2 types of "purinoceptors" have been identified by the use of pharmacologic agonists and antagonists. Purine-evoked responses have been identified in the gastrointestinal and urinary tracts.

Other nonadrenergic, noncholinergic fibers have the anatomic characteristics of sensory fibers and contain peptides (see the list above under **Cotransmitters**) that are stored in and released from the fiber terminals. These sensory fibers have been termed "sensory-efferent" or "sensory-local effector" fibers because, when activated by a sensory input, they are capable of releasing transmitter peptides from the sensory ending itself, from local axon branches, and from collaterals that terminate in the autonomic ganglia. These peptides are potent agonists at many autonomic effector tissues.

## DRUG LIST

The following drugs or metabolites are mentioned in this chapter. It is important to know which ones occur in the normal ANS and, for those that do, what their functions are. For those that are not normally present in the ANS, it is important to know the effects of their administration.

| | |
|---|---|
| Acetylcholine | 3-Methoxy-4-hydroxymandelic acid (VMA)[1] |
| Amphetamine | Metyrosine (α-methyl tyrosine)[1] |
| Atropine | Neostigmine |
| Botulinum toxin[1] | Norepinephrine |
| Cocaine | Propranolol |
| Dopa | Reserpine |
| Dopamine | Saxitoxin[1] |
| Epinephrine | Tetrodotoxin[1] |
| Metanephrine[1] | Tyramine |

[1]Should be learned with this chapter, since they are not discussed in detail in succeeding chapters. The other drugs will be covered in later chapters

## QUESTIONS

**DIRECTIONS (items 1–7):** Each numbered item or incomplete statement in this section is followed by answers or by completions of the statement. Select the ONE lettered answer or completion that is BEST in each case.

**1.** In the autonomic regulation of blood pressure,
**(A)** cardiac output is maintained constant at the expense of other hemodynamic variables
**(B)** elevation of blood pressure results in elevated aldosterone secretion
**(C)** baroreceptor nerve endings increase their firing rate when arterial pressure increases
**(D)** stroke volume and mean arterial blood pressure are the primary direct determinants of cardiac output
**(E)** the heart rate always increases when the cardiac output decreases

**2.** Alpha$_1$ receptors are associated with
**(A)** cardioacceleration
**(B)** vasodepression (vasodilatation)
**(C)** pupillary dilatation
**(D)** bronchodilatation
**(E)** all of the above

**3.** Probable effects of giving a "pure" arteriolar vasodilator (one that does not act on autonomic receptors) would be
**(A)** tachycardia and increased cardiac contractility
**(B)** tachycardia and decreased cardiac output
**(C)** decreased mean arterial pressure and decreased cardiac contractility
**(D)** no change in mean arterial pressure and decreased cardiac contractility
**(E)** no change in mean arterial pressure and increased salt and water excretion by the kidneys

**4.** Full activation of the sympathetic nervous system, as in maximal exercise, can produce all of the following responses EXCEPT
(A) mydriasis
(B) increased renal blood flow
(C) decreased intestinal motility
(D) bronchodilatation
(E) increased heart rate (tachycardia)

**5.** Mr Brown has recently had a successful cardiac transplant operation in which his badly damaged and failing heart was replaced by a healthy donor organ. Which of the following drugs would be expected to have the SMALLEST effect on his (transplanted) heart function, as compared with the function of a normal heart?
(A) Tyramine
(B) Norepinephrine
(C) Propranolol
(D) Bethanechol
(E) Atropine

**6.** "Nicotinic" sites include all of the following EXCEPT
(A) parasympathetic ganglia
(B) sympathetic ganglia
(C) skeletal muscle
(D) excitatory receptors on Renshaw cells in the spinal cord
(E) bronchial smooth muscle

**7.** The anticholinergic effects of botulinum toxin
(A) are caused by acetylcholine receptor blockade
(B) occur in preganglionic nerve endings
(C) occur in the effector cells (eg, smooth muscle)
(D) are treated with choline infusions
(E) are not seen at somatic motor nerve endings at skeletal muscle

**DIRECTIONS (items 8–10):** For the following 3 questions, use the accompanying diagram. Assume that the diagram can represent either the parasympathetic or the sympathetic nervous system. Select the ONE lettered answer that is best in each case.

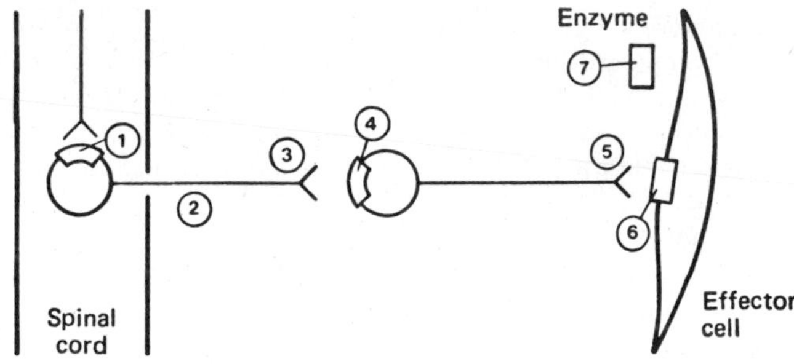


**8.** Which of the following drugs acts at site ③?
(A) Tyramine
(B) Reserpine
(C) Botulinum toxin
(D) 6-Hydroxydopamine
(E) Cocaine

**9.** Acetylcholine does NOT interact at which of the following sites in the diagram?
(A) Site ②
(B) Site ④
(C) Site ⑤
(D) Site ⑥
(E) Site ⑦

**10.** Atropine is a useful drug for inducing dilatation of the pupil and paralysis of accommodation. These effects of atropine occur at which of the following sites on the diagram?
(A) Site ③
(B) Site ④
(C) Site ⑤
(D) Site ⑥
(E) Site ⑦

## ANSWERS

**1.** Baroreceptors increase their firing rate with increased blood pressure. The answer is **(C).** (If you chose a different answer, review the components of the autonomic and hormonal feedback loops for the maintenance of blood pressure [Fig 6–2]).

**2.** Mydriasis can be caused by contraction of the radial fibers of the iris; these smooth muscle cells have alpha receptors. All the other responses are beta-mediated (Table 6–1). The answer is **(C).**

**3.** Because of the baroreceptor reflex, a directly acting drug that causes a drop in total peripheral resistance will induce a reflex increase in sympathetic outflow and a decrease in parasympathetic tone. As a result, the heart rate and cardiac force will increase. The answer is **(A).**

**4.** Sympathetic autonomic outflow causes constriction of the renal resistance vessels and a fall in renal blood flow. This is the typical response to severe exercise or hypotension. The answer is **(B).**

**5.** Cardiac transplantation requires cutting of all postsynaptic sympathetic and presynaptic parasympathetic nerves to the heart. As a result, sympathetic postganglionic nerve endings will degenerate and stores of norepinephrine will be depleted. A drug that acts by releasing stored norepinephrine (an indirectly acting sympathomimetic) would have a greatly reduced effect on a transplanted heart. The answer is **(A).**

**6.** Both types of ganglia and the neuromuscular junction have nicotinic cholinoceptors. Bronchial smooth muscle contains muscarinic receptors. The Renshaw cell was one of the first central neurons shown to respond to ACh (review the physiology of the spinal cord). The answer is **(E).**

**7.** Botulinum toxin impairs all types of cholinergic transmission, including preganglionic nerve endings and somatic motor nerve endings. It does so by altering the packaging of transmitter in vesicles within cholinergic nerve endings, resulting in impaired ACh release. Synthesis of the transmitter is not impaired, so infusion of choline is of no value. The answer is **(B).**

**8.** Each of these agents has a different mechanism of action, yet all but one act on the sympathetic postganglionic nerve terminal (site ⑤). Site ③ is a cholinergic nerve ending. The answer is **(C).**

**9.** Acetylcholine acts at both the nicotinic ganglionic receptor (site ④) and the muscarinic receptors on effector cells (site ⑥) and presynaptic nerve endings (site ⑤). It also interacts with acetylcholinesterase (site ⑦). It does not influence electrical transmission in axons (site ②). The answer is **(A).**

**10.** In the simplified diagram, the muscarinic receptors blocked by atropine are located only at the smooth muscle effector cells and postganglionic nerve terminals. This type of receptor is also found in ganglia, but very high concentrations of atropine are required to block it. Block of presynaptic muscarinic receptors would not allow mydriasis and cycloplegia. The answer is **(D).**

# 7 Cholinoceptor-Activating & Cholinesterase-Inhibiting Drugs

## OBJECTIVES

**Define the following terms:**

- Parasympathomimetic
- Cholinomimetic alkaloids
- Direct-acting cholinomimetics
- Indirect-acting cholinomimetics
- Choline esters
- Cyclospasm
- Short- and long-acting cholinesterase inhibitors
- Nicotinic agonists
- Muscarinic agonists
- Organophosphates
- Organophosphate aging
- Cholinergic crisis
- Myasthenic crisis

**You should be able to:**

- List the locations and types of acetylcholine receptors in the major organ systems (CNS, eyes, heart, vessels, bronchi, gut, genitourinary tract, skeletal muscle, exocrine glands).
- Describe the effects of acetylcholine on the major organs.
- Relate the different pharmacokinetic properties of the various choline esters and cholinomimetic alkaloids to their chemical properties.
- List the major clinical uses of cholinomimetic agonists.
- Describe the pharmacodynamic differences between direct- and indirect-acting cholinomimetic agents.
- List the major signs and symptoms of (1) acute nicotine toxicity and (2) organophosphate insecticide poisoning.

## CONCEPTS

Acetylcholinelike agonists (cholinomimetics) are subdivided in 2 ways: on the basis of their **spectrum of action** (ie, whether they are muscarinic or nicotinic) and on the basis of their **mechanism of action** (ie, whether they act directly at the acetylcholine [ACh] receptor [cholinoceptor] or indirectly through inhibition of cholinesterase). ACh may be considered the prototype direct-acting drug at both muscarinic and nicotinic receptors. Neostigmine is a prototype for the indirect-acting cholinesterase inhibitors.

### DIRECT-ACTING CHOLINOMIMETIC AGONISTS

This subclass comprises a group of choline esters (ACh, methacholine, carbachol, and bethanechol) and a second group of naturally occurring alkaloids (muscarine, pilocarpine, nicotine, and lobeline). The members differ in their spectrum of action (amount of muscarinic versus nicotinic stimulation) and in their pharmacokinetics (Table 7–1). Both factors influence their clinical use.

**A. Classification:** Muscarinic agonists are **parasympathomimetic;** ie, they mimic the actions of parasympathetic nerve stimulation. Several subgroups of muscarinic receptors have been identified (Table 7–2), but selective agonists for these subtype receptors are not available for clinical use. Nicotinic agonists are rarely classified on the basis of whether ganglionic or neuromuscular stimulation predominates because agonist selectivity is limited. However, relatively selective antagonists are available.

**B. Molecular Mechanisms of Action:** Several molecular mechanisms of muscarinic action have

**Table 7–1.** Cholinomimetics: Pharmacokinetics and spectrum of action.

| Drug | Spectrum of Action[1] | Pharmacokinetic Features |
|---|---|---|
| Direct-acting | | |
| Acetylcholine | B | Rapidly hydrolyzed by cholinesterase (ChE), 5–30 sec duration of action |
| Bethanechol | M | Resistant to ChE, orally active, poor lipid solubility, 30 min–2 h duration of action |
| Carbachol | B | Like bethanechol |
| Pilocarpine | M | Not an ester, orally active, good lipid solubility, 30 min–2 h duration of action |
| Nicotine | N | Like pilocarpine, duration 1–6 h |
| Indirect-acting | | |
| Edrophonium | B | Alcohol, quaternary amine, poor lipid solubility, orally inactive, 5–15 min duration of action |
| Neostigmine | B | Carbamate, quaternary amine, poor lipid solubility, orally active, 30 min–2 h duration of action |
| Physostigmine | B | Carbamate, tertiary amine, lipid soluble, 30 min–2 h duration of action |
| Pyridostigmine, ambenonium | B | Carbamates, quaternary amines, 2–6 h duration of action |
| Echothiophate | B | Phosphate, modest lipid solubility, 2–7 day duration of action |
| Parathion | B | Phosphate, high lipid solubility, 7–30 day duration of action |

[1]M = muscarinic, N = nicotinic, B = both muscarinic and nicotinic.

been defined (Table 7–2). One involves coupling of muscarinic receptors to phospholipase C, a membrane-bound enzyme that results in the release of the second messengers inositol-1,4,5-trisphosphate ($IP_3$) and diacylglycerol (DAG). DAG modulates the action of protein kinase C, an enzyme important in secretion, whereas $IP_3$ evokes the release of calcium from intracellular storage sites and results in contraction. A second mechanism couples muscarinic receptors to adenylyl cyclase through the inhibitory $G_i$ coupling protein. A third mechanism couples the receptor directly to potassium channels in the heart and elsewhere; muscarinic agonists cause opening of the channel.

The mechanism of nicotinic action has been clearly defined as a direct coupling of the nicotinic receptor to the opening of channels that are poorly selective for sodium and potassium (ACh channels) on ganglion cells and the neuromuscular end-plate. The receptor is located on the channel protein. Depolarization of the cell results.

**C. Tissue & Organ Effects:** The tissue and organ level effects are summarized in Table 7–3. Note that vasodilation is not parasympathomimetic (it is not evoked by parasympathetic nerve discharge, even though directly acting cholinomimetics do cause vasodilation). This action results

**Table 7–2.** Identified or cloned cholinoceptors.

| Receptor Type | Other Names | Postreceptor Mechanisms |
|---|---|---|
| $M_1$ | $M_{1a}$ | $IP_3$ cascade |
| $M_2$ | $M_{2a}$, cardiac $M_2$ | Inhibition of cAMP production |
| $M_3$ | $M_{2b}$, glandular $M_2$ | $IP_3$ cascade |
| $m_4$ | | Inhibition of cAMP production1 |
| $m_5$ | | $IP_3$, DAG cascade[1] |
| $N_M$ | End-plate receptor | Na,K depolarizing channel |
| $N_N$ | Ganglion receptor | Na,K depolarizing channel |

[1]Functional receptors have not been incontrovertibly identified, but genes have been.

**Table 7–3.** Effects of direct-acting cholinoceptor stimulants. Only the direct effects are indicated: homeostatic responses to these direct actions may be important.[1]

| Organ | Response |
|---|---|
| Eye | |
| Sphincter muscle of iris | Contraction (miosis). |
| Ciliary muscle | Contraction for near vision. |
| Heart | |
| Sinoatrial node | Decrease in rate (negative chronotropy). |
| Atria | Decrease in contractile strength (negative inotropy). Decrease in refractory period. |
| Atrioventricular node | Decrease in conduction velocity (negative dromotropy). |
| Ventricles | Small decrease in contractile strength. |
| Blood vessels | |
| Arteries | Dilatation (via EDRF). |
| Veins | Dilatation (via EDRF). |
| Lung | |
| Bronchial muscle | Contraction (bronchoconstriction). |
| Bronchial glands | Stimulation. |
| Gastrointestinal tract | |
| Motility | Increase. |
| Sphincters | Relaxation. |
| Secretion | Stimulation. |
| Urinary bladder | |
| Detrusor | Contraction. |
| Trigone and sphincter | Relaxation. |
| Glands | |
| Sweat, salivary, lacrimal, nasopharyngeal | Secretion. |

[1]Reproduced, with permission, from Katzung BG (editor): *Basic & Clinical Pharmacology,* 5th ed. Appleton & Lange, 1992.

from the release of endothelium-derived relaxing factor (EDRF; probably nitric oxide) in the vessels, mediated by uninnervated muscarinic receptors on the endothelial cells. Note also that the *baroreceptor reflex* is evoked by decreased blood pressure and will result in strong compensatory sympathetic discharge to the heart and, often, tachycardia.

The tissue and organ level effects of nicotinic ganglionic stimulation will depend on the autonomic innervation of the organ involved. The vessels are dominated by sympathetic innervation; therefore, nicotinic receptor activation results in vasoconstriction mediated by sympathetic postganglionic nerve discharge. The gut is dominated by parasympathetic control; nicotinic drugs increase motility and secretion because of increased parasympathetic postganglionic neuron discharge. Skeletal neuromuscular end-plate activation by direct-acting nicotinic drugs results in fasciculations and spasm of the muscles involved. Prolonged activation results in paralysis (see Chapter 26) and is an important hazard of exposure to both nicotine-containing and organophosphate insecticides.

**D. Clinical Use:** The major clinical applications of the muscarinic agonists are predictable from a consideration of organ effects and the diseases that benefit from an increase in cholinergic activity. They are summarized in Table 7–4. Direct-acting nicotinic agonists have no therapeutic applications; indirect-acting agents are superior (see below).

**E. Toxicity:** The signs and symptoms of overdosage are readily predicted from the general pharmacology of ACh.

1. **Muscarinic effects.** These include CNS stimulation (uncommon with direct-acting agonists), miosis, spasm of accommodation, bronchoconstriction, increased gastrointestinal and genitourinary smooth muscle activity, increased secretory activity (sweat glands, airway, gastrointestinal tract), vasodilation, and bradycardia if administered as an intravenous bolus (reflex tachycardia otherwise).

**Table 7–4.** Clinical applications and underlying actions of some cholinoceptor agonists.

| Drug | Application | Action |
|---|---|---|
| Direct-acting agonists | | |
| Bethanechol | Postoperative and neurogenic ileus and urinary retention | Activates bowel and bladder smooth muscle |
| Carbachol, pilocarpine | Glaucoma | Activate ciliary muscle of eye |
| Indirect-acting agonists | | |
| Neostigmine | Postoperative and neurogenic ileus and urinary retention | Increases efficiency of cholinergic transmission in bowel and bladder smooth muscle |
| Neostigmine, pyridostigmine, ambenonium, edrophonium | Myasthenia gravis, reversal of neuromuscular blockade | Increase efficiency of cholinergic transmission in skeletal muscle end-plates |
| Physostigmine, echothiophate | Glaucoma | Increase efficiency of cholinergic transmission in ciliary muscle of eye |

2. **Nicotinic effects.** These include CNS stimulation, ganglionic stimulation, and neuromuscular end-plate depolarization leading to fasciculations and paralysis.

## INDIRECT-ACTING AGONISTS

**A. Classification & Prototypes:** The indirect-acting cholinomimetic drugs fall into 2 major chemical classes: carbamic acid esters (**carbamates;** neostigmine is a prototype) and phosphoric acid esters (phosphates, **organophosphates;** echothiophate is a prototype). Edrophonium is a special case; it is not an ester and has a short duration of action.

**B. Mechanisms of Action:** Both carbamate and organophosphate inhibitors bind to the enzyme and are quickly hydrolyzed. The alcohol portion of the molecule is then released. The acidic portion (carbamate or phosphate) is released slowly compared with that of ACh (acetate).

1. **Carbamates** are hydrolyzed, and the carbamate is slowly released by cholinesterase over a period of 2–8 hours.
2. **Organophosphates** are long-acting drugs; they form an extremely stable complex with the enzyme and are released over periods of days to weeks.

**C. Effects:** These agents act by inhibiting cholinesterase and result in an increase in the concentration and half-life of ACh in the synapses in which it is released physiologically. Therefore, indirect agents have muscarinic or nicotinic effects, depending on which organ system is under consideration. They do not have therapeutic actions at sites where ACh is not normally released, eg, the endothelium of blood vessels.

**D. Clinical Use:** The major clinical applications of the indirect-acting cholinomimetics include both muscarinic and nicotinic effects. These effects are predictable based on a consideration of the organs and the diseases that benefit from an increase in cholinergic activity. They are summarized in Table 7–4. The carbamates, which include neostigmine, physostigmine, ambenonium, and pyridostigmine, are more commonly used in therapeutics than are organophosphates. Some carbamates (eg, carbaryl) are used in agriculture as insecticides. Three organophosphates used in medicine are echothiophate (an antiglaucoma drug), malathion (a scabicide), and metrifonate (an anthelmintic).

**E. Toxicity:** In addition to their therapeutic uses, the indirect-acting agents have importance because of accidental exposures to toxic amounts of pesticides. A case of intoxication is described in Case 1 (Appendix III). The most toxic of these drugs (eg, parathion) are rapidly fatal if exposure is not immediately recognized and treated. Treatment is described in Chapter 8. After first binding to cholinesterase, most organophosphate inhibitors can be removed from the enzyme by the use of "regenerator" compounds such as pralidoxime (see Chapter 8). However, if the enzyme-inhibitor binding is allowed to persist, aging (a further chemical change) occurs and regenerator drugs are no longer able to remove the inhibitor. Because of their toxicity, organophosphates are used extensively in agriculture as insecticides and anthelmintic agents; examples include malathion, parathion, and dichlorvos. Some of these agents (eg, malathion, dichlorvos) are relatively safe because they are metabolized rapidly to inactive products in mammals (and birds) but not in insects. Some are pro-drugs (eg, malathion, parathion) and must be metabolized to the active product (malaoxon and paraoxon, respectively). The signs and symptoms of poisoning are the same as those described for the direct-acting agents, with the following exceptions: Vasodilation is a late and uncommon effect; bradycardia is more common than tachycardia; CNS stimulation is common with organophosphate and physostigmine overdosage and includes convulsions, followed by respiratory and cardiovascular depression.

## DRUG LIST

The following drugs are important members of the group discussed in this chapter. Prototype agents should be learned in detail; the major variants should be known well enough to list the factors that distinguish them from the prototypes and from each other.

| Subclass | Prototype | Major Variants |
|---|---|---|
| Direct-acting drugs | | |
| Muscarinic agonists | Acetylcholine | Muscarine, carbachol, bethanechol, pilocarpine |
| Nicotinic agonists | Acetylcholine | Nicotine, carbachol, succinylcholine |
| Indirect-acting drugs (cholinesterase inhibitors) | | |
| Alcohol | Edrophonium | |
| Carbamates | Neostigmine | Pyridostigmine, physostigmine, carbaryl |
| Organophosphates | Echothiophate | Parathion, DFP, malathion, dichlorvos |

## QUESTIONS

**DIRECTIONS (items 1–10):** Each numbered item or incomplete statement in this section is followed by answers or by completions of the statement. Select the ONE lettered answer or completion that is BEST in each case.

**1.** Physostigmine and bethanechol in small doses have similar effects on all of the following EXCEPT
**(A)** neuromuscular junction (skeletal muscle)
**(B)** salivary glands
**(C)** ureteral tone
**(D)** sweat glands
**(E)** gastric secretion

**2.** Parathion has all of the following characteristics EXCEPT:
**(A)** It is less persistent in the environment than DDT
**(B)** It is more toxic to humans than malathion
**(C)** It is inactivated by conversion to paraoxon
**(D)** It is very lipid-soluble and is well absorbed through the skin and lungs
**(E)** Toxicity, if treated early, may be partly reversed by pralidoxime

**3.** In the treatment of myasthenia gravis, the best agent for distinguishing between myasthenic crisis (insufficient therapy) and cholinergic crisis (excessive therapy) is
**(A)** atropine
**(B)** physostigmine
**(C)** echothiophate
**(D)** pralidoxime
**(E)** edrophonium

**4.** The cause of death in organophosphate "nerve gas" poisoning would probably be
**(A)** gastrointestinal bleeding
**(B)** hypertension
**(C)** respiratory failure
**(D)** congestive heart failure
**(E)** cardiac arrhythmia

**5.** Pyridostigmine and neostigmine may cause all of the following EXCEPT
**(A)** reversible inhibition of acetylcholinesterase
**(B)** spasm of accommodation
**(C)** constipation
**(D)** bronchoconstriction
**(E)** weakness of skeletal muscle

**6.** Both parasympathetic nerve stimulation and a slow infusion of bethanechol increase the
**(A)** heart rate
**(B)** bladder tone
**(C)** both **(A)** and **(B)** are correct
**(D)** neither **(A)** nor **(B)** is correct

**7.** In the human eye, echothiophate can cause all of the following EXCEPT
**(A)** miosis
**(B)** ciliary spasm
**(C)** reversal of the cycloplegic action of atropine
**(D)** decrease in the incidence of cataracts
**(E)** reduction in intraocular pressure

**8.** In the comparison of bethanechol and pilocarpine, all of the following are correct EXCEPT:
**(A)** Both are hydrolyzed by cholinesterase
**(B)** Both may cause tachycardia
**(C)** Both may cause bronchoconstriction
**(D)** Both activate muscarinic receptors
**(E)** Both may increase gastrointestinal motility

**9.** Typical symptoms of cholinesterase inhibitor toxicity include all of the following EXCEPT
**(A)** nausea, vomiting, diarrhea
**(B)** salivation, sweating
**(C)** miosis
**(D)** paralysis of skeletal muscles
**(E)** paralysis of accommodation

**10.** Actions of cholinoceptor agonists and their clinical effects include
**(A)** cyclospasm and improved aqueous humor drainage in glaucoma
**(B)** decreased gastrointestinal motility with resulting gastrointestinal stasis (ileus)
**(C)** improved neuromuscular transmission and accelerated recovery from neuromuscular blockade
**(D)** improved neuromuscular transmission and prevention of cholinergic crisis of myasthenia
**(E)** both **(A)** and **(C)** are correct

## ANSWERS

**1.** Because physostigmine acts on the enzyme cholinesterase, which is present at *all* cholinergic synapses, it will increase acetylcholine effects at both the nicotinic and muscarinic junctions. Bethanechol, on the other hand, is a direct-acting agent that is selective for muscarinic junctions. The answer is **(A)**.

2. The "-thion" organophosphates (those containing the P=S bond) are activated, not inactivated, by conversion to P=O derivatives. The answer is **(C).**

3. Since short-acting drugs are usually preferable for diagnostic use, the best agent is the shortest-acting cholinesterase inhibitor, edrophonium. The answer is **(E).**

4. Respiratory failure, from neuromuscular paralysis or central nervous system depression, is by far the most important cause of death in acute cholinesterase inhibitor toxicity. The answer is **(C).**

5. Cholinesterase inhibition is typically associated with increased (never decreased) bowel activity. Skeletal muscle weakness is an important sign of excessive cholinesterase inhibition (cholinergic crisis). The answer is **(C).**

6. Choice **(A)** is not correct because the vagus slows the heart. The answer is **(B).**

7. The long-acting cholinesterase inhibitors are associated with an increased incidence of cataracts in patients receiving these drugs for glaucoma. All the other effects are typical muscarinic actions. The answer is **(D).**

8. Neither bethanechol nor pilocarpine is hydrolyzed by acetylcholinesterase. The answer is **(A).**

9. Questions referring to cholinesterase inhibitor toxicity are very common. Skeletal muscle paralysis results from prolonged depolarization of neuromuscular end-plates (depolarizing blockade). Cholinomimetics cause cyclospasm, the opposite of paralysis of accommodation (cycloplegia). The answer is **(E).**

10. Cholinesterase inhibitors may either improve or impair neuromuscular transmission. Cholinergic crisis is caused by too much acetylcholine at the end-plate. Cholinomimetics never decrease gastrointestinal motility; in fact, they may be used to reverse postoperative ileus. The answer is **(E).**

# Cholinoceptor Blockers & Cholinesterase Regenerators

# 8

## OBJECTIVES

**Define the following terms:**

- Anti-motion-sickness agent
- Antimuscarinic delirium
- Atropine fever
- Atropine flush
- Cholinesterase regenerator
- Cycloplegic
- Depolarizing blockade
- Miotic
- Mydriatic
- Nondepolarizing blockade
- Organophosphate aging
- Orthostatic hypotension
- Parasympatholytic
- Pharmacokinetic selectivity

**You should be able to:**

- Describe the effects of atropine on the major organ systems (CNS, eyes, heart, vessels, bronchi, gut, genitourinary tract, exocrine glands, skeletal muscle).
- List the signs, symptoms, and treatment of atropine poisoning.
- List the major clinical indications and contraindications for the use of muscarinic antagonists.
- Describe the autonomic effects of the ganglion-blocking nicotinic antagonists.
- List one antimuscarinic agent promoted for each of the following special uses: mydriasis and cycloplegia, parkinsonism, peptic ulcer, and asthma.

## CONCEPTS

The cholinoceptor antagonists are readily grouped into subclasses on the basis of their spectrum of action (ie, the receptors they block, whether they are muscarinic or nicotinic).

### MUSCARINIC ANTAGONISTS

**A. Classification & Pharmacokinetics:**

1. **Muscarinic antagonists** can be further subdivided on the basis of their pharmacokinetics, especially their ability to distribute into the CNS. A major determinant of this property is the presence or absence of a permanently charged (quaternary) amine group in the drug. This is because charged molecules are more polar and therefore less likely to penetrate a lipid barrier such as the blood-brain barrier.
   a. **Pharmacokinetics of atropine.** Atropine is the prototype antimuscarinic drug. It is an alkaloid found in *Atropa belladonna* and many other plants. Because it is a tertiary amine, it is relatively lipid-soluble and readily crosses membrane barriers. It is well distributed into the CNS and other organs and is eliminated partially by metabolism in the liver and partially by renal excretion. The dominant elimination half-life is approximately 2 hours, and the duration of action of normal doses is 4–8 hours, except in the eyes, where the effects last for up to 72 hours.
   b. **Pharmacokinetics of other muscarinic blockers.** In ophthalmology, topical activity (ability to enter the eye after conjunctival administration) and duration of action are important in determining the usefulness of several antimuscarinic drugs. A similar ability to cross lipid barriers is important for the agents used in parkinsonism. In contrast, the drugs used for their antisecretory or antispastic actions in the gut, the genitourinary tract, and the bronchi are selected for minimum CNS activity and often incorporate quaternary amine groups to limit penetration through the blood-brain barrier.

2. **Receptor subgroups.** The division of muscarinic receptors into subgroups is still tentative, and the antagonists currently approved for clinical use are not very selective for any single type. However, pirenzepine is considered moderately selective for the $M_1$ subgroup and has entered clinical trials for the treatment of peptic ulcer.

**B. Mechanism of Action:** The antimuscarinic agents act like competitive (surmountable) pharmacologic antagonists, and their blocking effects can be overcome by increased concentrations of muscarinic agonists.

**C. Effects:** The peripheral actions of muscarinic blockers are mostly predictable effects derived from cholinoceptor blockade (Table 8–1). The CNS effects are less predictable. Those seen at therapeutic concentrations include sedation, reduction of motion sickness, and, as noted above, reduction of some signs of parkinsonism. Cardiovascular effects at therapeutic doses include an initial reduction of heart rate caused by stimulation of the central vagal nucleus, followed by the tachycardia and decreased atrioventricular conduction time predicted by peripheral vagal blockade.

**D. Clinical Use:** The muscarinic blockers have several therapeutic applications in the eyes, the gut, the urinary bladder, and the bronchi. In addition, several effects in the brain are important. These are summarized in Table 8–1.

1. **Eyes.** Antimuscarinic drugs used to dilate the pupil and to paralyze accommodation include atropine, homatropine, cyclopentolate, and tropicamide.
2. **Gut.** Atropine, methscopolamine, and propantheline have long been used in acid-peptic disease to reduce acid secretion, but they are not as effective as are $H_2$ blockers such as cimetidine, and they cause more adverse effects. Pirenzepine is a newer, perhaps more selective, $M_1$ muscarinic blocker that may be more useful in treating peptic ulcer. Muscarinic blockers can also be used to reduce cramping and hypermotility in transient diarrheas.
3. **Bladder.** Atropine, methscopolamine, and similar agents may be used to reduce urgency in mild cystitis.
4. **CNS.** Scopolamine is a standard therapy for motion sickness; new drugs are measured against it. Benztropine, biperiden, and trihexyphenidyl are representative of several antimuscarinic agents used to treat parkinsonism. They are not as effective as L-DOPA (see Chapter 27).
5. **Airways.** Parenteral atropine has long been used to reduce airway secretions during surgery. Ipratropium is a quaternary antimuscarinic agent used by inhalation to reduce bronchoconstriction in asthma.

**E. Toxicity:**

1. **Predictable toxicities.** Antimuscarinic actions lead to several important and potentially dangerous effects. In young children, these effects result in hyperthermia or "atropine fever"; they are caused by blockade of thermoregulatory sweating. In the elderly, important targets include the eyes (glaucoma) and the bladder (urinary retention). Dry mouth, constipation, and blurred vision are more common and less threatening adverse effects in all age groups.
2. **Toxicities not predictable from peripheral autonomic actions:**
   a. **CNS effects.** CNS toxicity includes sedation, amnesia, and delirium or hallucinations; it may progress to convulsions. Central muscarinic receptors are probably involved.
   b. **Cardiovascular effects.** At toxic doses, intraventricular conduction may be blocked; this

**Table 8–1.** Organ effects and clinical applications of muscarinic antagonists.

| Organ | Effect | Clinical Applications |
|---|---|---|
| CNS | Reduces motion sickness<br>Extrapyramidal effect | Motion sickness<br>Parkinson's disease |
| Eye | Cycloplegia<br>Mydriasis | Refraction in infants<br>Retinal examination, breakage of adhesions |
| Gastrointestinal tract | Reduces secretion<br>Reduces motility | Treatment of acid-peptic disease, excess salivation<br>Treatment of temporary cramping, diarrhea |
| Genitourinary tract | Reduces bladder wall tone | Treatment of temporary cramping and urgency |
| Bronchi | Relaxes airway smooth muscle | Asthma |

is probably not mediated by muscarinic blockade, and it is difficult to treat. Dilation of the cutaneous vessels of the head, neck, and trunk also occurs at these doses; the resulting "atropine flush" may be diagnostic of overdose with the drug.

## NICOTINIC ANTAGONISTS

**A. Classification & Prototypes:** Nicotinic receptor antagonists are divided into ganglion-blocking drugs and neuromuscular-blocking drugs.

1. **Ganglion-blocking drugs.** Blockers of ganglionic nicotinic receptors are now of largely academic interest, although they were important historically for introducing the era of successful therapy of hypertension. Hexamethonium (C6), mecamylamine, and several other ganglion blockers were extensively used for this disease. Unfortunately, the adverse effects of ganglion blockade are so severe (both sympathetic and parasympathetic divisions are blocked) that few patients are able to tolerate these drugs for long periods. At present, trimethaphan, a short-acting agent, is the only ganglion blocker important in therapy. Its action is like that of a competitive pharmacologic antagonist. It is poorly lipid-soluble and has a short half-life. It is inactive orally but is used intravenously for the therapy of severe accelerated hypertension (malignant hypertension). Because ganglion blockers markedly reduce venous tone, they produce postural hypotension as a major mechanism of pressure reduction.
2. **Neuromuscular-blocking drugs.** Neuromuscular-blocking drugs are important for producing complete skeletal muscle relaxation in surgery, and new ones are frequently introduced. They are discussed in depth in Chapter 26.
   a. **Nondepolarizing group.** Tubocurarine is the prototype. It produces a competitive block at the end-plate, causing flaccid paralysis that lasts 30–60 minutes (longer if large doses have been given). Pancuronium, atracurium, and vecuronium are shorter-acting nondepolarizing blockers. Gallamine is an older drug that is only rarely used in the USA.
   b. **Depolarizing group.** Succinylcholine, a nicotinic agonist, is the only member of this group used in the USA. It produces fasciculations during induction of paralysis, and patients may complain of muscle pain after its use. The drug is hydrolyzed by pseudocholinesterase (plasma cholinesterase) and has a half-life of a few minutes in persons with normal plasma cholinesterase activity.

## CHOLINESTERASE REGENERATORS

The cholinesterase regenerators form a special class of agents that are not receptor antagonists but are chemical antagonists. They are oximes and have an extremely high affinity for the phosphorus atom in organophosphate insecticides—if aging has not occurred. Because the affinity of the oxime group for phosphorus exceeds that of the enzyme active site, these agents are able to displace the enzyme from the inhibitor, thus regenerating the active enzyme. Pralidoxime, the oxime currently available in the USA, is often used in the emergency department to treat patients exposed to drugs such as parathion.

# DRUG LIST

The following drugs are important members of the groups discussed in this chapter. Prototype agents should be learned in detail; the major variants should be known well enough to list the factors that distinguish them from the prototypes and from each other; and the other significant agents should be recognized as belonging to a specific subclass.

| Subclass | Prototype | Major Variants | Other Significant Agents |
|---|---|---|---|
| Muscarinic antagonists | Atropine | Scopolamine, propantheline, pratropium, pirenzepine | Homatropine, methscopolamine, tropicamide |
| Nicotinic antagonists | Curare, hexamethonium | Pancuronium, (nicotine),[1] trimethaphan | Atracurium, vecuronium, (succinylcholine),[1] mecamylamine |
| Cholinesterase regenerator | Pralidoxime | | |

[1]An agonist that causes blockade by prolonged depolarization of the membrane with which the cholinoceptor is associated.

## QUESTIONS

**DIRECTIONS (items 1–12):** Each numbered item or incomplete statement in this section is followed by answers or by completions of the statement. Select the ONE lettered answer or completion that is BEST in each case.

**1.** In children, the most dangerous toxic effect of the belladonna alkaloids is
**(A)** hypertension
**(B)** hallucinations
**(C)** hyperthermia
**(D)** dehydration
**(E)** intraventricular heart block

**2.** Which of the following pairs of drugs and properties is correct?
**(A)** Atropine: Poorly absorbed after oral administration
**(B)** Cyclopentolate: Well absorbed from conjunctival sac
**(C)** Scopolamine: Short duration of action when used as an anti-motion-sickness agent
**(D)** Ipratropium: Well absorbed, long elimination half-life
**(E)** Benztropine: Quaternary, poor CNS penetration

**3.** Atropine overdosage may cause all of the following EXCEPT
**(A)** mental aberrations
**(B)** relaxation of gastrointestinal smooth muscle
**(C)** decrease in gastric secretion
**(D)** pupillary constriction
**(E)** increase in cardiac rate

**4.** All of the following can be blocked by atropine pretreatment EXCEPT
**(A)** vagal bradycardia (lowering of cardiac rate caused by vagal stimulation)
**(B)** tachycardia induced by infusion of acetylcholine
**(C)** sweating induced by injection of pilocarpine
**(D)** increased blood pressure induced by nicotine poisoning
**(E)** salivation induced by neostigmine

**5.** In using antimuscarinic drugs in ophthalmology,
**(A)** atropine is longer-acting than cyclopentolate and more efficacious than methscopolamine
**(B)** excess antimuscarinic effect is more easily reversed with physostigmine than with neostigmine
**(C)** both **(A)** and **(B)** are correct
**(D)** neither **(A)** nor **(B)** is correct

**DIRECTIONS (items 6 and 7):** Two new synthetic drugs (*X* and *Y*) are to be studied for their cardiovascular effects. They are given to 3 anesthetized animals while the blood pressure is recorded. The first animal has received no pretreatment, the second has received an effective dose of a ganglion blocker, and the third has received an effective dose of a muscarinic antagonist. The net changes induced by the new drugs (not by the blocking drugs) are shown in the graph below.

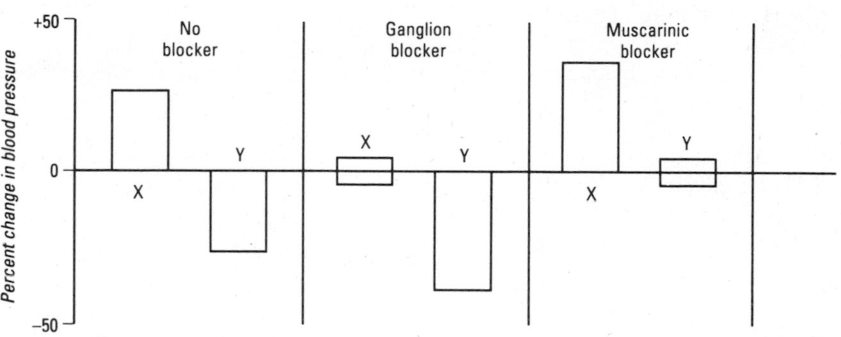


**Graph 8–1.**

6. Drug *X* is probably a drug similar to
   (A) acetylcholine
   (B) nicotine
   (C) epinephrine
   (D) atropine
   (E) hexamethonium

7. Drug *Y* is probably a drug similar to
   (A) acetylcholine
   (B) nicotine
   (C) pralidoxime
   (D) edrophonium
   (E) hexamethonium

8. Ganglion-blocking drugs have all of the following properties EXCEPT:
   (A) They cause constipation
   (B) They cause orthostatic hypotension
   (C) They impair sexual function
   (D) They increase maximal exercise heart rate
   (E) They cause cycloplegia

9. All of the following may cause cycloplegia (paralysis of accommodation) when used topically in the eye EXCEPT
   (A) atropine
   (B) physostigmine (eserine)
   (C) tropicamide
   (D) cyclopentolate
   (E) scopolamine

10. Atropine therapy in the elderly may be hazardous because
    (A) atropine can elevate intraocular pressure in patients with glaucoma
    (B) atropine frequently causes ventricular tachycardia
    (C) urinary retention may be precipitated in women
    (D) the elderly are particularly prone to developing dangerous hyperthermia
    (E) atropine often causes excessive vasodilation and hypotension in the elderly

**11.** When a dose-response study of atropine is carried out in young adults, which of the following effects may be observed?
**(A)** Bradycardia
**(B)** Tachycardia
**(C)** CNS stimulation, eg, hallucinations
**(D)** CNS depression, eg, sedation
**(E)** All of the above

**12.** Accepted therapeutic indications for the use of antimuscarinic drugs include all of the following EXCEPT
**(A)** Parkinson's disease
**(B)** hypertension
**(C)** traveler's diarrhea
**(D)** motion sickness
**(E)** cystitis

## ANSWERS

**1.** Choices **(B)**, **(C)**, and **(E)** are possible effects of the atropine group. However, in children the most dangerous effect is hyperthermia. Deaths with body temperatures in excess of 42 °C have occurred after the use of atropine-containing eye drops in children. The answer is **(C).**

**2.** Atropine is very well absorbed. Scopolamine has a long duration of action. Ipratropium is poorly absorbed from the airways into the circulation and has a short elimination half-life. Benztropine is lipid-soluble and penetrates into the CNS well. Only **(B)** is correct.

**3.** Pupillary dilatation is a characteristic atropine effect, as indicated by the origin of the name belladonna ("beautiful lady") from the ancient cosmetic use of extracts of the plant to dilate the pupils. The answer is **(D).**

**4.** Atropine blocks muscarinic receptors and inhibits parasympathomimetic effects. Nicotine can induce both parasympathomimetic and sympathomimetic effects, by virtue of its ganglion-stimulating action. Hypertension reflects sympathetic discharge and therefore would not be blocked by atropine. The answer is **(D).**

**5.** Atropine is considerably longer-acting (about 48–72 hours) than cyclopentolate (about 1 hour). Physostigmine penetrates the surface of the eye better than neostigmine—it is a tertiary amine. The answer is **(C).**

**6.** Drug ***X*** causes an increase in blood pressure that is blocked by a ganglion blocker but not by a muscarinic blocker. The pressor response is actually increased by pretreatment with a muscarinic blocker, suggesting that compensatory vagal discharge might have blunted the full response. This description fits a ganglion stimulant such as nicotine. It does not fit epinephrine, since the pressor effects of epinephrine are produced at alpha receptors, not in the ganglia. The answer is **(B).**

**7.** Drug ***Y*** causes a decrease in blood pressure that is blocked by a muscarinic blocker but not by a ganglion blocker. Therefore, the depressor effect must be evoked at a site distal to the ganglia. In fact, the drop in blood pressure is actually greater in the presence of ganglion blockade, suggesting that compensatory sympathetic discharge might have blunted the full depressor action of drug ***Y*** in the untreated animal. The description fits a direct-acting muscarinic stimulant such as acetylcholine (given in high dosage). Indirect-acting cholinomimetics (cholinesterase inhibitors) would not produce this pattern because the vascular muscarinic receptors involved in the depressor response are not innervated. The answer is **(A).**

**8.** Ganglion blockers can increase the resting heart rate, because that is determined largely by vagal tone. However, they will decrease the maximum exercise rate, since acceleration to the maximum level requires an increase of sympathetic tone. The answer is **(D).**

**9.** All antimuscarinic agents are, in theory, capable of causing cycloplegia. Physostigmine, on the other hand, is an indirect-acting cholinomimetic. The answer is **(B).**

**10.** The elderly have a much higher incidence of glaucoma than do younger people (and may be unaware of the disease until late in its course). Antimuscarinic agents may increase intraocular pressure in individuals with glaucoma. Elderly men have a much higher probability than women of developing urinary retention, because they have a high incidence of prostatic hypertrophy. Cardiac and hyperthermic reactions to atropine are not common in the elderly. The answer is **(A).**

**11.** All of the effects may be observed in a group of subjects (or even in a single subject, though not at the same time). The answer is **(E).**

**12.** Hypertension is not responsive to antimuscarinic agents. The answer is **(B).**

# Adrenoceptor Stimulants 9

## OBJECTIVES

**Define the following terms:**

- Anorexiant
- Catecholamine
- Decongestant
- Direct, indirect agonist
- Mydriatic
- Phenylisopropylamine
- Selective alpha agonist, beta agonist
- Sympathomimetic
- Reuptake inhibitor

**You should be able to:**

- List tissues that contain significant numbers of $\alpha_1$ or $\alpha_2$ receptors.
- List tissues that contain significant numbers of $\beta_1$ or $\beta_2$ receptors.
- Describe the major organ system effects of a pure alpha agonist, a pure beta agonist, and a mixed alpha and beta agonist, and give examples of each type of drug.
- Describe a clinical situation in which the effects of an indirect sympathomimetic would differ from those of a direct agonist.
- List the major clinical applications of the adrenoceptor agonists.

## CONCEPTS

**A. Classification & Prototypes:** The adrenoceptor agonists are subdivided in 2 ways: by spectrum of action and by mode of action.

**1. Spectrum of action:** The adrenoceptors are classified as alpha or beta receptors; both groups are further subdivided into 2 (or more) subgroups. Epinephrine may be considered a single prototype with effects at all receptor types ($\alpha_1$, $\alpha_2$, $\beta_1$, and $\beta_2$). Alternatively, separate prototypes, phenylephrine (alpha) and isoproterenol (beta), may be defined. The distribution of these receptors is set forth in Table 9–1.

2. **Mode of action:** The adrenoceptor agonists may directly activate their receptors, or they may act indirectly to increase the release of endogenous catecholamines. Blockade of metabolism (ie, block of catechol-O-methyltransferase [COMT] and monoamine oxidase [MAO]) has little direct effect on autonomic activity, but MAO inhibition does increase the stores of catecholamines in storage vesicles and may potentiate the action of indirect-acting sympathomimetics. Phenylisopropylamines such as amphetamine cause the release of stored catecholamines and are therefore mainly indirect in their mode of action. They are also relatively resistant to metabolism by MAO. Tyramine, although not a phenylisopropylamine, is an indirect-acting sympathomimetic but is readily metabolized by MAO. Another form of indirect action is that of cocaine, which prevents reuptake of catecholamines by nerve terminals and increases the synaptic concentration of released transmitter. Tricyclic antidepressants have a similar effect.
3. **Chemistry and pharmacokinetics:** The endogenous adrenoceptor agonists (epinephrine, norepinephrine, and dopamine) are catecholamines and are metabolized by COMT and MAO as noted above. As a result, they are inactive when given by the oral route. After their release from nerve endings, they are again taken up into nerve endings and into perisynaptic cells; they have a short duration of action. The phenylisopropylamines are resistant to MAO, and noncatecholamines are resistant to COMT; these agents are orally active, and their effects last much longer than do those of parenteral catecholamines.

## B. Mechanism of Action:

1. **Smooth muscle $\alpha_1$-receptor** effects are mediated primarily by activation of the phosphoinositide cascade, liberating inositol-1,4,5-trisphosphate and diacylglycerol. Calcium is released in smooth muscle cells, and enzymes are activated. Direct gating of calcium channels may also play a role in increasing the intracellular calcium concentration.
2. **Alpha$_2$-receptor activation** results in inhibition of adenylyl cyclase via the coupling protein $G_i$.
3. **Beta receptors (both $\beta_1$ and $\beta_2$)** stimulate adenylyl (formerly called adenylate) cyclase via the coupling protein $G_s$ and increase cAMP concentration in the cell.
4. **Dopamine $D_1$ receptors** activate adenylyl cyclase in neurons and vascular smooth muscle. (Dopamine $D_2$ receptors are located primarily in the brain.)

**Table 9–1.** Distribution of adrenoceptor subtypes.[1]

| Type | Tissue | Actions |
|---|---|---|
| $\alpha_1$ | Most vascular smooth muscle | Contraction |
| | Pupillary dilator muscle | Contraction (dilates pupil) |
| | Pilomotor smooth muscle | Erects hair |
| | Rat liver | Glycogenolysis |
| $\alpha_2$ | Postsynaptic CNS adrenoceptors | Probably multiple |
| | Platelets | Aggregation |
| | Adrenergic and cholinergic nerve terminals | Inhibition of transmitter release |
| | Some vascular smooth muscle | Contraction |
| | Fat cells | Inhibition of lipolysis |
| | Pancreatic B cells | Inhibition of insulin release |
| $\beta_1$ | Heart, fat cells,[2] CNS | Activation of adenylyl cyclase, stimulation of the heart |
| | Pancreatic B cells | Increase insulin release |
| $\beta_2$ | Respiratory, uterine, and vascular smooth muscle | Activation of adenylyl cyclase, relaxation of smooth muscle |
| Dopamine$_1$ | Renal and other splanchnic vessels, CNS | Activation of adenylyl cyclase |
| Dopamine$_2$ | Nerve terminals, CNS | ? Inhibition of adenylyl cyclase |

[1]Modified and reproduced, with permission, from Katzung BG (editor): *Basic & Clinical Pharmacology,* 5th ed. Appleton & Lange, 1992.
[2]Newer evidence suggests that beta receptors controlling lipolysis may be a third type of receptor, ie, $\beta_3$.

## C. Organ System Effects:

1. **Alpha$_1$ agonists** increase smooth muscle tone in various organs. Because they increase blood pressure, they often evoke a compensatory reflex bradycardia.
2. **Alpha$_2$ agonists** (eg, clonidine) cause vasoconstriction when administered intravenously or topically (eg, as a nasal spray); however, when given orally, they accumulate in the CNS and cause hypotension as described in Chapter 11.
3. **Beta$_1$ stimulants** increase cardiac rate and force, and facilitate atrioventricular conduction. They also increase renin secretion and stimulate lipolysis.
4. **Beta$_2$ stimulants** dilate skeletal muscle blood vessels and bronchi. They also decrease uterine and bladder tone.
5. **Dopamine and its analogs** cause vasodilation in the splanchnic and renal vascular beds by activating $D_1$ receptors. In the CNS, they increase extrapyramidal activity and have complex behavioral effects (through both $D_1$ and $D_2$ receptors [see Chapters 27 and 28]).
6. **Indirect-acting phenylisopropylamines** stimulate the CNS, producing alertness, elevation of mood, and anorexia, in addition to weak peripheral epinephrinelike effects.

## D. Clinical Use (Table 9–2):

1. **Cardiovascular applications:**
   a. Conditions in which an increase in blood flow is desired (heart failure, most types of shock): $\beta_1$ agonists are useful.
   b. Conditions in which a decrease in blood flow or increase in blood pressure is desired (local hemostatic or decongestant applications, spinal shock, *temporary* maintenance of blood pressure under emergency conditions): $\alpha_1$ agonists are useful.
2. **Other applications:**
   a. Conditions in which smooth muscle relaxation is needed (asthma, premature labor): $\beta_2$ agonists are used.
   b. Conditions in which CNS stimulation is desired (narcolepsy, obesity, hyperkinetic attention deficit disorder): centrally active, indirect-acting sympathomimetics are used.

## E. Toxicity:

1. **Catecholamines:** Because of their limited penetration into the CNS, these drugs have little central toxicity when given systemically. In the periphery, their adverse effects are extensions of their pharmacologic alpha or beta actions: excessive vasoconstriction, cardiac arrhythmias, cardiac necrosis, and pulmonary edema or hemorrhage.

**Table 9–2.** Pharmacokinetics and clinical applications of sympathomimetics.

| Drug | Oral Activity | Duration of Action | Clinical Applications |
|---|---|---|---|
| **Catecholamines** | | | |
| Epinephrine | No | Minutes | Anaphylaxis, glaucoma, asthma; used as a vasoconstrictor adjunct to local anesthetics. |
| Norepinephrine | No | Minutes | Used as a vasoconstrictor. |
| Isoproterenol | No | Minutes | Asthma, atrioventricular block. |
| Dopamine | No | Minutes | Shock. |
| Dobutamine | No | Minutes | Shock, congestive heart failure. |
| **Other sympathomimetics** | | | |
| Amphetamine | Yes | Hours | Narcolepsy, obesity. |
| Ephedrine | Yes | Hours | Asthma (obsolete); used as a vasoconstrictor. |
| Phenylephrine | Yes | Hours | Used as a vasoconstrictor (systemic or nasal decongestion) and as a mydriatic. |
| Albuterol, terbutaline, ritodrine, metaproterenol | Yes | Hours | Asthma, preterm labor. |
| Oxymetazoline, xylometazoline | Yes | Hours | Used as nasal decongestants. |
| Phenmetrazine | Yes | Hours | Attention deficit disorder. |
| Cocaine | Some | Minutes to hours | Used as a local anesthetic with vasoconstrictor action. |

2. **Other sympathomimetics:** The phenylisopropylamines may produce mild to severe CNS toxicity, depending on dosage. In small doses they induce nervousness, anorexia, and insomnia; in higher doses they may cause anxiety, aggressiveness, or paranoid behavior. Rarely, convulsions occur. Peripherally acting agents (eg, the $\beta_2$ agonists used in asthma) have peripheral toxicity that is predictable on the basis of the receptors they activate. Thus, $\alpha_1$ agonists cause hypertension, $\beta_1$ agonists cause tachycardia and more serious arrhythmias, and $\beta_2$ agonists cause skeletal muscle tremor. It is important to note that none of these drugs is perfectly selective; eg, at high doses, $\beta_1$-selective agents have $\beta_2$ actions and vice versa. Cocaine is particularly important as a drug of abuse: its major toxicities include cardiac arrhythmias or infarct and convulsions. A fatal outcome is far more common with acute cocaine overdose than with any other sympathomimetic.

## DRUG LIST

The following drugs are important members of the group discussed in this chapter. Prototype agents should be learned in detail; the major variants should be known well enough to list the factors that distinguish them from the prototypes and from each other, and the other significant agents should be recognized as belonging to a specific subclass.

| Subclass | Prototype | Major Variants | Other Significant Agents |
|---|---|---|---|
| General agonists | | | |
| Direct | Epinephrine | | |
| Indirect | Tyramine | | Amphetamine, ephedrine, methylphenidate, phenylpropanolamine |
| Reuptake inhibitors | Cocaine | Amphetamine | |
| Selective agonists | | | |
| $\alpha_1, \alpha_2, \beta_1$ | | Norepinephrine | |
| $\alpha_2 > \alpha_1$ | | Clonidine | $\alpha$-Methylnorepinephrine |
| $\alpha_1 > \alpha_2$ | | Phenylephrine | Methoxamine, metaraminol |
| $\beta_1 = \beta_2$ | | Isoproterenol | |
| $\beta_1 > \beta_2$ | | Dobutamine | Prenalterol |
| $\beta_2 > \beta_1$ | | Terbutaline | Albuterol, metaproterenol, ritodrine |
| Dopamine receptor | | Dopamine | Bromocriptine, apomorphine |

## QUESTIONS

**DIRECTIONS (items 1–10):** Each numbered item or incomplete statement in this section is followed by answers or by completions of the statement. Select the ONE lettered answer or completion that is BEST in each case.

1. Dilation of vessels in muscle, constriction of cutaneous vessels, and positive inotropic and chronotropic effects on the heart are all actions of
   **(A)** metaproterenol
   **(B)** norepinephrine
   **(C)** acetylcholine
   **(D)** epinephrine
   **(E)** isoproterenol

2. A long-acting indirect sympathomimetic agent sometimes used by the oral route is
(A) epinephrine
(B) ephedrine
(C) dobutamine
(D) isoproterenol
(E) phenylephrine

3. When pupillary dilation, but not cycloplegia, is desired, a good choice is
(A) homatropine
(B) pilocarpine
(C) isoproterenol
(D) tropicamide
(E) phenylephrine

4. Which of the following act(s) primarily on a receptor located on the membrane of the autonomic effector cell?
(A) Cocaine
(B) Tyramine
(C) Clonidine
(D) Epinephrine
(E) All of the above

5. When a moderate pressor dose of norepinephrine is given after pretreatment with a large dose of atropine, which of the following is most probable response to the norepinephrine?
(A) A decrease in heart rate caused by direct cardiac effect
(B) A decrease in heart rate caused by indirect reflex effect
(C) An increase in heart rate caused by direct cardiac action
(D) An increase in heart rate caused by indirect reflex action
(E) No change in heart rate

6. Which of the following may stimulate the central nervous system?
(A) Sympathomimetic drugs
(B) Antimuscarinic drugs
(C) Both (A) and (B)
(D) Neither (A) nor (B)

7. Selective $\beta_2$ stimulants frequently cause
(A) skeletal muscle tremor
(B) tachycardia in direct proportion to bronchodilation
(C) vasodilation in the skin
(D) increased cGMP in mast cells
(E) all of the above

8. Epinephrine increases the concentration of all of the following EXCEPT
(A) glucose in the blood
(B) free fatty acids in the blood
(C) lactate in the blood
(D) cAMP in the heart
(E) triglycerides in the fat cells

9. Phenylephrine
(A) increases skin temperature
(B) causes miosis in the eye
(C) constricts small vessels in the nasal mucosa
(D) increases gastric secretion and motility
(E) all of the above

**10.** Beta$_2$-selective stimulants are effective in
**(A)** Raynaud's syndrome
**(B)** delayed or insufficiently strong labor
**(C)** ischemic ulcers of the skin
**(D)** asthma
**(E)** coronary insufficiency manifested by angina

## ANSWERS

**1.** The actions describe the effects of activating alpha, $\beta_1$, and $\beta_2$ receptors. Of the drugs listed, only epinephrine has all of these actions. The answer is **(D).**

**2.** Phenylephrine and ephedrine are the only orally effective agents listed. Phenylephrine has a direct action and relatively short duration. Although oral ephedrine is almost obsolete, this drug still appears on examinations. The answer is **(B).**

**3.** Antimuscarinics (homatropine and tropicamide) are mydriatic and cycloplegic; alpha-sympathomimetic agonists are only mydriatic. The answer is **(E).**

**4.** The indirectly acting agents (cocaine and tyramine) act on the uptake or release of catecholamines by the nerve terminal; clonidine acts primarily on the $\alpha_2$ receptor of the presynaptic nerve terminal. The answer is **(D).**

**5.** Atropine will prevent the normal reflex bradycardia, since that requires integrity of the vagal pathway. The direct action of norepinephrine on the sinus node will be unmasked. The answer is **(C).**

**6.** Phenylisopropylamines such as amphetamine are traditional stimulants with a spectrum of effects from mild alertness to paranoid schizophrenia and convulsions; antimuscarinic agents are capable of inducing hallucinations and convulsions. The answer is **(C).**

**7.** Tremor is a common $\beta_2$ effect. If the tachycardia (a $\beta_1$ action) was proportionate to the bronchodilating effect, the drug could not be called $\beta_2$-selective. (It is true that, at high doses, such drugs become less selective.) Blood vessels in the skin have almost exclusively alpha (vasoconstrictor) receptors. The answer is **(A).**

**8.** Epinephrine increases the concentration of free fatty acids by activating lipolysis of triglycerides in fat cells. The answer is **(E).**

**9.** Choice **(A)** is incorrect; cutaneous vasoconstriction reduces skin temperature. Choice **(B)** is wrong; phenylephrine is a good mydriatic. Alpha-agonists in ordinary dosage have little effect on the gut but may inhibit it. The answer is **(C).**

**10.** The absence of $\beta_2$ receptors in the cutaneous vascular bed makes beta agonists useless in conditions involving reduced skin blood flow. Furthermore, ischemic ulcers are usually associated with structural occlusion of vessels that is not reversible with vasodilators. Beta adrenoceptors increase the cardiac rate and force, and increase the myocardial oxygen demand; they are generally contraindicated in angina. Uterine and bronchiolar smooth muscle are relaxed by $\beta_2$ agonists. The answer is **(D).**

# Adrenoceptor Blockers 10

## OBJECTIVES

**Define the following terms:**

- Competitive blocker
- Covalently bound inhibitor
- Epinephrine reversal
- Familial tremor
- Hypertrophic cardiomyopathy
- Intrinsic sympathomimetic activity (ISA)
- Irreversible blocker
- Membrane-stabilizing activity (MSA)
- Open-angle glaucoma
- Orthostatic hypotension
- Partial agonist
- Pheochromocytoma
- Presynaptic receptor
- Raynaud's phenomenon

**You should be able to:**

- Describe the effects of phentolamine on hemodynamic responses to epinephrine and norepinephrine.
- Compare the effects of propranolol, metoprolol, and pindolol.
- Compare the pharmacokinetics of propranolol, atenolol, esmolol, and nadolol.
- Describe the clinical indications and toxicities of typical alpha- and beta-blockers.

## CONCEPTS

Alpha- and beta-blocking agents differ markedly in their clinical applications. They are considered separately.

### ALPHA-BLOCKING DRUGS

**A. Classification:** Subdivisions of the alpha-blockers are based on selective affinity for $\alpha_1$ versus $\alpha_2$ receptors. A second feature used in classifying the alpha-blocking drugs is their duration of action and reversibility.

1. **Phenoxybenzamine** is the prototype long-acting, irreversible alpha-blocker. It is only slightly $\alpha_1$-selective.
2. **Phentolamine (nonselective) and tolazoline (slightly $\alpha_2$-selective)** are competitive (reversible) blocking agents.
3. **Prazosin** is a selective, reversible $\alpha_1$-blocker. **Terazosin** and **doxazosin** are newer drugs with similar properties. The advantage of $\alpha_1$ selectivity is discussed below.

**B. Pharmacokinetics:** These drugs are all active by the oral as well as parenteral routes. Phenoxybenzamine has a very long duration of action—about 48 hours—because it binds covalently to its receptor. Phentolamine and tolazoline have durations of action of 2–4 hours when used orally and 20–40 minutes when given parenterally. Prazosin acts for 8–10 hours.

**C. Mechanism of Action:** As noted above, phenoxybenzamine binds covalently to the alpha receptor, thereby ensuring an irreversible (insurmountable) blockade. The other agents are competitive pharmacologic antagonists—ie, their effects can be surmounted by increased concentrations of agonist. This difference may be important in the treatment of pheochromocytoma, in which massive releases of catecholamines from the tumor might overcome a reversible blockade.

**D. Effects:**

1. **Nonselective blockers:** These agents cause a predictable blockade of alpha-mediated re-

sponses to sympathetic nervous system discharge and exogenous sympathomimetics (ie, the responses listed in Table 9–1). The most important effects of nonselective alpha-blockers are those on the cardiovascular system; however, the application of nonselective alpha-blockers is limited by the baroreceptor reflex response *(tachycardia)* and other adverse effects. **Epinephrine reversal,** a predictable result of the use of alpha-blocking drugs, refers to an alteration in the direction of blood pressure change when epinephrine is given, from the normal pressor effect (brought about by alpha-mediated vasoconstriction) to a depressor effect (brought about by beta-mediated vasodilation) in a subject pretreated with an alpha-blocker. The effect is occasionally seen as a toxic effect of drugs for which alpha blockade is an adverse effect (eg, phenothiazine tranquilizers and antihistamines).

2. **Selective alpha-blockers:** Because prazosin blocks vascular $\alpha_1$ more than it blocks the $\alpha_2$ receptors associated with cardiac sympathetic nerve endings, it does not lead to the marked reflex tachycardia that accompanies the vasodilation produced by nonselective blockers.

**E. Clinical Use:** Nonselective alpha-blockers have limited clinical applications. The best documented of these applications are in presurgical management of pheochromocytoma and as antidotes in accidental overdosage with alpha agonists. Some patients with Raynaud's disease respond partially to phentolamine. Prazosin and other $\alpha_1$-selective blockers are used to treat hypertension (see Chapter 11).

**F. Toxicity:** The most important toxic effect of overdosage is simple extension of the alpha-blocking effects. Oral administration of all of these drugs can cause nausea and vomiting. Some patients experience an exaggerated hypotensive response to the first dose of prazosin. Therefore, the first dose is usually small and is taken just before going to bed.

## BETA-BLOCKING DRUGS

### A. Classification & Pharmacokinetics

1. **Subgroups and mechanisms:** All of the clinically available beta-blockers are competitive antagonists. Propranolol is the prototype. Drugs in this group are usually classified on the basis of partial agonist activity, local anesthetic action, and $\beta_1$ versus $\beta_2$ selectivity (Table 10–1).
   - **a.** Partial agonist activity ("intrinsic sympathomimetic activity," pindolol, acebutolol) may be an advantage in treating patients with asthma.
   - **b.** Local anesthetic activity ("membrane-stabilizing action") is a disadvantage when beta-blockers are used topically in the eye. It is absent from timolol, betaxolol, and levobunolol.
   - **c.** $\beta_1$-receptor selectivity ($\beta_1$ block > $\beta_2$), a property of metoprolol, atenolol, and acebutolol, may be an advantage when treating patients with asthma. Butoxamine, a $\beta_2$-selective drug, is used only in research.
   - **d.** Labetalol is an unusual agent with combined alpha- and beta-blocking action. This drug has 4 stereoisomers; the alpha-blocking activity resides in the *SR* enantiomer and the beta-blocking action in the *RR* enantiomer. The other 2 enantiomers (*RS* and *SS*) are practically inactive.

**Table 10–1.** Properties of several beta receptor-blocking drugs.[1]

| | Selectivity | Partial Agonist Activity | Local Anesthetic Activity | Elimination Half-Life (hours) | Approximate Bioavailability (percent) |
|---|---|---|---|---|---|
| Acebutolol | $\beta_1$ | Yes | Yes | 3–4 | 50 |
| Atenolol | $\beta_1$ | No | No | 6–9 | 40 |
| Esmolol | $\beta_1$ | No | No | 10 min | – |
| Labetalol | None | No | No | 5 | 30 |
| Metoprolol | $\beta_1$ | No | Yes | 3–4 | 50 |
| Nadolol | None | No | No | 14–24 | 33 |
| Pindolol | None | Yes | Yes | 3–4 | 90 |
| Propranolol | None | No | Yes | 3.5–6 | 30[2] |
| Timolol | None | No | No | 4–5 | 50 |

[1]Reproduced, with permission, from Katzung BG (editor): *Basic & Clinical Pharmacology,* 5th ed. Appleton & Lange, 1992.
[2]Bioavalilability is dose-dependent.

**Table 10–2.** Effects and clinical applications of beta-blocking drugs.

| Drug | Application | Effect |
|---|---|---|
| Propranolol, metoprolol, timolol | Hypertension | Reduced cardiac output, reduced renin secretion |
| Propranolol, nadolol | Angina pectoris | Reduced cardiac rate and force |
| Propranolol | Hypertrophic cardiomyopathy | Reduced cardiac rate and force |
| Propranolol, metoprolol, timolol | Myocardial infarct prophylaxis | Reduced ectopic focus facilitation in the heart |
| Propranolol, esmolol, acebutolol | Supraventricular tachycardia | Slowed atrioventricular nodal conduction |
| Propranolol | Migraine | Unknown |
| Propranolol | Familial tremor | Reduced beta-mediated neuromuscular facilitation |
| Propranolol | Thyroid storm | Reduced cardiac rate and force |
| Timolol, betaxolol, levobunolol | Glaucoma | Reduced aqueous humor formation |

2. **Pharmacokinetics:** The systemic beta-blocking agents have been developed for chronic oral use, but bioavailability varies widely (Table 10–1). Esmolol is a short-acting beta-blocker that is used only parenterally.

**B. Effects & Clinical Use:** Most of the organ-level effects of beta-blockers (Table 10–2) are predictable from blockade of the beta receptor-mediated effects of sympathetic discharge. Effects of beta blockade not previously emphasized (and not recognized until beta-blockers became widely used) include reduction of aqueous humor formation in the eye and reduction of skeletal muscle tremor. The cardiovascular and ophthalmic applications are extremely important.

**C. Toxicity:** Cardiovascular adverse effects are extensions of the beta blockade induced by these agents and include bradycardia, atrioventricular blockade, and congestive heart failure. Patients with diseases of the airways may suffer asthmatic attacks. Premonitory symptoms of hypoglycemia, eg, from insulin overdosage, may be masked. CNS adverse effects include sedation, fatigue, and sleep alterations. Atenolol and nadolol are claimed to have less marked CNS action because they do not enter the CNS as readily as other beta-blockers do.

## DRUG LIST

The following drugs are important members of the group discussed in this chapter. Prototype agents should be learned in detail; the major variants should be known well enough to list the factors that distinguish them from the prototypes and from each other, and the other significant agents should be recognized as belonging to a specific subclass.

| Subclass | Prototype | Major Variants | Other Significant Agents |
|---|---|---|---|
| α-Blockers | Phenoxybenzamine | Phentolamine, prazosin, yohimbine ($\alpha_2$) | Labetalol, ergotamine |
| β-Blockers | Propranolol | Metoprolol, timolol, pindolol, esmolol, butoxamine ($\beta_2$) | Nadolol, atenolol, labetalol |

## QUESTIONS

**DIRECTIONS (items 1–10):** Each numbered item or incomplete statement in this section is followed by answers or by completions of the statement. Select the ONE lettered answer or completion that is BEST in each case.

**1.** Which of the following effects of epinephrine would be blocked by phentolamine but not by metoprolol?
**(A)** Relaxation of bronchial smooth muscle
**(B)** Cardiac stimulation
**(C)** Contraction of the radial smooth muscle in the iris
**(D)** Increase of the cAMP level in skeletal muscle
**(E)** Relaxation of the uterus

**2.** Phentolamine and tolazoline
**(A)** are beta-blockers
**(B)** induce vasospasm when administered in large doses
**(C)** cause tachycardia
**(D)** cause hypertension
**(E)** block both alpha and beta receptors

**3.** Propranolol is useful in all of the following EXCEPT
**(A)** hypertension
**(B)** familial tremor
**(C)** idiopathic hypertrophic subaortic cardiomyopathy
**(D)** angina
**(E)** partial atrioventricular heart block

**4.** Adverse effects that limit the use of adrenoceptor blockers include
**(A)** bronchoconstriction from alpha-blockers
**(B)** congestive heart failure from beta-blockers
**(C)** sleep disturbances from alpha-blockers
**(D)** impaired blood sugar response with alpha-blockers
**(E)** increased intraocular pressure with beta-blockers

**5.** Phenoxybenzamine is used in the treatment of all of the following EXCEPT
**(A)** pheochromocytoma
**(B)** carcinoid
**(C)** Raynaud's disease
**(D)** essential hypertension

**6.** Pretreatment with phentolamine blocks all of the following EXCEPT
**(A)** vasoconstriction induced by norepinephrine
**(B)** increased cardiac contractile force induced by norepinephrine
**(C)** bradycardia induced by phenylephrine
**(D)** pilomotor erection ("gooseflesh")
**(E)** mydriasis induced by phenylephrine

**7.** Propranolol pretreatment will block
**(A)** norepinephrine-induced bradycardia
**(B)** methacholine-induced tachycardia
**(C)** nicotine-induced hypertension
**(D)** norepinephrine-induced inhibition of insulin secretion
**(E)** all of the above

**8.** Regarding beta-blocking drugs,
**(A)** timolol lacks the local anesthetic potency of propranolol
**(B)** nadolol lacks the $\beta_2$-blocking action
**(C)** pindolol is a beta antagonist with high membrane-stabilizing (local anesthetic) activity
**(D)** metoprolol blocks $\beta_2$ receptors selectively
**(E)** all of the above

**9.** Which of the following bind(s) covalently to the site specified?
**(A)** Atenolol—beta receptor
**(B)** Labetalol—alpha and beta receptors
**(C)** Pindolol—beta receptor
**(D)** Phenoxybenzamine—alpha receptor
**(E)** None of the above

**10.** Mr Augen is a 60-year-old man with glaucoma. Your therapy for him might include
**(A)** topical epinephrine
**(B)** topical pilocarpine
**(C)** topical timolol
**(D)** oral acetazolamide
**(E)** all of the above

**DIRECTIONS (items 11–14):** Four new synthetic drugs (designated ***W, X, Y,*** and ***Z***) are to be studied for their cardiovascular effects. They are given to 4 anesthetized animals while the heart rate is recorded. The first animal has received no pretreatment, the second has received an effective dose of hexamethonium, the third has received an effective dose of atropine, and the fourth has received an effective dose of phenoxybenzamine. The net changes induced by the new drugs (not by the blocking drugs) are shown in Graph 10–1.

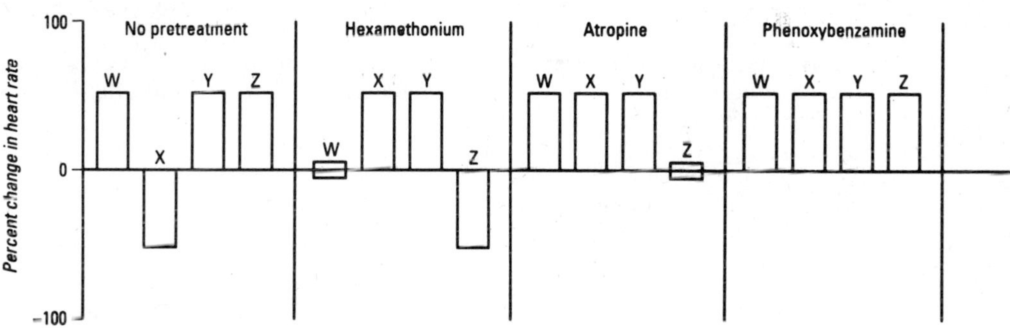


**Graph 10–1.**

**11.** Drug ***W*** is probably
**(A)** a drug similar to acetylcholine
**(B)** a vasodilator that does not affect ANS receptors
**(C)** a drug similar to norepinephrine
**(D)** a drug similar to isoproterenol
**(E)** a drug similar to edrophonium

**12.** Drug ***X*** is probably
**(A)** a drug similar to acetylcholine
**(B)** a vasodilator that does not affect ANS receptors
**(C)** a drug similar to norepinephrine
**(D)** a drug similar to isoproterenol
**(E)** a drug similar to edrophonium

**13.** Drug *Y* is probably
(A) a drug similar to acetylcholine
(B) a vasodilator that does not affect ANS receptors
(C) a drug similar to norepinephrine
(D) a drug similar to isoproterenol
(E) a drug similar to edrophonium

**14.** Drug *Z* is probably
(A) a drug similar to acetylcholine
(B) a vasodilator that does not affect ANS receptors
(C) a drug similar to norepinephrine
(D) a drug similar to isoproterenol
(E) a drug similar to edrophonium

## ANSWERS

**1.** Contraction of the pupillary dilator muscle is blocked by phentolamine but not by metoprolol. All the other effects are mediated by beta receptors. The answer is **(C)**.

**2.** These alpha-blockers cause hypotension and reflex tachycardia. The answer is **(C)**.

**3.** Atrioventricular block is an important contraindication to the use of beta-blockers. The answer is **(E)**.

**4.** Congestive heart failure is the adverse effect. Each of the other choices reverses the correct pairing of receptor subtype (alpha versus beta) with effect. The answer is **(B)**.

**5.** Phenoxybenzamine is not useful in essential hypertension because it causes tachycardia and marked orthostatic hypotension. It is used in Raynaud's disease, but its efficacy in this application is controversial. The answer is **(D)**.

**6.** Phenylephrine induces bradycardia through the baroreceptor reflex. Blockade of its vasoconstrictor effect will prevent the bradycardia. Pilomotor erection is mediated by alpha receptors. The answer is **(B)**.

**7.** The beta-blocker will not block the vagal slowing induced by norepinephrine hypertension. Nicotine-induced hypertension and norepinephrine-induced inhibition of insulin secretion are mediated by alpha receptors. The answer is **(B)**.

**8.** Nadolol is a nonselective beta-blocker, and metoprolol is a selective $\beta_1$-blocker. Timolol is useful in glaucoma because it does not anesthetize the cornea. The answer is **(A)**.

**9.** The answer is **(D)**, phenoxybenzamine.

**10.** All of the drugs listed are used in glaucoma. Acetazolamide is discussed in Chapter 15. The answer is **(E)**.

**11.** Drug ***W*** causes tachycardia that is blocked by ganglion blockade; therefore, it is probably a compensatory reflex tachycardia. Two of the choices may cause a pure reflex tachycardia: the nonautonomic vasodilator and acetylcholine. However, the reflex tachycardia evoked by acetylcholine is blocked by atropine (see the answer to question 14). Thus, drug ***W*** must be a nonautonomic vasodilator. The answer is **(B)**.

**12.** Drug ***X*** causes reduction of the heart rate, but this is converted into a tachycardia by hexamethonium and atropine—ie, the bradycardia is a vagal reflex. Phenoxybenzamine also reverses the bradycardia to a tachycardia, suggesting that alpha receptors are needed to induce the reflex bradycardia and that drug ***X*** has beta-agonist actions. The choices that evoke a vagal reflex bradycardia but can also cause a direct tachycardia are limited; the answer is **(C).**

**13.** Drug ***Y*** causes a direct tachycardia that is not significantly influenced by any of the blockers; the answer is **(D).**

**14.** Drug ***Z*** causes tachycardia that is converted to a bradycardia by hexamethonium and blocked completely by atropine. This indicates that the tachycardia is a reflex evoked by a direct vascular effect that is blocked by atropine, ie, muscarinic vasodilation. The answer is **(A).**

# Part III. Cardiovascular Drugs

# Drugs Used in Hypertension 11

## OBJECTIVES

**Define the following terms:**

- Baroreceptor reflex
- Calcium channel blockade
- Catecholamine pump
- End-organ damage
- Essential hypertension
- False transmitter
- Malignant hypertension
- Orthostatic hypotension
- Postganglionic neuron blocker
- Rebound hypertension
- Reflex tachycardia
- Reuptake of transmitter
- Stepped care
- Sympatholytic, sympathoplegic
- Transmitter vesicle
- Vasomotor center

**You should be able to:**

- List the 4 major groups of antihypertensive drugs and give examples of drugs in each group.
- Describe the homeostatic responses to each of the 4 major types of antihypertensive drugs.
- List the major sites of action of sympathoplegic drugs and give examples of drugs that act at each site.
- List the major toxicities of the prototype antihypertensive agents.
- Describe the reasons for the low incidence of detection of hypertension and the inadequate compliance of patients with treatment regimes once hypertension is diagnosed.

## CONCEPTS

This group of drugs is organized around a clinical indication—the need to treat a disease—rather than a receptor type. As a result, the drugs covered in this chapter are much more heterogeneous than are those in preceding chapters on autonomic drugs. They include diuretics, sympathoplegics, vasodilators, and angiotensin antagonists.

The strategies for treating high blood pressure are based on the determinants of arterial pressure (see Figure 6–2). These strategies include reduction of blood volume, sympathetic tone, vascular smooth muscle tone, and angiotensin concentration. Because of the baroreceptor reflex, the compensatory homeostatic responses to these drugs may be significant.

### DIURETICS

These drugs are covered in greater detail in Chapter 15 but are mentioned in this chapter because of their importance in hypertension. Diuretics lower blood pressure by reducing the blood volume and by exerting a direct vascular effect that is not yet understood. Diuretics important for treating hypertension are the thiazides (eg, **hydrochlorothiazide**) and the loop diuretics (eg, **furosemide**). Homeostatic compensatory responses are minimal (Table 11–1).

### SYMPATHOPLEGICS

Sympathoplegic agents interfere with sympathetic nerve function in several ways. The result is a reduction in one or more of the following: venous tone, heart rate, contractile force of the heart, cardiac

**Table 11–1.** Compensatory homeostatic responses to antihypertensive drugs and their major adverse effects. Drugs are listed in the order presented in the text.

| Class & Drug | Compensatory Responses | Adverse Effects |
|---|---|---|
| Diuretics | | |
| Hydrochlorothiazide | Minimal | Hypokalemia; slight hyperlipidemia, hyperuricemia. |
| Sympathoplegics | | |
| Veratrum alkaloids | Salt & water retention | Vomiting, diarrhea. |
| Clonidine | Salt & water retention | Dry mouth; sedation; severe rebound hypertension if drug is stopped suddenly. |
| Methyldopa | Salt & water retention | Sedation; positive Coombs reaction. |
| Ganglion-blockers | Salt & water retention | Severe orthostatic hypotension; blurred vision; constipation; sexual dysfunction. |
| Reserpine (low doses) | Minimal | Sedation; depression; nasal stuffiness; diarrhea. |
| Guanethidine | Salt & water retention | Orthostatic and exercise hypotension; sexual dysfunction; diarrhea. |
| Prazosin | Salt & water retention | First-dose orthostatic hypotension; dizziness; headache. |
| β-Blockers | Minimal | Sleep alterations; sedation; impotence; congestive heart failure; asthma. |
| Vasodilators | | |
| Hydralazine | Salt & water retention, tachycardia | Nausea; headache; flushing; lupus erythematosuslike syndrome. |
| Minoxidil | Salt & water retention; tachycardia | Hirsutism; pericardial effusion. |
| Nifedipine | Salt & water retention | Constipation; nausea; dizziness; flushing. |
| Nitroprusside | Salt & water retention | Cyanide toxicity (releases CN). |
| Angiotensin-converting enzyme inhibitors | | |
| Captopril | Minimal | Renal decompensation in patients with renal artery disease; bone marrow suppression (rare). |

output, and total peripheral resistance. Compensatory homeostatic responses and adverse effects are significant for some of these agents (Table 11–1). Sympathoplegics are subdivided by anatomic site of action (Fig 11–1).

**A. Drugs That Act On Baroreceptors:** The **veratrum alkaloids** sensitize the carotid sinus baroreceptors, reduce sympathetic outflow, and increase parasympathetic outflow. They produce various adverse effects and are obsolete.

**B. Drugs That Act in the CNS:** Alpha$_2$-selective agonists (eg, **clonidine, methyldopa**) cause a decrease in sympathetic outflow by a mechanism that is not yet completely understood. They accumulate in the CNS when given orally. Methyldopa is a pro-drug; it is converted to α-methylnorepinephrine in the brain. Both agents can reduce cardiac output and vascular resistance. The major homeostatic response is salt retention.

**C. Ganglion-Blocking Drugs:** Nicotinic blockers (eg, **trimethaphan**) are very efficacious but are used only in hypertensive emergencies and other acute situations because of their severe adverse effects. Orthostatic hypotension is a prominent feature of their action and can be exploited by raising the head of the patient's bed to reduce supine blood pressure. Trimethaphan has a short duration of action (minutes) and is given by continuous intravenous infusion. The major homeostatic response is salt retention.

**D. Postganglionic Sympathetic Nerve Terminal Blockers:** Drugs that deplete the sympathetic nerve terminal of norepinephrine transmitter stores (eg, **reserpine**), prevent release of these stores, or have both actions (eg, **guanethidine**) are useful antihypertensive drugs. The major homeostatic response is salt retention. In high dosage, both of these agents produce a high incidence of adverse effects. If used at all, reserpine is given in low doses as an adjunct to other agents. Reserpine readily enters the CNS; guanethidine does not. Both have long durations of

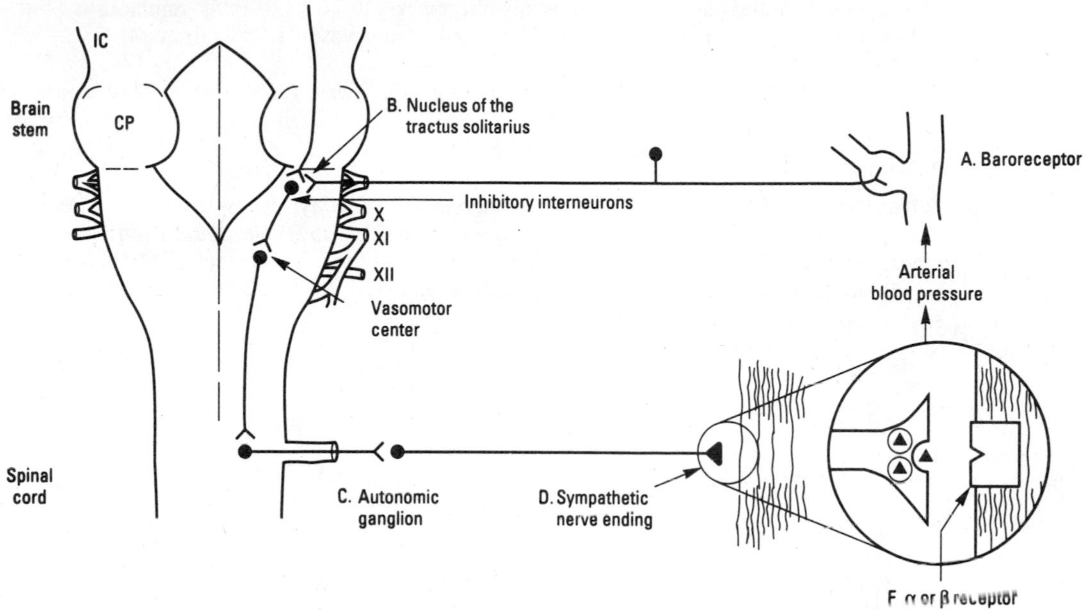


**Figure 11–1.** Baroreceptor reflex arc and sites of action of sympathoplegic drugs.

action (days to weeks). **MAO inhibitors,** although no longer used to treat hypertension, are of interest because they cause the formation of a **false transmitter (octopamine)** in sympathetic postganglionic neuron terminals. This substance is stored in vesicles along with increased amounts of norepinephrine. Normal nerve action potentials release the weak false transmitter with norepinephrine, resulting in diminished vascular and cardiac responses. However, large doses of indirect-acting sympathomimetics (eg, the tyramine in a meal of fermented foods) may cause the release of large amounts of stored norepinephrine and result in a hypertensive crisis.

**E. Adrenoceptor Blockers: Prazosin** (or another $\alpha_1$-selective agent) or one of many beta-blockers is often used. Alpha-blockers reduce vascular resistance. The nonselective alpha-blockers **(phentolamine, phenoxybenzamine)** are of no value in treating chronic hypertension. Homeostatic responses to such alpha-blockers include salt retention and tachycardia. Alpha$_1$-selective adrenoceptor blockers are relatively free of many of the severe adverse effects of the nonselective alpha-blockers and postganglionic nerve terminal sympathoplegic agents. Beta-blockers (eg, **propranolol**) initially reduce cardiac output, but after a few days their action appears to include a decrease in vascular resistance as a significant effect. The latter effect may result from reduced angiotensin levels (beta-blockers reduce renin release from the kidney). The beta-blockers are among the most heavily used antihypertensive drugs.

Beta-blockers are associated with slightly elevated triglyceride and diminished high-density lipoprotein levels in the blood; other potential adverse effects are listed in Table 11–1.

## VASODILATORS

Drugs that dilate blood vessels by acting directly on smooth muscle cells through nonautonomic mechanisms are useful in treating many hypertensive patients. Homeostatic responses include salt retention and tachycardia and may be marked (Table 11–1).

**A. Hydralazine & Minoxidil:** These agents have more effect on arterioles than on veins when used in hypertension. They are suitable for chronic therapy. Although hydralazine can cause a lupuslike syndrome, this is uncommon at dosage levels below 200 mg/day. Minoxidil is extremely efficacious and is therefore reserved for severe hypertension. Although the mechanism of action of hydralazine is unknown, minoxidil appears to be a pro-drug: minoxidil sulfate is a potassium channel opener that hyperpolarizes and relaxes vascular smooth muscle.

**B. Calcium Channel-Blocking Agents:** These (eg, **diltiazem, nifedipine**, and **verapamil**) are effective vasodilators and are suitable for chronic use in hypertension of any severity. Their mechanism of action is discussed in Chapter 12.

**C. Nitroprusside & Diazoxide:** These agents are used only in hypertensive emergencies. Nitroprusside is a short-acting agent (a few minutes) that must be infused intravenously. Its mechanism of action is probably similar to that of the nitrates: It increases cGMP concentrations in smooth muscle. Diazoxide is given as intravenous boluses and has a duration of action of several hours.

### ANGIOTENSIN ANTAGONISTS

The useful members of this group (**ACE inhibitors,** eg, **captopril**) inhibit the enzyme variously known as kininase II, peptidyl dipeptidase, and angiotensin-converting enzyme (ACE). The result is a reduction in blood levels of angiotensin II and aldosterone and probably an increase in blood levels of endogenous vasodilators of the kinin family (eg, bradykinin). ACE inhibitors have a low incidence of serious adverse effects in adults with normal renal function. However, they cause renal damage in the fetus during the second and third trimesters. Homeostatic compensation is minimal. A second type of angiotensin antagonist is represented by **saralasin,** which competitively inhibits angiotensin II at its receptor site (saralasin is a partial agonist). This drug is a polypeptide used only in academic research settings.

## CLINICAL USE

Hypertension is difficult to discover because it produces no symptoms until late in its course, when end-organ damage (to the kidneys, heart, cerebral vessels, and retina) occurs. Because of the lack of symptoms, patients may be unconvinced of the need for medication, and remain noncompliant, unless careful education is carried out.

**A. Stepped Care:** Until recently, the most important aspect of modern hypertension therapy was the concept of using multiple drugs to minimize individual drug toxicities. This approach is still used in patients with severe hypertension. Typically, drugs are added to a patient's regimen in stepwise fashion (stepped care), each additional agent chosen from a different subgroup with further escalation stopped as soon as adequate blood pressure control has been achieved. The usual steps include (1) life-style measures such as salt restriction and weight reduction, (2) diuretics, (3) sympathoplegics, (4) vasodilators, and (5) ACE inhibitors. The ability of drugs in steps 2 and 3 to control the homeostatic responses induced by the others should be noted (eg, propranolol reduces the tachycardia induced by hydralazine).

**B. Monotherapy:** It has been found in large clinical studies that many patients do well on a single drug (eg, an ACE inhibitor, calcium channel blocker, or $\alpha_1$-blocker). This approach to the treatment of mild and moderate hypertension has become more popular than stepped care because of its simplicity, improved patient compliance, and relatively low incidence of toxicity.

**C. Malignant Hypertension:** Malignant hypertension is an accelerated phase of severe hypertension with rapidly progressing damage to end organs and rising blood pressure. This condition may be signaled by deterioration of renal function, encephalopathy, and retinal hemorrhages or by angina, stroke, or myocardial infarction. Malignant hypertension must be managed on an emergency basis in the hospital. Powerful vasodilators (nitroprusside or diazoxide) are combined with diuretics (furosemide if necessary) and beta-blockers to lower blood pressure to the 140–160/90–110 range promptly (within a few hours). Further reduction can then be pursued more slowly.

## DRUG LIST

The following drugs are important members of the group discussed in this chapter. Prototype agents should be learned in detail; the major variant and the other significant agents should be known well enough to list the factors that distinguish them from the prototypes and from each other.

| Subclass | Prototype | Major Variants | Other Significant Agents |
|---|---|---|---|
| Diuretics | Hydrochlorothiazide or furosemide (See Diuretics) | | |
| Sympathoplegics | | | |
| Carotid sinus | | | Veratrum alkaloids |
| CNS action | Methyldopa | Clonidine | Guanabenz |
| Ganglion blockers | Trimethaphan | | Hexamethonium, mecamylamine |
| Postganglionic neuron blockers | Guanethidine, reserpine, MAO inhibitors | | Guanadrel |
| Receptor blockers | | | |
| Alpha | Prazosin | | Terazosin |
| Beta | Propranolol | | Metoprolol, atenolol, etc |
| Combined alpha and beta | Labetalol | | |
| Vasodilators | Hydralazine, nifedipine, nitroprusside | | Minoxidil, verapamil |
| Angiotensin antagonists | Captopril, saralasin | | Enalapril, lisinopril |

## QUESTIONS

**DIRECTIONS (items 1–10):** Each numbered item or incomplete statement in this section is followed by answers or by completions of the statement. Select the ONE lettered answer or completion that is BEST in each case.

**1.** A college friend consults you regarding the suitability of the therapy his doctor has prescribed for hypertension. He complains of postural and exercise hypotension ("dizziness"), some diarrhea, and problems with ejaculation during sex. Which of the following is most likely to produce these effects?
**(A)** Propranolol
**(B)** Guanethidine
**(C)** Prazosin
**(D)** Hydralazine
**(E)** Captopril

**2.** Each of the following can cause bradycardia EXCEPT
**(A)** clonidine
**(B)** propranolol
**(C)** reserpine
**(D)** hydralazine
**(E)** guanethidine

**3.** In comparing methyldopa and guanethidine,
**(A)** guanethidine, but not methyldopa, results in salt and water retention if used without a diuretic
**(B)** guanethidine is less efficacious in severe hypertension
**(C)** guanethidine causes fewer central nervous system adverse effects such as sedation
**(D)** methyldopa causes more orthostatic hypotension
**(E)** guanethidine causes more immunologic adverse effects (eg, hemolytic anemia)

**4.** Captopril and enalapril do all of the following EXCEPT
(A) increase renin concentration in the blood
(B) inhibit an enzyme
(C) competitively inhibit angiotensin at its receptor
(D) decrease the angiotensin II concentration in the blood
(E) increase sodium and decrease potassium levels in the urine

**5.** Which of the following reduces the release of norepinephrine from the sympathetic nerve terminal in response to normal vasomotor center discharge?
(A) Hydralazine
(B) Prazosin
(C) Minoxidil
(D) Reserpine
(E) Propranolol

**6.** Postural hypotension is a common adverse effect of all of the following types of drugs EXCEPT
(A) those that cause venodilation
(B) those that cause ganglionic blockade
(C) those that cause alpha-receptor blockade
(D) those that cause excessive diuresis and decreased blood volume
(E) those that cause beta-receptor blockade

**7.** Urinary retention in an elderly man is most likely to result from
(A) trimethaphan
(B) reserpine
(C) hydralazine
(D) guanethidine
(E) propranolol

**8.** Important although uncommon adverse effects of vasodilators include all of the following EXCEPT
(A) lupus erythematosus with hydralazine
(B) reduced cardiac output or atrioventricular block with verapamil
(C) precipitation of severe gout with prazosin
(D) pericardial abnormalities with minoxidil
(E) cyanide toxicity with nitroprusside

**9.** Comparison of guanethidine and propranolol shows that
(A) both increase heart rate
(B) both diminish central sympathetic outflow
(C) both decrease cardiac output
(D) both produce orthostatic hypotension
(E) none of the above

**10.** Reserpine, an alkaloid derived from the root of *Rauwolfia serpentina,*
(A) has been used in large doses to control hyperglycemia
(B) can cause psychiatric depression
(C) can decrease gastrointestinal secretion and motility
(D) often causes a reflex increase in heart rate when it lowers blood pressure
(E) is the safest of the sympathoplegic agents

## ANSWERS

**1.** Guanethidine is the only one of the 3 sympathoplegics listed here that is likely to cause the marked adverse effects described. Captopril and hydralazine are not sympathoplegics and are therefore not associated with the adverse effects described. The answer is **(B).**

**2.** Any sympathoplegic can, in sufficient dosage, cause bradycardia. Conversely, any vasodilator can induce tachycardia and, unless it is also sympathoplegic or a calcium channel blocker, will never lower the heart rate. The answer is **(D).**

**3.** Guanethidine causes many peripheral adverse effects but is poorly distributed into the CNS, so it is relatively free of CNS effects. The answer is **(C).**

**4.** These converting *enzyme* inhibitors act on the enzyme, not on the angiotensin receptor. The plasma renin level may increase as a result of the homeostatic response to reduced angiotensin II level. The answer is **(C).**

**5.** Drugs that act on smooth muscle (hydralazine and minoxidil) and sympathoplegics that act distal to the CNS vasomotor center (prazosin and propranolol) actually increase sympathetic outflow to a significant degree via the baroreceptor reflex. However, reserpine depletes transmitter stores, despite the increase in central sympathetic outflow. The answer is **(D).**

**6.** Beta-blocking drugs do not cause orthostatic hypotension. The answer is **(E).**

**7.** This parasympatholytic effect will occur only with the ganglion blocker. The answer is **(A).**

**8.** Beta-blockers, not alpha-blockers, are associated with an increase in serum uric acid levels. (Even with beta-blockers, gout is uncommon and usually easily managed.) The answer is **(C).**

**9.** Neither drug increases the heart rate or reduces central sympathetic outflow. Propranolol does not cause orthostatic hypotension. The answer is **(C).**

**10.** Reserpine is of no value in hyperglycemia. It does not induce reflex tachycardia, because it lowers blood pressure by reducing sympathetic neurotransmitter release in the heart as well as the vessels. The answer is **(B).**

# 12 Vasodilators & the Treatment of Angina

## OBJECTIVES

**Define the following terms:**

- Angina of effort
- Classic angina
- Atherosclerotic angina
- Vasospastic angina
- Variant angina
- Prinzmetal's angina
- Coronary vasodilator
- Peripheral vasodilator
- "Monday disease"
- Nitrate tolerance
- Tachyphylaxis
- Unstable angina
- Preload
- Afterload
- Intramyocardial fiber tension
- Double product
- Myocardial revascularization

**You should be able to:**

- List the major determinants of cardiac oxygen consumption.
- List the strategies for relief of anginal pain.
- Contrast the therapeutic and adverse effects of nitrates, beta-blockers, and calcium channel blockers when used for angina.
- Contrast the effects of medical therapy and surgical therapy of angina.

## CONCEPTS

### PATHOPHYSIOLOGY OF ANGINA

A. **Determinants of Cardiac Oxygen Requirement:** The treatment of coronary insufficiency is based on physiologic factors that control the myocardial oxygen requirement. The major determinant is myocardial fiber tension; ie, the higher the tension, the greater the oxygen requirement. Several variables contribute to fiber tension:
   1. **Preload** (a function of blood volume and venous tone).
   2. **Cardiac contractility** (a function of sympathetic outflow to the heart).
   3. **Afterload** (arterial blood pressure, a function of peripheral vascular resistance).
   4. **Heart rate,** which contributes to time-integrated fiber tension (at high heart rates, fibers spend more time at systolic tension levels) and, inversely, to the time available for coronary flow (coronary blood flow is low or nil during systole). Blood pressure and heart rate may be multiplied to yield the double product, a measure of cardiac oxygen requirement. Effective drugs reduce the double product in patients with atherosclerotic angina.

B. **Types of Angina:** There are 2 major causes of the disease:
   1. **Atherosclerotic occlusion** of the coronaries, which produces classic angina, also known as angina of effort.
   2. **Reversible vasospastic reduction** of coronary flow; also known as angioplastic angina, variant angina, or Prinzmetal's angina.
   3. **A third type of angina,** *unstable* or *crescendo* angina, combines the features of both atherosclerotic plaques and vasospasm and adds platelet aggregation to the causes of diminished coronary flow. Unstable angina is thought to be the immediate precursor of a myocardial infarction and is treated as a medical emergency.

C. **Therapeutic Strategies:** The same primary defect causes anginal pain in all types of angina: Coronary oxygen delivery is inadequate for the myocardial oxygen requirement. This can be corrected in 2 ways: by increasing oxygen delivery or by reducing oxygen requirement. Pharmacologic therapies include the nitrates, the calcium channel blockers, and the beta-blockers. All 3 groups reduce oxygen requirement in atherosclerotic angina, and nitrates and calcium channel blockers (but not beta-blockers) can increase oxygen delivery—by reducing spasm—in the vasospastic form. Myocardial revascularization surgically corrects coronary obstruction either by bypass grafting or by angioplasty (enlargement of the lumen by means of a special catheter).

## NITRATES

**A. Classification & Pharmacokinetics: Nitroglycerin** (the active ingredient in dynamite) is the most important of the nitrates and is available in forms that provide a range of durations of action from 15 minutes (sublingual) to 8–10 hours (transdermal) (Table 12–1). Because treatment of acute attacks and prevention of attacks are both important aspects of therapy, the pharmacokinetics of these different dosage forms are clinically significant.

Nitroglycerin (glyceryl trinitrate) is rapidly denitrated in the liver—first to the dinitrate (glyceryl dinitrate), which has significant vasodilating effect, and then to the mononitrate, which is much less active. Because of the high enzyme activity in the liver, the first-pass effect for nitroglycerin is high—about 90%. The efficacy of oral (swallowed) nitroglycerin probably results from the high levels of glyceryl dinitrate in the blood. The effects of sublingual nitroglycerin are mainly the result of the unchanged drug.

Other nitrates are similar to nitroglycerin in their pharmacokinetics and pharmacodynamics. After nitroglycerin, **isosorbide dinitrate** is the most extensively used. Several other nitrates are available for oral use and, like the oral nitroglycerin preparation, have a relatively long duration of action. **Amyl nitrite** is a volatile and rapidly acting vasodilator that was used to treat angina by the inhalational route but is now rarely prescribed.

**B. Mechanism of Action:** The nitrates release nitric oxide (NO) in smooth muscle; this causes an increase of cGMP and leads to smooth muscle relaxation.

**C. Organ System Effects:**

1. **Cardiovascular.** Smooth muscle relaxation leads to peripheral vasodilation, which results in reduced cardiac size and cardiac output through reduced preload, and reduced afterload. These decreases contribute to reduction in myocardial fiber tension and oxygen consumption. Thus, the primary mechanism of therapeutic benefit in atherosclerotic angina is reduction of the oxygen requirement, not necessarily an increase in coronary flow. A significant reflex tachycardia is predictable.
2. **Other organs.** There is a minor effect on the smooth muscle of the bronchi, gastrointestinal tract, and genitourinary tract, but these effects are too small to be clinically significant. There are no significant effects on other tissues.

**D. Clinical Uses:** As previously noted, nitroglycerin is available in several formulations. The standard form for treatment of acute anginal pain is the sublingual tablet, which has a duration of action of 15–30 minutes. Oral (swallowed) nitroglycerin has a duration of 2–4 hours. Sustained-release oral forms have a somewhat longer duration (Table 12–1). Transdermal formulations (ointment or patch) can maintain blood levels for up to 24 hours. However, tolerance develops after about 8 hours, markedly diminishing the effectiveness thereafter.

**Table 12–1.** Pharmacokinetically distinct forms of nitrate and nitrite drugs used in angina.

| Category | Example | Duration of Action |
|---|---|---|
| Very short | Amyl nitrite | 3–5 min |
| Short | Sublingual nitroglycerin or isosorbide | 10–30 min (isosorbide has a somewhat longer half-life than nitroglycerin) |
| Intermediate | Oral sustained-release nitroglycerin or isosorbide | 6–8 h |
| Long | Transdermal nitroglycerin (ointment or patch) | 8–10 h (blood levels may persist for 24 h, but tolerance limits the duration of action) |

**E. Toxicity of Nitrates & Nitrites:** The most common toxic effects of nitrates are the responses evoked by vasodilation. These include tachycardia, orthostatic hypotension, and throbbing headache from meningeal vasodilatation. Nitrites are of potential importance as toxicologic hazards (causing methemoglobinemia), and the same effect has potential antidotal action in cyanide poisoning. The nitrates do not cause methemoglobinemia. In the past, the nitrates were responsible for several occupational diseases in munitions plants in which workplace contamination by these volatile chemicals was severe. The most common of these diseases was **"Monday disease,"** or the alternating development of tolerance (during the work week) and loss of tolerance (over the weekend) for the vasodilating action, resulting in headache, tachycardia, and dizziness every Monday.

## CALCIUM CHANNEL-BLOCKING DRUGS

**A. Classification & Pharmacokinetics:** Three major types of calcium channel blockers are approved for use in angina in the USA; they are typified by **diltiazem, nifedipine,** and **verapamil.** They differ markedly in structure, but all are orally active and most have half-lives of 3–6 hours. Several newer dihydropyridine drugs are closely related to nifedipine and possess the same properties. **Nimodipine** is a member of the dihydropyridine family with similar properties, but it is approved only for the management of stroke associated with subarachnoid hemorrhage.

**B. Mechanism of Action:** These drugs block voltage-dependent calcium channels, especially the calcium channels in cardiac and smooth muscle. By decreasing calcium influx during action potentials in a frequency- and voltage-dependent manner, they reduce systolic intracellular calcium concentration and muscle contractility.

**C. Effects:** These agents relax blood vessels and, to a lesser extent, the uterus, bronchi, and gut. The rate and contractility of the heart are reduced by diltiazem and verapamil. Nifedipine and other dihydropyridines evoke greater vasodilation, and the resulting sympathetic reflex prevents bradycardia and may actually increase the heart rate. All of the calcium channel blockers reduce blood pressure.

**D. Clinical Use:** These drugs are effective as prophylactic therapy in both types of angina, but they are particularly useful in treating the vasospastic form, and nifedipine can also be used to abort an attack. In atherosclerotic angina, they are particularly valuable when combined with nitrates (Table 12–2). In addition to well-established uses in angina, hypertension, and supraventricular tachycardia, these agents are being tried in migraine, preterm labor, stroke, and Raynaud's disease. As noted above, nimodipine is approved for use in hemorrhagic stroke.

**E. Toxicity:** The calcium channel blockers cause constipation, edema, nausea, flushing, and dizziness. More serious adverse effects include congestive heart failure, atrioventricular blockade, and sinus node depression.

## BETA-BLOCKING DRUGS

**A. Classification:** These drugs are described in detail in Chapter 10. All beta-blockers are effective in treating atherosclerotic angina.

**B. Mechanism of Action:** See Chapter 10.

**C. Effects:** Actions include both beneficial effects (decreased heart rate, cardiac force, blood pressure) and detrimental effects (increased heart size, longer ejection period).

**D. Clinical Use:** Beta-blockers are used only for prophylactic therapy of angina; they are of no value in an acute attack. They are effective in preventing exercise-induced angina but have poor results against the vasospastic form. The combination of beta-blockers with nitrates is useful because several adverse reflex effects evoked by the nitrates (tachycardia, increased cardiac force) are prevented or reduced by beta blockade (Table 12–2).

**E. Toxicity:** See Chapter 10.

**Table 12–2.** Effects of nitrates alone and with beta-blockers or calcium channel blockers in angina pectoris.[1]

| | Nitrates Alone[2] | β-Blockers or Calcium Channel Blockers[2] | Combined Nitrates With β-Blockers or Calcium Channel Blockers |
|---|---|---|---|
| Heart rate | *Reflex increase* | Decrease[3] | Decrease |
| Arterial pressure | Decrease | Decrease | Decrease |
| End-diastolic volume | Decrease | *Increase* | None or decrease |
| Contractility | *Reflex increase* | Decrease[3] | None |
| Ejection time | Decrease | *Increase* | None |

[1]Reproduced, with permission, from Katzung BG (editor): *Basic & Clinical Pharmacology,* 5th ed. Appleton & Lange, 1992.
[2]Undesirable effects are shown in *italics.*
[3]Nifedipine may cause a reflex *increase* in heart rate and cardiac contractility.

### NONPHARMACOLOGIC THERAPY

Both coronary artery bypass grafting (CABG) and percutaneous transluminal coronary angioplasty (PTCA) have become important therapeutic modalities in severe angina. These are the only methods capable of consistently increasing coronary flow in atherosclerotic angina

## DRUG LIST

The following drugs are important members of the group discussed in this chapter. Prototype agents should be learned in detail; the major variants should be known well enough to list the factors that distinguish them from the prototypes and from each other, and the other significant agents should be recognized as belonging to a specific subclass.

| Subclass | Prototype | Major Variants | Other Significant Agents |
|---|---|---|---|
| Nitrates | Nitroglycerin | Different dosage forms | Isosorbide dinitrate, amyl nitrite |
| Calcium channel blockers | Nifedipine | Verapamil | Diltiazem |
| Beta-blockers | Propranolol | | Metoprolol, etc |

## QUESTIONS

**DIRECTIONS (items 1–10):** Each numbered item or incomplete statement in this section is followed by answers or by completions of the statement. Select the ONE lettered answer or completion that is BEST in each case.

**1.** Nitroglycerin, either directly or through reflexes, results in all of the following EXCEPT
**(A)** tachycardia
**(B)** decreased cardiac force
**(C)** increased venous capacitance
**(D)** decreased intramyocardial fiber tension
**(E)** decreased afterload

**2.** The antianginal effect of propranolol may be attributed to all of the following EXCEPT
(A) block of exercise-induced tachycardia
(B) reduced resting heart rate
(C) decreased cardiac force
(D) increased end-diastolic ventricular volume
(E) decreased systolic fiber tension

**3.** The major direct determinant of myocardial oxygen consumption is
(A) heart rate
(B) diastolic blood pressure
(C) cardiac output
(D) blood volume
(E) myocardial fiber tension

**4.** An adverse effect common to nitroglycerin, guanethidine, and trimethaphan is
(A) orthostatic hypotension
(B) throbbing headache
(C) bradycardia
(D) impaired sexual function
(E) lupus erythematosus syndrome

**5.** Nitroglycerin in moderate doses may produce all of the following EXCEPT
(A) meningeal vasodilatation
(B) reflex tachycardia
(C) increased cardiac force
(D) methemoglobinemia
(E) sympathetic discharge

**6.** Epidemiologic surveys suggest that workers exposed to high levels of nitrates in the workplace have
(A) a high incidence of methemoglobinemia on the job
(B) an increased incidence of angina on Mondays as compared with other days
(C) a high incidence of cyanide poisoning in the workplace
(D) an increased incidence of headaches on Mondays as compared with other days
(E) all of the above

**7.** A drug that often causes tachycardia when given in ordinary doses is
(A) isosorbide dinitrate
(B) verapamil
(C) guanethidine
(D) propranolol
(E) diltiazem

**8.** Effective drugs for the prophylaxis of angina of effort over 4- to 6-hour periods include all of the following EXCEPT
(A) transdermal nitroglycerin
(B) amyl nitrite
(C) diltiazem
(D) nadolol
(E) oral isosorbide dinitrate

**9.** Drugs that may precipitate angina when used for other indications include all of the following EXCEPT
(A) hydralazine
(B) terbutaline
(C) isoproterenol
(D) guanethidine
(E) cocaine

**10.** When using nitrates in combination with other drugs for the treatment of angina,
**(A)** the actions of beta-blockers and nitrates on cardiac size are additive
**(B)** the actions of calcium channel blockers and nitrates on cardiac force are antagonistic
**(C)** the actions of calcium channel blockers and nitrates on vascular tone are antagonistic
**(D)** the actions of beta-blockers and nitrates on heart rate are additive
**(E)** the actions of calcium channel blockers and beta blockers on cardiac force are antagonistic

## ANSWERS

**1.** Nitroglycerin increases cardiac force because the decrease in blood pressure evokes a reflex increase in sympathetic discharge. The answer is **(B)**.

**2.** Propranolol has all the effects listed, but the increase in end-diastolic volume is not advantageous—it tends to increase oxygen consumption. The answer is **(D)**.

**3.** The answer is **(E)**, fiber tension. The other variables contribute to this determinant.

**4.** These drugs all reduce venous return sufficiently to cause some degree of postural hypotension (not very prolonged for nitroglycerin). Throbbing headache is a problem only with the nitrates, bradycardia only with guanethidine, sexual problems only with sympathoplegics (trimethaphan and guanethidine), and lupus with none of them. The answer is **(A)**.

**5.** Methemoglobinemia never occurs with the doses of nitrates used to treat angina. (The nitrites are much more likely to cause methemoglobinemia.) The answer is **(D)**.

**6.** Nitrites, not nitrates, cause methemoglobinemia in adults. Headache, not angina, has an increased incidence upon returning to work on Monday. Neither nitrates nor nitrites are related to causation of cyanide poisoning, but nitrites are used as one part of the antidote for cyanide intoxication. The answer is **(D)**.

**7.** Isosorbide (like all the nitrates) causes reflex tachycardia, but all the other drugs lower the heart rate. The answer is **(A)**.

**8.** The calcium channel blockers and the beta-blockers are generally effective in reducing the number of attacks of angina of effort and have durations of 4–8 hours. Oral and transdermal nitrates have similar durations. Amyl nitrite has the shortest duration of action (1–5 minutes) of any drug used in angina. The answer is **(B)**.

**9.** In general, drugs that induce hypertension or tachycardia, whether directly or by reflex, tend to precipitate angina in individuals with coronary obstruction, unless cardiac work is greatly reduced (as in the case of the nitrates). The answer is **(D)**.

**10.** Beta-blockers (or calcium channel blockers) and nitrates have opposite effects on heart size (nitrates decrease size). The actions of calcium channel blockers and nitrates on vascular tone are similar (both decrease it). The answer is **(B)**.

# 13 Cardiac Glycosides & Congestive Heart Failure

## OBJECTIVES

**Define the following terms:**

- Atrioventricular node
- Bigeminy
- Cardenolide
- Congestive heart failure
- ECG deflections: P, QRS, T waves
- ECG intervals: PR, QT, QRS duration; ST segments
- End-diastolic fiber length
- Premature ventricular beats
- Sinus node
- Sodium pump ($Na^+$,$K^+$-ATPase)
- Sodium-calcium exchange
- Ventricular function curve
- Ventricular tachycardia

**You should be able to:**

- Describe the process of excitation-contraction coupling in cardiac muscle.
- Describe the strategies and list the major drug groups used in the treatment of congestive heart failure.
- Describe the probable mechanism of action of digitalis.
- Describe the nature and mechanism of the toxic effects of digitalis on the heart.
- List some positive inotropic drugs that have been investigated as digitalis substitutes.

## CONCEPTS

### PATHOPHYSIOLOGY OF CONGESTIVE HEART FAILURE & TREATMENT STRATEGIES

**A. Pathophysiology:** Congestive heart failure has a well-defined pathophysiology, although the underlying biochemical pathology is not understood. The fundamental physiologic defect, a decrease in cardiac contractility, is best shown by the ventricular function curve (Frank-Starling curve, Fig 13–1). The result of this defect is that cardiac output is inadequate for the needs of the body. The homeostatic responses of the body to depressed cardiac output (mediated mainly by the sympathetic nervous system) increase the load on the heart; the increased load contributes to a further decline in cardiac function. The ventricular function curve reflects some of these deleterious homeostatic responses and may also be used to demonstrate the response to drugs. Responses include the following:

1. **Tachycardia:** An early compensatory response, mediated by increased sympathetic tone.
2. **Increased peripheral vascular resistance:** An early compensatory response, mediated by increased sympathetic tone.
3. **Retention of salt and water by the kidney:** An early compensatory response, mediated by the renin-angiotensin-aldosterone system and by increased sympathetic outflow. Salt and water retention results in edema and pulmonary congestion.
4. **Cardiomegaly:** A compensatory structural response.
5. **Shortness of breath and decreased exercise tolerance.**

**B. Therapeutic Strategies in Congestive Heart Failure:** Traditional therapies for congestive heart failure have emphasized either direct treatment of the depressed heart with positive inotropic drugs or removal of retained salt and water with diuretics. Recent studies have shown that reduction of preload or afterload with vasodilators can also be helpful, especially in acute or complicated congestive failure. In chronic heart failure, angiotensin-converting enzyme (ACE) inhibitors are extremely useful.

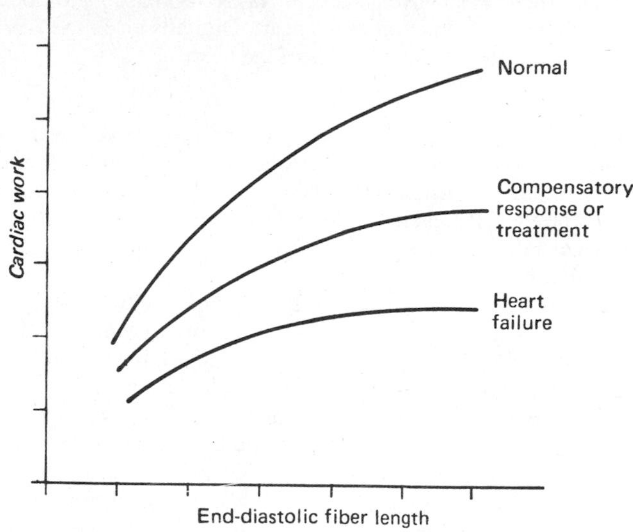


**Figure 13–1.** Ventricular function (Frank-Starling) curve. The abscissa can be any measure of preload—fiber length, filling pressure, pulmonary capillary wedge pressure, etc. The ordinate is a measure of useful external cardiac work—stroke volume, cardiac output, etc.

## DIGITALIS GLYCOSIDES

**A. Classification, Prototypes, & Pharmacokinetics:** All cardiac glycosides include a steroid nucleus and a lactone ring; most also have one or more sugar residues. The sugar residues constitute the glycoside portion of the molecule, and the steroid nucleus plus lactone ring make up the "genin" portion. The cardiac glycosides are often called "digitalis" because the 2 agents most commonly used in the USA (digoxin and digitoxin) come from the digitalis (foxglove) plant. However, many digitalislike drugs come from other plants, and a few come from animals. Ouabain is a shorter-acting glycoside that is not derived from foxglove. Many other drugs have positive inotropic effects (the primary action of digitalis), but these other agents are not cardiac glycosides if they lack the first 2 structural features (steroid nucleus plus lactone ring). The pharmacokinetics of digoxin and digitoxin are summarized in Table 13–1.

**B. Mechanism of Action:** Inhibition of cell membrane $Na^+$,$K^+$-ATPase by digitalis is well documented and may be assumed to be the biochemical mechanism of action of digitalis. The translation of this effect into an increase in cardiac contractility involves the $Na^+$-$Ca^{2+}$ exchange mechanism. Inhibition of $Na^+$,$K^+$-ATPase results in an increase in intracellular sodium levels. The increased sodium level tips the balance of sodium-calcium exchange in the direction of moving more calcium into the cell. An increased intracellular calcium level increases contractile force. Other mechanisms of action have been proposed, but they are probably not as important as

**Table 13–1.** Pharmacokinetic parameters of typical cardiac glycosides in adults. Digoxin is the most commonly used agent.

| | Digoxin | Digitoxin |
|---|---|---|
| Oral availability (%) | 60–85 | 100 |
| Half-life in body (hours) | 40 | 168 |
| Primary organs of elimination | Kidney | Liver, kidney |
| Clearance (mL/min/70 kg) | 130 | 3.2 |
| Volume of distribution (L/70 kg) | 640 | 36 |
| Therapeutic plasma concentration (ng/mL) | 0.5–1.5 | 10–25 |
| Typical maintenance dose (mg/d/70 kg) | 0.125–0.5 | 0.05–0.2 |

the ATPase effect. The consequences of $Na^+$,$K^+$-ATPase inhibition are seen in both the mechanical and the electrical function of the heart. Digitalis also modifies autonomic outflow, and this action affects the electrical properties of the heart.

## C. Effects:

1. **Mechanical effects:** The increase in contractility evoked by digitalis results in increased ventricular ejection, decreased end-systolic and end-diastolic size, increased cardiac output, and increased renal perfusion. These beneficial effects permit a decrease in the compensatory responses previously described. The decrease in sympathetic tone is especially beneficial.
2. **Electrical effects:** These include both early responses and toxic (adverse) responses. They are summarized in Table 13–2.
   a. **Early responses.** Increased PR interval, caused by slowing of atrioventricular conduction velocity, and flattening of the T wave are often seen. The effect of digitalis on the atrioventricular node is largely parasympathetic in origin and can be partially blocked by atropine. It includes an increase in the atrioventricular nodal refractory period. Inversion of the T wave and ST depression may occur later.
   b. **Toxic responses.** Increased automaticity, caused by intracellular calcium overload, is the most important manifestation of toxicity. It results from delayed afterdepolarizations, which may evoke extrasystoles, tachycardia, or fibrillation in any part of the heart. In the ventricles, the extrasystoles are recognized as premature ventricular beats (PVBs). When PVBs are coupled to normal beats in a 1:1 fashion, the rhythm is called bigeminy.

## D. Clinical Use:

1. **Congestive heart failure.** Digitalis is the traditional positive inotropic agent used in the treatment of congestive heart failure. However, other agents (diuretics, ACE inhibitors, vasodilators) may be equally effective and less toxic in some patients. Because the half-lives of both of the commonly used digitalis glycosides are greater than 1 day, the drugs accumulate in the body and dosing regimens must be carefully designed and monitored.
2. **Atrial fibrillation.** It is desirable in this condition to reduce the conduction velocity or in-

**Table 13–2.** Actions of digitalis on cardiac electrical function.[1]

| Effect | Atria[2] | Atrioventricular Node[2] | Ventricles, Purkinje System[2] |
|---|---|---|---|
| Direct | Shortens refractory period. | Increases refractory period. | Shortens refractory period, or no significant effect. |
| | No significant effect on conduction velocity. | Decreases conduction velocity. | Decreases conduction velocity. |
| | Decreases normal automaticity; increases abnormal automaticity. | Increases or decreases normal automaticity; increases abnormal automaticity. | Increases or decreases normal automaticity; ***increases abnormal automaticity.*** |
| Indirect (ANS)<br>1. Vagal | ***Shortens refractory period.***<br>Decreases sinoatrial rate. | ***Increases refractory period.***<br>***Decreases conduction velocity.*** | No major effect. |
| 2. Sympathetic (toxic doses) | Increases sinoatrial rate. | Shortens refractory period.<br>Junctional extrasystoles. | ***Increases abnormal automaticity.*** |
| Effect on ECG and rhythm<br>Early | P wave changes. | ***Lengthens PR interval.*** | ST depression, T wave inversion |
| Progressive toxicity | Premature atrial beats. | Second- or third-degree block. | ***Ventricular premature depolarizations.*** |
| | Atrial fibrillation. | Junctional tachycardia. | Bigeminy, ***ventricular tachycardia, ventricular fibrillation.*** |

[1]Reproduced, with permission, from Katzung BG (editor): *Basic & Clinical Pharmacology,* 5th ed. Appleton & Lange, 1992.
[2]The most important effects are in boldface italic.

rease the refractory period of the atrioventricular node so that the rate of ventricular excitation is decreased. The parasympathomimetic actions of digitalis effectively accomplish this.

**E. Treatment of Digitalis Toxicity:** The treatment of digitalis toxicity is important because toxicity is common and dangerous. A case of severe intoxication is described in Case 2 (Appendix I).

1. Correction of potassium deficiency is useful in chronic digitalis intoxication. Mild toxicity may often be managed by omitting one or 2 doses of digitalis and giving oral $K^+$ supplements. Severe acute intoxication (as in suicidal overdoses) usually causes marked hyperkalemia and should not be treated with supplemental potassium.
2. Antiarrhythmic drugs may be useful if increased automaticity is prominent. Agents that do not severely impair cardiac contractility (eg, lidocaine) are favored. Severe acute digitalis overdose usually causes suppression of all pacemaker cells, and such patients should always receive a transvenous pacemaker while in the intensive care unit.
3. Digoxin antibodies (Fab fragments) are available commercially and should always be used if other therapies appear to be failing. They are effective for both digoxin and digitoxin overdose and may save otherwise terminally poisoned patients.

## OTHER DRUGS USED IN CONGESTIVE HEART FAILURE

The major agents used with or as alternatives to digitalis in treating congestive heart failure include diuretics, ACE inhibitors, $\beta_1$-selective sympathomimetics, phosphodiesterase inhibitors, and vasodilators.

**A. Diuretics:** The most important agent for immediate reduction of pulmonary congestion and severe edema is furosemide. Thiazides such as hydrochlorothiazide are often used in the management of chronic failure even before digitalis is considered. The pharmacologic characteristics of these drugs are discussed in Chapter 15.

**B. Angiotensin-Converting Enzyme Inhibitors:** These agents are at least as effective as digitalis in the management of chronic heart failure. Although they have no direct positive inotropic action, ACE inhibitors reduce aldosterone secretion, vascular resistance, and salt and water retention. They reduce symptoms and appear to prolong life. They are now considered among the first-line drugs for chronic heart failure, along with diuretics and digitalis.

**C. $\beta_1$-Selective Adrenoceptor Agonists:** Dobutamine and prenalterol are useful in some cases of acute failure. However, they are not satisfactory for chronic failure.

**D. Phosphodiesterase Inhibitors:** Amrinone and milrinone are the major representatives of this infrequently used group, although theophylline (in the form of aminophylline) was used in the past. These drugs increase cAMP levels by inhibiting its breakdown by phosphodiesterase and cause an increase in intracellular calcium levels similar to that produced by beta-adrenoceptor agonists. They also cause vasodilation, which may be responsible for a major part of their beneficial effect.

**E. Vasodilators:** Pure vasodilator therapy (hydralazine, nitroglycerin, nitroprusside) is used frequently for acute severe congestive failure. The use of these vasodilator drugs is based on the reduction in cardiac size and improved efficiency that can be realized with proper adjustment of venous return and resistance to ventricular ejection. Vasodilator therapy can be dramatically effective, especially in cases in which increased afterload is a major factor in causing the failure (eg, hypertension in an individual who has just had an infarction).

## DRUG LIST

The following drugs are important members of the group discussed in this chapter. **Prototype agents should be learned in detail; the major variant and the other significant agents should be known well enough to list the factors that distinguish them from the prototypes and from each other.**

| Subclass | Prototype | Major Variants | Other Significant Agents |
|---|---|---|---|
| Digitalis | Digoxin | Digitoxin | Ouabain |
| Positive inotropic digitalis substitutes | Dobutamine, amrinone | | Prenalterol, milrinone, theophylline |
| Diuretics | Furosemide, hydrochlorothiazide | | |
| Vasodilators | Hydralazine, nitroprusside | | |
| ACE inhibitors | Captopril | | Enalapril |

## QUESTIONS

**DIRECTIONS (items 1–6):** Each numbered item or incomplete statement in this section is followed by answers or by completions of the statement. Select the ONE lettered answer or completion that is BEST in each case.

**1.** The primary mechanism of action of digitalis involves
**(A)** an increase of the action potential amplitude
**(B)** an increase in ATP synthesis
**(C)** a modification of the actin molecule
**(D)** an increase in systolic intracellular calcium levels
**(E)** a block of sodium-calcium exchange

**2.** All of the following may be useful in the therapy of failure with high end-diastolic pressure and pulmonary edema EXCEPT
**(A)** nitroprusside
**(B)** digoxin
**(C)** ouabain
**(D)** propranolol
**(E)** dobutamine

**3.** Important effects of digitalis on the heart include
**(A)** increased force of contraction
**(B)** decreased atrioventricular conduction velocity
**(C)** increased ectopic automaticity
**(D)** decreased ejection time
**(E)** all of the above

**4.** All of the following characteristics of the cardiac glycosides are correct EXCEPT:
**(A)** Digoxin has a half-life of about 40 hours
**(B)** Digitoxin and digoxin both increase intracellular calcium
**(C)** Digitoxin has a significant enterohepatic circulation with a very long half-life
**(D)** Digoxin is heavily used because it is less toxic than the other glycosides
**(E)** Digitoxin inhibits $Na^+$,$K^+$-ATPase

**5.** Drugs that cause clinically useful or physiologically important positive inotropic effects include all of the following EXCEPT
 **(A)** amrinone
 **(B)** captopril
 **(C)** digoxin
 **(D)** dobutamine
 **(E)** norepinephrine

**6.** Effects of digitalis on electrical functions of the heart include all of the following EXCEPT
 **(A)** prolonged atrioventricular refractory period
 **(B)** lowered sinoatrial nodal rate
 **(C)** increased atrial rate in atrial flutter
 **(D)** decreased ventricular rate in atrial flutter
 **(E)** decreased ectopic automaticity

**DIRECTIONS (items 7–10):** Items 7–10 consist of lettered headings followed by a set of numbered phrases. For each numbered phrase, select the ONE lettered heading that is most closely associated with it. Each lettered heading may be selected once, more than once, or not at all.

 **(A)** Enalapril
 **(B)** Furosemide
 **(C)** Potassium
 **(D)** Dobutamine
 **(E)** Digoxin

**7.** Administration would tend to decrease or reverse a mild to moderate digitalis-induced arrhythmia

**8.** Useful in chronic congestive failure but has no direct positive inotropic action

**9.** Beta$_1$-selective agent sometimes used in acute congestive failure

**10.** Effective pulmonary vasodilator

## ANSWERS

**1.** The action potential is not increased in height but is often reduced in duration. There is no evidence that digitalis changes ATP levels or modifies the actin molecule. Digitalis does not block the sodium-calcium exchange but changes its function by changing intracellular sodium. The answer is **(D)**.

**2.** Propranolol is contraindicated. All the other agents are actually used in congestive heart failure by virtue of positive inotropic or vasodilator effects. The answer is **(D)**.

**3.** All are correct. The answer is **(E)**.

**4.** Digoxin is more popular because it has a shorter half-life than digitoxin. It is not less toxic. The answer is **(D)**.

**5.** Captopril and other ACE inhibitors are very useful in congestive heart failure but have no direct inotropic action. The answer is **(B)**.

**6.** The atrial flutter rate is often increased by digitalis because the drug decreases the atrial refractory period. The ventricular rate is typically decreased in this arrhythmia, because digitalis increases atrioventricular blockade. Increased, not decreased, ectopic automaticity is a very common and important effect of the digitalis glycosides. The answer is **(E)**.

7. A decreased serum potassium level tends to exacerbate digitalis toxicity, since the ion competes with digitalis at the $Na^+$,$K^+$-ATPase site of action. Therefore, potassium is often administered to patients with mild to moderate digitalis intoxication. The answer is **(C).**

8. ACE inhibitors are useful in treating congestive failure because they reduce vascular resistance and sodium retention. The answer is **(A).**

9. Dobutamine is a $\beta_1$-selective agonist sometimes used in acute failure. The answer is **(D).**

10. Although used mainly as a diuretic, furosemide is also an effective dilator of pulmonary blood vessels. For this reason it is especially effective in acute failure with pulmonary congestion. The answer is **(B).**

# 14 Antiarrhythmic Drugs

## OBJECTIVES

**Define the following terms:**

- Abnormal automaticity
- Action potential
- Atrial, ventricular fibrillation
- Calcium channel blockers
- Conduction velocity, time
- Group I, II, III, and IV drugs
- Local anesthetics
- Reentrant arrhythmia
- Refractory period
- Selective depression
- Sodium channel blockers
- Supraventricular tachycardia
- Ventricular tachycardia

**You should be able to:**

- Describe the distinguishing features of the 4 major groups of antiarrhythmic drugs and adenosine.
- List 2 or 3 of the most important drugs in each of the 4 groups.
- List the major toxicities of the drugs in the preceding item.
- Describe the mechanism of selective depression by local anesthetic antiarrhythmic agents.
- Explain how hyperkalemia, hypokalemia, or an antiarrhythmic drug can cause an arrhythmia.

## CONCEPTS

Cardiac arrhythmias are the most common cause of death in patients who have had a myocardial infarction. They are also the most serious manifestation of digitalis toxicity.

### PATHOPHYSIOLOGY

A. **What is an Arrhythmia?** Normal cardiac function is dependent on generation of an impulse in the normal pacemaker (the sinoatrial [SA] node) and on its conduction through the atrial muscle, the atrioventricular (AV) node, and the Purkinje conduction system to the ventricular muscle (Fig 14–1). Normal pacemaking and conduction require normal action potentials (dependent on

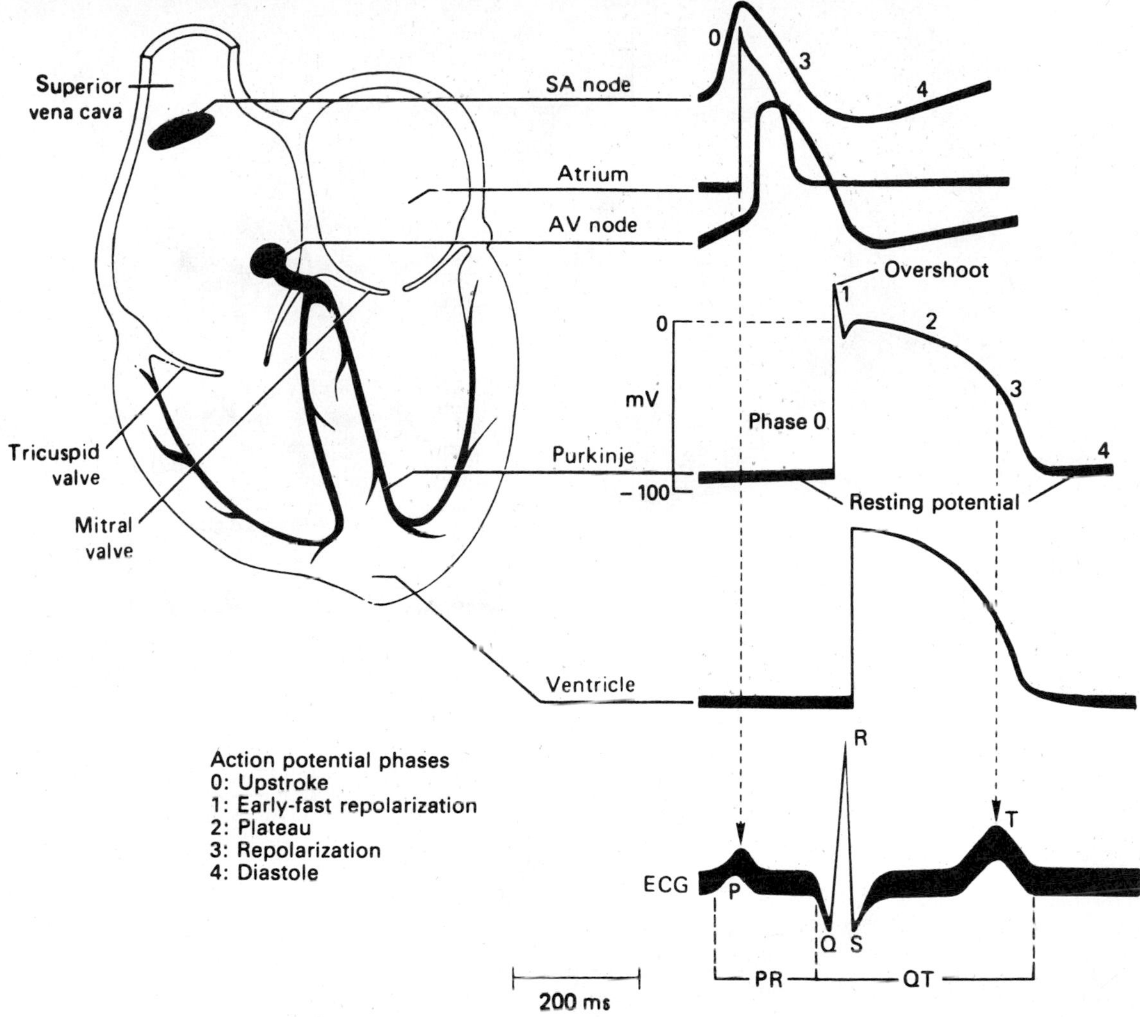


**Figure 14–1.** Schematic representation of the heart and normal cardiac electrical activity (intracellular recordings from areas indicated and ECG). The ECG is the body surface manifestation of the depolarization and repolarization waves of the heart. The P wave is generated by atrial depolarization, the QRS wave by ventricular muscle depolarization, and the T wave by ventricular repolarization. Thus the PR interval is a measure of the conduction time from atrium to ventricle and the QRS duration indicates the time required for all of the ventricular cells to be activated (ie, the intraventricular conduction time). The QT interval reflects the duration of the ventricular action potential.

sodium, calcium, and potassium channel activity), under appropriate autonomic control. Arrhythmias are therefore defined by exclusion—ie, *any rhythm that is not a normal sinus rhythm (NSR) is an arrhythmia.* Examples of electrocardiogram (ECG) recordings of normal sinus rhythm and some common arrhythmias are shown in Fig 14–2. The effects of the major antiarrhythmic drugs are summarized in Table 14–1.

**B. Arrhythmogenic Mechanisms: Abnormal automaticity** and **reentrant conduction** are the 2 major arrhythmogenic mechanisms for non-NSR rhythms. A few of the clinically important arrhythmias are atrial flutter, atrial fibrillation (AF), atrioventricular nodal reentry (a common type of supraventricular tachycardia [SVT]), premature ventricular beats (PVBs), ventricular tachycardia (VT), and ventricular fibrillation (VF).

**C. Drug Group Classification:** These agents are often classified by using a system loosely based on the channel or receptor involved. This system specifies 4 groups, usually denoted by Roman numerals I through IV:

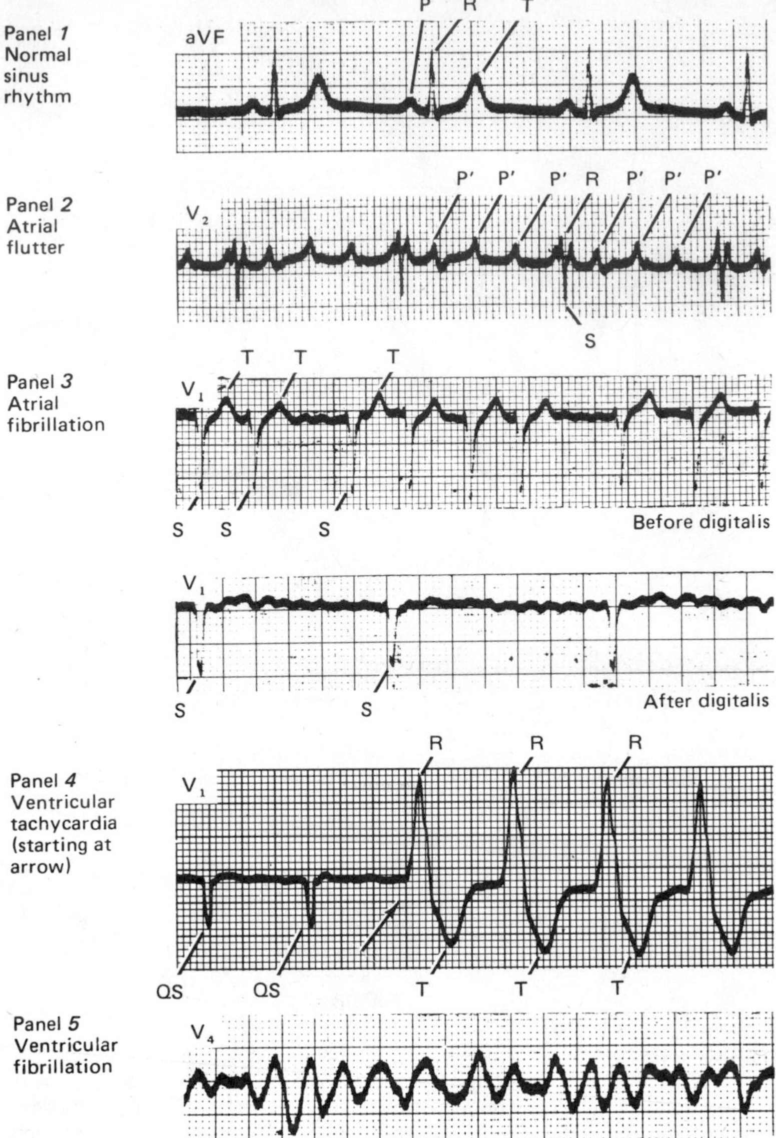


**Figure 14–2.** Typical ECGs of normal sinus rhythm and some common arrhythmias. Major waves (P, Q, R, S, and T) are labeled in each ECG record except in panel 5, in which electrical activity is completely disorganized and none of these deflections are recognizable. (Modified and reproduced, with permission, from Goldman MJ: *Principles of Clinical Electrocardiography,* 11th ed. Lange, 1982.)

**I.** Sodium channel blockers
**II.** Beta adrenoceptor blockers
**III.** Drugs that prolong the action potential (potassium channel blockers)
**IV.** Calcium channel blockers

Adenosine and potassium ions are important antiarrhythmic agents that fall outside these traditional groupings.

**D. Therapeutic Mechanism:** A useful channel-blocking antiarrhythmic drug binds to its receptor much more readily when the channel is open or inactivated than when it is fully repolarized and

**Table 14–1.** Membrane actions of antiarrhythmic drugs.[1]

| Drug | Block of Sodium Channels: Normal Cells | Block of Sodium Channels: Depolarized Cells | Refractory Period: Normal Cells | Refractory Period: Depolarized Cells | Calcium Channel Blockade | Effect on Pacemaker Activity | Sympatholytic Action |
|---|---|---|---|---|---|---|---|
| Adenosine (Adenocard) | 0 | 0 | 0 | 0 | 0 | 0 | + |
| Amiodarone (Cordarone) | + | +++ | ↑↑ | ↑↑↑ | + | ↓↓ | + |
| Bretylium (Bretylol) | 0 | 0 | ↑↑↑ | ↑↑↑ | 0 | ↑↓[2] | ++ |
| Disopyramide (Norpace) | + | +++ | ↑ | ↑↑ | + | ↓↓ | 0 |
| Encainide (Enkaid) | + | +++ | 0 | ↑ | 0 | ↓↓ | 0 |
| Esmolol (Brevibloc) | 0 | + | 0 | NA[3] | 0 | ↓↓ | +++ |
| Flecainide (Tambocor) | + | +++ | 0 | ↑ | 0 | ↓↓ | 0 |
| Imipramine (investigational) | + | + | ↑ | ↑↑ | 0 | ↓↓ | 0 |
| Lidocaine (Xylocaine) | 0 | +++ | ↓ | ↑↑ | 0 | ↓↓ | 0 |
| Mexiletine (Mexitil) | 0 | +++ | 0 | ↑↑ | 0 | ↓↓ | 0 |
| Moricizine (Ethmozine) | + | + | ↓ | ↓ | 0 | ↓↓ | 0 |
| Phenytoin (Dilantin) | 0 | + | ↓ | ↑ | + | ↓ | + |
| Procainamide (Pronestyl, others) | + | +++ | ↑ | ↑↑↑ | 0 | ↓ | + |
| Propafenone (Rythmol) | + | + | ↑ | ↑↑ | + | ↓↓ | + |
| Propranolol (Inderal) | 0 | + | ↓ | ↑↑ | 0 | ↓↓ | +++ |
| Quinidine (many trade names) | + | + | ↑ | ↑↑ | 0 | ↓↓ | + |
| Sotalol (investigational) | 0 | 0 | ↑↑ | ↑↑↑ | 0 | ↓↓ | +++ |
| Tocainide (Tonocard) | 0 | +++ | 0 | ↑↑ | 0 | ↓↓ | 0 |
| Verapamil (Calan, Isoptin) | 0 | + | 0 | ↑ | +++ | ↓↓ | + |

[1]Reproduced, with permission, from Katzung BG (editor): *Basic & Clinical Pharmacology,* 5th ed. Appleton & Lange, 1992.
[2]Bretylium may transiently increase pacemaker rate by causing catecholamine release.
[3]Data not available.

recovered from its previous activity. Ion channels in arrhythmic tissue spend more time in the open or inactivated states than do channels in normal tissue. Therefore, antiarrhythmic drugs block channels in abnormal tissue more effectively than they block channels in normal tissue. As a result, antiarrhythmic channel blockers are **state-dependent** in their action. Because of the difference in blocking ability, they have a **selectively** depressant effect on tissue that is depolarizing frequently (eg, during a fast tachycardia) or is relatively depolarized during rest (eg, by anoxia). This is particularly true of sodium and calcium channel blockers.

## GROUP I (LOCAL ANESTHETICS)

### A. Prototypes:

1. **Group IA (prolong action potential and QT interval).** The prototype group IA agent is quinidine. Other group IA drugs include amiodarone, procainamide, and disopyramide.
2. **Group IB (shorten action potential).** The prototype group IB drug is lidocaine. Mexiletine and tocainide are other group IB agents.
3. **Group IC (no effect on action potential duration or QT interval).** The prototype group IC drug is flecainide. Encainide and propafenone are also members of this group.

### B. Pharmacokinetics:

1. **Quinidine** is orally active and has a half-life of 6 hours.
2. **Lidocaine** is not orally active (because of high first-pass metabolism) and has a half-life of 1 to 2 hours.
3. **Flecainide** is orally active and has a half-life of 18–20 hours.
4. **Amiodarone** is unusual in having a prolonged half-life (several weeks).

**C. Cardiac Effects:** All group I drugs block conduction in depolarized tissue and slow or abolish abnormal pacemakers wherever these processes depend on sodium channels.

1. **Quinidine** affects both atrial and ventricular arrhythmias. It increases action potential (AP) duration and the effective refractory period (ERP). The increase in AP duration generates an increase in the QT interval (Fig 14–1).
2. **Lidocaine** affects Purkinje and ventricular tissue and has little effect on atrial tissue. It reduces AP duration and has little effect on (or reduces) the ERP in normal cells.
3. **Flecainide** has no effect on ventricular AP duration and the QT interval.

**D. Clinical Use:**

1. **Quinidine** is used in all types of arrhythmias, especially chronic ones requiring outpatient treatment.
2. **Lidocaine** is useful in acute ventricular arrhythmias, especially those following myocardial infarction. It is usually given intravenously, but intramuscular administration is also possible.
3. **Flecainide** is effective in both atrial and ventricular arrhythmias, but is approved only for refractory ventricular tachycardias that tend to progress to ventricular fibrillation at unpredictable times, resulting in "sudden death."
4. **Amiodarone** is effective in most types of arrhythmias, but because of its serious toxicity it is reserved for use in arrhythmias that are resistant to other drugs.

**E. Toxicity:** All antiarrhythmics can depress cardiac contractility and may *cause* arrhythmias in susceptible patients.

1. **Quinidine** causes cinchonism (headache, tinnitus), cardiac depression, gastrointestinal upset, and allergic reactions (eg, thrombocytopenic purpura). **Procainamide** causes a reversible syndrome similar to lupus erythematosus. Disopyramide has marked antimuscarinic effects and may precipitate congestive heart failure.
2. **Lidocaine.** This drug causes typical local anesthetic toxicity (ie, CNS stimulation, including convulsions), cardiovascular depression (usually minor), and allergy (usually rashes but may extend to anaphylaxis).
3. **Flecainide.** This drug can exacerbate or precipitate arrhythmias (proarrhythmic effect). The group IC drugs are limited to last-resort applications in refractory ventricular tachycardias because of their marked tendency to cause arrhythmias.
4. **Amiodarone.** This drug causes thyroid dysfunction (hyper- or hypothyroidism), paresthesias, tremor, microcrystalline deposits in the cornea and skin, and pulmonary fibrosis. It is also considered a last-resort drug.

## GROUP II (BETA-BLOCKERS)

**A. Prototype:** The prototype is **propranolol.** Its mechanism of action in arrhythmias may include some local anesthetic (membrane-stabilizing) effect but relies primarily on beta blockade and suppression of abnormal pacemakers. Arrhythmias that depend on abnormal pacemakers are particularly common during digitalis toxicity and in the first 24 months after myocardial infarction.

**B. Other Group II Drugs:** These include **esmolol,** a very short-acting beta-blocker for intravenous administration that is used almost exclusively as an antiarrhythmic in acute surgical arrhythmias. **Metoprolol** is commonly used as a prophylactic drug in patients who have had a myocardial infarction. Amiodarone also has beta-blocking effects.

## GROUP III (POTASSIUM CHANNEL BLOCKERS)

**A. Prototype:** The prototype is **bretylium.** Group III drugs appear to act by prolonging the action potential. This increases the ERP and reduces the ability of the heart to respond to rapid tachycardias and early extrasystoles. Bretylium is used parenterally.

**B. Mechanism of Action:** The AP prolongation is probably caused by blockade of potassium channels, which are responsible for the repolarization of the AP.

C. **Clinical Use:** Bretylium is used rarely and only in the treatment of refractory post-myocardial infarction arrhythmias, especially recurrent ventricular fibrillation. Amiodarone is an important agent that also prolongs the AP and is therefore sometimes classified as a group III drug. It also belongs to other groups, since it also blocks sodium channels, beta receptors, and calcium channels. Quinidine and N-acetylprocainamide (NAPA), the metabolite of procainamide, also significantly prolong the AP.

## GROUP IV (CALCIUM CHANNEL BLOCKERS)

A. **Prototype:** The prototype is **Verapamil.** Diltiazem is also an effective antiarrhythmic drug, but nifedipine is not.

B. **Mechanism & Effects:** These calcium channel blockers are effective in arrhythmias that must traverse calcium-dependent cardiac tissue (eg, the atrioventricular node).

C. **Clinical Use:** Calcium channel blockers were drugs of choice in atrioventricular nodal reentry (also known as nodal tachycardia and supraventricular tachycardia) until adenosine became available; they are quite effective in this type of arrhythmia. These drugs are orally active; verapamil is also available for parenteral use (and when used as an antiarrhythmic is usually given intravenously). The most important toxicity relates to excessive pharmacologic effect, since cardiac contractility can be significantly depressed. Amiodarone has some calcium channel blocking activity.

## UNCLASSIFIED ANTIARRHYTHMIC DRUGS

A. **Adenosine:** Adenosine is a normal component of the body, but when given as an intravenous bolus it markedly slows conduction in the atrioventricular node. It is extremely effective in abolishing atrioventricular nodal arrhythmias and has become the drug of choice for these conditions. It has an extremely short half-life (about 15 seconds). Toxicity includes flushing and hypotension, but because of the short half-life these effects do not limit the use of the drug.

B. **Potassium Ions:** Potassium depresses ectopic pacemakers, including those caused by digitalis toxicity. Hypokalemia is associated with increased incidence of arrhythmias, especially in patients receiving digitalis. Conversely, excessive potassium levels depress conduction and can cause reentry arrhythmias. Therefore, when treating arrhythmias, serum potassium levels should be measured and, if abnormal, normalized. Patients with hyperkalemia are more sensitive to the cardiac depressant effects of antiarrhythmic drugs.

## DRUG LIST

The following drugs are important members of the group discussed in this chapter. Prototype agents should be learned in detail; the major variants should be known well enough to list the factors that distinguish them from the prototypes and from each other; and the other significant agents should be recognized as belonging to a specific subclass.

| Subclass | Prototype | Major Variants | Other Significant Agents |
|---|---|---|---|
| Group IA | Quinidine | Amiodarone | Procainamide, disopyramide |
| Group IB | Lidocaine | | Mexiletine, tocainide |
| Group IC | Flecainide | | Encainide, propafenone |
| Group II | Propranolol | Esmolol | Metoprolol |
| Group III | Bretylium | Amiodarone | |
| Group IV | Verapamil | | Diltiazem |
| Unclassified | Adenosine | Potassium | |

## QUESTIONS

**DIRECTIONS (items 1–9):** Each numbered item or incomplete statement in this section is followed by answers or by completions of the statement. Select the ONE lettered answer or completion that is BEST in each case.

**1.** All of the following statements are accurate EXCEPT:
**(A)** Quinidine may cause cardiac arrest in patients with atrioventricular block
**(B)** Quinidine increases cardiac contractility
**(C)** Quinidine prolongs the effective refractory period
**(D)** Quinidine may induce thrombocytopenia
**(E)** Quinidine may induce tinnitus

**2.** In treating quinidine overdose, rational therapy would be to
**(A)** give KCl
**(B)** give digitalis
**(C)** give a calcium chelator such as EDTA
**(D)** administer nitroprusside
**(E)** administer sodium lactate

**3.** Lidocaine typically
**(A)** reduces abnormal automaticity
**(B)** reduces the resting potential
**(C)** increases the action potential duration
**(D)** increases the PR interval
**(E)** increases contractility

**4.** A computer programmer attending a meeting in your city comes to your office because of a possible drug reaction. She has been taking an antiarrhythmic drug by mouth, but the identity of the agent is unknown. Which of the following is LEAST likely?
**(A)** If she has a thyroid abnormality, the drug may be amiodarone
**(B)** If she has a purpuric rash, the drug may be quinidine
**(C)** If she has tinnitus and diarrhea, the drug may be lidocaine
**(D)** If she has marked antimuscarinic signs, the drug may be disopyramide
**(E)** If she has signs of lupus erythematosus, the drug may be procainamide

**5.** All of the following can be used for chronic therapy EXCEPT
(A) esmolol
(B) disopyramide
(C) amiodarone
(D) verapamil
(E) procainamide

**6.** The antiarrhythmic of choice in most cases of supraventricular tachycardia (nodal tachycardia) is
(A) propranolol
(B) quinidine
(C) flecainide
(D) amiodarone
(E) adenosine

**7.** Antiarrhythmic substances that must be given parenterally include
(A) quinidine
(B) flecainide
(C) verapamil
(D) lidocaine
(E) metoprolol

**8.** Drugs that can abolish reentry arrhythmias include
(A) quinidine
(B) lidocaine
(C) amiodarone
(D) verapamil
(E) all of the above

**9.** Recognized adverse effects of quinidine include all of the following EXCEPT
(A) cinchonism
(B) constipation
(C) thrombocytopenic purpura
(D) displacement of digoxin from its binding sites with possible digoxin toxicity
(E) angioneurotic edema

**DIRECTIONS (items 10–14):** Items 10–14 consist of lettered headings followed by a set of numbered phrases. For each numbered phrase, select the ONE lettered heading that is most closely associated with it. Each lettered heading may be selected once, more than once, or not at all.

(A) Quinidine
(B) Adenosine
(C) Amiodarone
(D) Verapamil
(E) Lidocaine

**10.** Blocks sodium channels and decreases action potential duration

**11.** Slows conduction through the atrioventricular node by an action on calcium channels

**12.** May cause pulmonary fibrosis; has a very long half-life

**13.** Blocks sodium channels and prolongs action potential duration; duration of action is 6–8 hours

**14.** Very useful in supraventricular tachycardia; half-life is 10–15 seconds

## ANSWERS

1. In clinical situations, quinidine often diminishes cardiac contractility and output. It never increases these variables. The answer is **(B)**.

2. Quinidine, like other local anesthetics, acts from inside the cell. Intracellular acidosis causes trapping of higher concentrations of this weak base inside the membrane. Administration of an alkalizing agent such as sodium lactate reduces acidosis. In addition, the movement of hydrogen ions out of the cell will be balanced by the transfer of potassium ions into it. This will increase the resting membrane potential and reduce the intensity of local anesthetic effects. The answer is **(E)**.

3. All of the sodium channel-blocking antiarrhythmic drugs reduce abnormal automaticity. None of them reduce resting potential or increase contractility. Lidocaine has very little effect on the electrocardiogram in normal sinus rhythm. The answer is **(A)**.

4. Lidocaine is not taken on an outpatient basis. Furthermore, lidocaine in toxic parenteral doses may produce CNS adverse effects, but these usually consist of paresthesias, light-headedness, and convulsions. The answer is **(C)**.

5. Esmolol is an ester that is rapidly metabolized even when given intravenously; it is inactive by the oral route. Therefore, it would not be suitable for chronic therapy. The answer is **(A)**.

6. Calcium channel blockers are effective in supraventricular tachycardias. However, adenosine is just as effective in most supraventricular tachycardias and is less toxic. The answer is **(E)**.

7. Only lidocaine must be given parenterally. The answer is **(D)**.

8. All are correct. Since the question does not specify which types of ionic channels are involved in the arrhythmia, both sodium and calcium channel blockers are legitimate answers. The answer is **(E)**.

9. Quinidine has a wide spectrum of adverse effects, but it causes increased, not decreased, gastrointestinal motility. The answer is **(B)**.

10. Group IB drugs typically block sodium channels and decrease the action potential duration. The answer is **(E)**.

11. Verapamil is the calcium channel blocker in this list. The answer is **(D)**.

12. Pulmonary fibrosis is a very important, potentially lethal, toxicity of amiodarone. The answer is **(C)**.

13. Quinidine and amiodarone both block sodium channels and prolong the action potential. The duration of amiodarone action, however, is several weeks. The answer is **(A)**.

14. The only drug in the list with a half-life of seconds is adenosine. The answer is **(B)**.

# Diuretic & Antidiuretic Agents 15

## OBJECTIVES

**Define the following terms:**

- Bicarbonate diuretic
- Diluting segment
- Hyperchloremic metabolic acidosis
- Hypokalemic metabolic alkalosis
- Nephrogenic diabetes insipidus
- Pituitary diabetes insipidus
- Potassium-sparing diuretic
- Uricosuric diuretic

**You should be able to:**

- List 5 major types of diuretics and relate them to their sites of action.
- Describe 2 drugs that reduce potassium loss during a sodium diuresis.
- Describe a therapy that will reduce calcium excretion in patients who have recurrent urinary stones.
- Describe a treatment for severe hypercalcemia in a patient with advanced carcinoma.
- Describe a method for reducing urine volume in nephrogenic diabetes insipidus.
- List the major applications and the toxicities of thiazides, loop diuretics, and potassium-sparing diuretics.

## CONCEPTS

### RENAL TRANSPORT & DIURETIC DRUG GROUPS

**A. Renal Transport Mechanisms:** The effects of the diuretic agents are predictable from a knowledge of the function of the segment of the nephron in which they act (Fig 15–1).

1. **Proximal convoluted tubule.** This segment carries out isosmotic reabsorption of amino acids, glucose, and cations. Bicarbonate reabsorption is favored over chloride reabsorption because the high concentration of carbonic anhydrase in this segment provides for rapid formation of $CO_2$, which is rapidly reabsorbed from the urine. This segment is responsible for 40–50% of the total reabsorption of sodium.
2. **Thick portion of the ascending limb of the loop of Henle.** This segment pumps sodium, potassium, and chloride out of the lumen into the interstitium of the kidney. It provides the concentration gradient for the countercurrent-concentrating mechanism in the kidney and is responsible for 30–40% of the sodium reabsorbed. It also carries out significant calcium and magnesium reabsorption.
3. **Distal convoluted tubule.** This segment, also called the diluting segment, actively pumps sodium and chloride out of the lumen of the nephron. It is responsible for approximately 10% of sodium reabsorption. Calcium is reabsorbed in this segment, under the control of parathyroid hormone (PTH).
4. **Collecting tubule.** The final segment of the nephron is the primary site of acidification of the urine and aldosterone-regulated reabsorption of sodium. It is responsible for reabsorbing approximately 2–4% of the total filtered sodium. Reabsorption of water, under the control of antidiuretic hormone (ADH), also occurs here.

**B. Classification:** Diuretics are classified according to their site or mode of action in the renal tubule. The **carbonic anhydrase inhibitors** and **osmotic diuretics** act principally in the proximal tubule. The **loop diuretics** act in the ascending limb of the loop of Henle. The **thiazide diuretics** act in the distal convoluted tubule. The **potassium-sparing diuretics** act in the collecting ducts. Most diuretics act from the luminal side of the nephron. Some of their effects are summarized in Table 15–1.

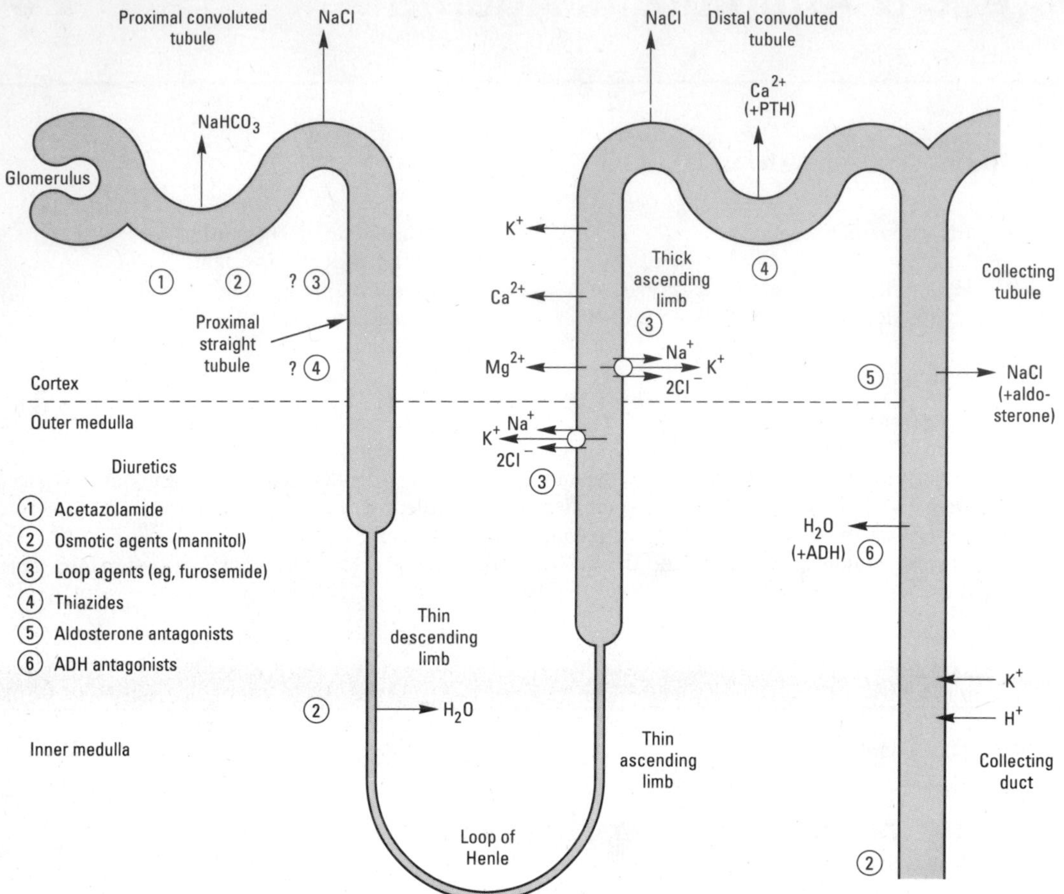


**Figure 15–1.** Tubule transport systems and sites of action of diuretics. (Reproduced, with permission, from Katzung BG [editor]: *Basic & Clinical Pharmacology,* 5th ed. Appleton & Lange, 1992.)

**Table 15–1.** Changes in urinary electrolyte patterns in response to diuretic drugs.[1]

| Agent | Urinary Electrolyte Patterns[2] | | |
|---|---|---|---|
| | NaCl | $NaHCO_3$ | $K^+$ |
| Carbonic anhydrase inhibitors | + | +++ | + |
| Loop agents | ++++ | − | + |
| Thiazides | + | + − | + |
| Loop agents plus thiazides | +++++ | + | + |
| $K^+$- sparing agents | + | − | - |

[1]Reproduced, with permission, from Katzung BG (editor): *Basic & Clinical Pharmacology,* 5th ed. Appleton & Lange, 1992.
[2]+ = increase, − = decrease.

## CARBONIC ANHYDRASE INHIBITORS

**A. Classification & Prototypes:** The prototype agent is acetazolamide. It is a sulfonamide derivative.

**B. Mechanism of Action:** Inhibition of carbonic anhydrase by acetazolamide slows the following reaction (site ① in Fig 15–1):

$$H^+ + HCO_3^- \rightarrow H_2O + CO_2$$

This reaction is necessary for maximal reabsorption of bicarbonate from the glomerular filtrate and for secretion of bicarbonate in other tissues. The inhibitory effect of acetazolamide occurs throughout the body.

**C. Effects:** The major renal effect is a bicarbonate diuresis (ie, sodium bicarbonate is excreted) in which body bicarbonate is depleted and a metabolic acidosis results. Because the bicarbonate is depleted, sodium bicarbonate excretion slows, even with continued diuretic administration, and the diuresis is self-limiting. In the eye, secretion of aqueous humor is reduced and a useful reduction in intraocular pressure can be achieved. This effect is not self-limiting.

**D. Clinical Use:** The major application of these agents is in the treatment of glaucoma. They must be used orally, but topical formulations are under study. Carbonic anhydrase inhibitors are also used to prevent development of acute mountain (high-altitude) sickness. The mechanism of action in this application is not well understood.

**E. Toxicity:** Drowsiness and paresthesias are reported. Alkalinization of the urine may cause precipitation of calcium salts and formation of renal stones. Renal potassium wasting may be marked. Patients with hepatic impairment may develop hepatic encephalopathy.

## LOOP DIURETICS

**A. Classification & Prototypes:** The prototype loop agent is **furosemide.** Furosemide and bumetanide are sulfonamide derivatives. **Ethacrynic acid** is a phenoxyacetic acid derivative; it is not a sulfonamide. The loop diuretics are relatively short-acting (diuresis usually occurs over the 4 hours following a dose).

**B. Mechanism of Action:** Loop diuretics inhibit a transporter of sodium, potassium, and chloride (site ③ in Fig 15–1) and reduce the lumen-positive potential across the tubule wall.

**C. Effects:** The loop of Henle is responsible for a large proportion of total renal sodium reabsorption; therefore, a full dose of a loop diuretic produces a massive sodium chloride diuresis. The concentrating ability of the nephron is reduced because the full activity of the loop of Henle is required to establish the hypertonic interstitium of the renal papilla that permits the final concentration of urine in the collecting tubule. The diluting capacity of the kidney is also reduced by these drugs because removal of most of the sodium chloride is needed at this site to make urine hypotonic. (The distal convoluted tubule is also a diluting segment.) Loss of the positive inside potential reduces reabsorption of divalent cations as well, and calcium excretion is significantly increased. Phenoxyacetic acid derivatives (eg, ethacrynic acid) are effective uricosuric drugs.

**D. Clinical Use:** The major application of loop diuretics is in the treatment of edematous states (eg, congestive heart failure and ascites). These drugs are particularly valuable in acute pulmonary edema, in which their separate pulmonary vasodilating action often plays a useful role. They are sometimes used in hypertension if the response to thiazides is inadequate, but their short duration of action is a disadvantage in this condition. A less common but important application is in the treatment of severe hypercalcemia (eg, that induced by certain cancers). This life-threatening situation can often be managed with large doses of furosemide coupled with parenteral electrolyte (sodium and potassium chloride) and volume supplementation.

**E. Toxicity:** Loop diuretics usually induce a hypokalemic metabolic alkalosis. Because large amounts of sodium are presented to the collecting tubules, wasting of potassium, which is excreted by the kidney in order to conserve sodium, may be severe. Because they are so efficacious, the loop diuretics can cause hypovolemia and cardiovascular complications. Ototoxicity is an important toxic effect of the loop agents.

## THIAZIDE DIURETICS

**A. Classification & Prototypes:** The prototype agent, **hydrochlorothiazide,** is a sulfonamide derivative. A few agents that lack the typical thiazide ring in their structure nevertheless have effects identical to those of thiazides and are therefore considered thiazidelike. **Indapamide** is a relatively new thiazidelike agent with a significant vasodilating effect. Thiazides are active by the oral route and have a duration of action of 6–12 hours.

**B. Mechanism of Action:** The major action of thiazides is to inhibit sodium chloride transport in the early segment of the distal convoluted tubule (site ④ in Fig 15–1), a site at which significant dilution of urine takes place. They thus reduce the diluting capacity (but not the concentrating ability) of the nephron.

**C. Effects:** In full doses, thiazides produce a moderate sodium and chloride diuresis. A hypokalemic metabolic alkalosis may occur. The normal lumen-negative electrical potential of this portion of the nephron is reduced, permitting more complete reabsorption of calcium. When thiazides are used with a loop diuretic, a synergistic effect with marked diuresis occurs. Thiazides reduce the blood pressure. Initially, the reduction reflects the reduction of blood volume, but with continued use, these agents appear to reduce vascular resistance. The vascular effect is modest but significant and is maximal at doses lower than the maximal diuretic dosage. Compared with older thiazides and thiazidelike agents, indapamide has a greater ratio of vasodilating-to-sodium diuretic effects.

**D. Clinical Use:** The major application of thiazides is in hypertension, for which their long duration of action and moderate intensity of action are particularly useful. Chronic therapy of edematous conditions such as congestive heart failure is another common application. Recurrent renal calcium stone formation can sometimes be controlled with thiazides.

**E. Toxicity:** A severe sodium diuresis with hyponatremia is an uncommon but dangerous early effect of thiazides. Chronic therapy is often associated with potassium wasting, since an increased sodium load is presented to the collecting tubules. Diabetic patients may have significant hyperglycemia. Serum uric acid and lipid levels are also increased in some individuals.

## POTASSIUM-SPARING DIURETICS

**A. Classification & Prototypes:** **Spironolactone** is a pharmacologic antagonist of aldosterone in the collecting tubules. **Triamterene** and **amiloride** act by a different mechanism in the collecting tubules. These drugs are active when given orally. Spironolactone has a slow onset and offset of action (24–72 hours). Triamterene and amiloride have durations of action of 12–24 hours.

**B. Mechanism of Action:** As previously noted, spironolactone is a direct inhibitor of aldosterone at the steroid receptor. It causes an increase in sodium clearance and a decrease in potassium excretion. Triamterene and amiloride are inhibitors of sodium flux in this portion of the tubule and have a similar result (site ⑤ in Fig 15–1).

**C. Effects:** These drugs increase sodium excretion by 3–5% and decrease potassium and hydrogen ion excretion; they may cause hyperchloremic metabolic acidosis.

**D. Clinical Use:** Hyperaldosteronism (eg, in cirrhosis) is an important indication for spironolactone. Potassium wasting caused by chronic therapy with loop or thiazide diuretics, if not controlled by dietary sodium restriction and potassium supplements, will usually respond to these drugs. The most common use is in the form of products that combine a thiazide with a potassium-sparing agent.

**E. Toxicity:** The most important toxic effect is hyperkalemia. These drugs should never be given with potassium supplements. Spironolactone may cause endocrine abnormalities, including gynecomastia and antiandrogenic effects.

## OSMOTIC DIURETICS

**A. Classification & Prototypes:** The prototype osmotic diuretic is **mannitol.** It is given intravenously.

**B. Mechanism of Action:** Because it is filtered at the glomerulus but poorly reabsorbed from the tubule, mannitol "holds" water in the lumen by virtue of its osmotic effect. The major location for this action is the proximal convoluted tubule (site ② in Fig 15–1), where the bulk of isosmotic reabsorption normally takes place. Reabsorption of water is also reduced in the descending limb of the loop of Henle and in the collecting tubule.

**C. Effects:** The volume of urine is increased. Most filtered solutes will be excreted in larger amounts unless they are actively reabsorbed. The net change in sodium excretion is unpredictable.

**D. Clinical Use:** These drugs are used to maintain high urine flow (eg, when renal blood flow is reduced and in conditions of solute overload from severe hemolysis or rhabdomyolysis). Mannitol (as well as several other osmotic agents) is useful in reducing intraocular pressure in acute glaucoma and intracranial pressure in neurologic conditions.

**E. Toxicity:** Removal of water from the intracellular compartment may cause hyponatremia and pulmonary edema. Headache, nausea, and vomiting are common.

## ANTIDIURETIC HORMONE AGONISTS & ANTAGONISTS

**A. Classification & Prototypes:** **Antidiuretic hormone** and **desmopressin** are prototype antidiuretic hormone (ADH) agonists. **Demeclocycline** and **lithium ions** are ADH antagonists.

**B. Mechanism of Action:** ADH facilitates water reabsorption from the collecting tubule by activation of adenylyl cyclase. The increased cAMP level opens or causes insertion of additional water channels in this part of the tubule. Demeclocycline and lithium inhibit the action of ADH at some point distal to the generation of cAMP.

**C. Effects:** ADH reduces urine volume and increases its concentration. ADH antagonists have the opposite effects.

**D. Clinical Use:** ADH and desmopressin are useful in pituitary diabetes insipidus. They are of no value in the nephrogenic form of the disease, but salt restriction, thiazides, and loop diuretics may be used. ADH antagonists are used in syndromes of inappropriate ADH secretion (eg, certain tumors that secrete ADH-like peptides).

**E. Toxicity:** In the presence of ADH and desmopressin, a large water load may cause dangerous hyponatremia. In children under 8 years of age, demeclocycline (like other tetracyclines) causes bone and teeth abnormalities.

## DRUG LIST

The following drugs are important members of the group discussed in this chapter. Prototype agents should be learned in detail; the major variants should be known well enough to list the factors that distinguish them from the prototypes and from each other; and the other significant agent should be recognized as belonging to a specific subclass.

| Subclass | Prototype | Major Variants | Other Significant Agents |
|---|---|---|---|
| Carbonic anhydrase inhibitor | Acetazolamide | | |
| Osmotic | Mannitol | | |
| Loop diuretic | Furosemide | Ethacrynic acid | |
| Thiazide and thiazidelike agents | Hydrochlorothiazide | Indapamide | |
| Potassium-sparing diuretics | Spironolactone | Triamterene | Amiloride |
| ADH agonists | Vasopressin (ADH) | Desmopressin | |
| ADH inhibitors | Demeclocycline | | |

## QUESTIONS

**DIRECTIONS (items 1–4):** Each numbered item or incomplete statement in this section is followed by answers or by completions of the statement. Select the ONE lettered answer or completion that is BEST in each case.

**1.** Which of the following has a rapid diuretic effect, plus smooth muscle effects that make it useful in the treatment of acute pulmonary edema?
**(A)** Furosemide
**(B)** Thiazide diuretic
**(C)** Spironolactone
**(D)** Triamterene
**(E)** Acetazolamide

**2.** The most useful agent in the treatment of recurrent calcium stones is
**(A)** mannitol
**(B)** furosemide
**(C)** spironolactone
**(D)** hydrochlorothiazide
**(E)** acctazolamide

**3.** When used chronically to treat hypertension, thiazide diuretics have all of the following properties or effects EXCEPT:
**(A)** They reduce blood volume or vascular resistance (or both)
**(B)** Their maximal effects on blood pressure occur at doses below the maximal diuretic dose
**(C)** They may cause an elevation of plasma uric acid and triglyceride levels
**(D)** They generally decrease the urinary excretion of calcium
**(E)** They cause ototoxicity

**4.** Which of the following drugs is correctly associated with site and maximal diuretic efficacy?
**(A)** Thiazides—distal convoluted tubule—10% of filtered $Na^+$
**(B)** Spironolactone—diluting segment—10%
**(C)** Ethacrynic acid—thick ascending limb—15%
**(D)** Indapamide—collecting duct—2%
**(E)** All of the above

**DIRECTIONS (items 5–10):** Items 5–10 consist of lettered headings followed by a set of numbered phrases. For each numbered phrase, select the ONE lettered heading that is most closely associated with it. Each lettered heading may be selected once, more than once, or not at all.

(A) Spironolactone
(B) Furosemide
(C) Triamterene
(D) Hydrochlorothiazide
(E) Acetazolamide

**5.** Causes self-limiting diuresis and may cause hyperchloremic metabolic acidosis

**6.** Has its major effect in the distal convoluted tubule

**7.** Reduces the formation of concentrated urine in water-deprived subjects

**8.** Useful in glaucoma and high-altitude sickness

**9.** Often used in hypertension; may elevate serum uric acid and lipid levels

**10.** Can reduce the action of aldosterone without blocking its receptors

## ANSWERS

**1.** Furosemide has a rapid onset of action, is very efficacious, and appears to have some direct smooth muscle-relaxing effects. The answer is **(A)**.

**2.** The thiazides are useful in the prevention of calcium stones because they inhibit the renal excretion of calcium. In contrast, the loop agents facilitate calcium excretion. The answer is **(D)**.

**3.** Thiazides do not cause ototoxicity, loop diuretics do. The answer is **(E)**.

**4.** Spironolactone acts in the collecting duct, not the diluting segment (the distal convoluted tubule). It is not capable of causing a 10% sodium diuresis. Ethacrynic acid is a loop diuretic and can produce a 30% increase in sodium excretion. Indapamide, a thiazidelike drug, acts in the distal convoluted tubule and the proximal tubule, not in the collecting duct. The answer is **(A)**.

**5.** Potassium-sparing diuretics and carbonic anhydrase inhibitors may cause a hyperchloremic metabolic acidosis. Only carbonic anhydrase inhibitors cause a self-limiting diuresis. The loop and thiazide agents tend to cause hypokalemic metabolic alkalosis. The answer is **(E)**.

**6.** The thiazides act in the distal convoluted tubule. The answer is **(D)**.

**7.** Loop agents and thiazides decrease the diluting capacity of the kidney. Only loop agents act directly to limit the concentrating ability of the kidney. The answer is **(B)**.

**8.** The carbonic anhydrase inhibitors are useful in both conditions. The answer is **(E)**.

**9.** The thiazides are the most commonly used diuretics in hypertension; they may increase serum lipid and uric acid levels. The answer is **(D)**.

**10.** Triamterene acts in the collecting tubule to block sodium channels generated by aldosterone. Spironolactone blocks the binding of aldosterone to its receptors. The answer is **(C)**.

# Part IV. Drugs With Important Actions on Smooth Muscle

# Histamine, Serotonin, & the Ergot Alkaloids 16

## OBJECTIVES

**Define the following terms:**

- Acid-peptic disease
- Autacoids
- Carcinoid
- Ergotism (''St. Anthony's Fire'')
- Gastrinoma
- IgE-mediated immediate reaction
- Oxytocic
- Prolactinoma
- Zollinger-Ellison syndrome

**You should be able to:**

- List the major organ system effects of histamine and serotonin.
- List 2 or 3 different antihistamines of the $H_1$ and $H_2$ types.
- List 2 antiserotonin drugs and their major applications.
- List the major organ system effects of the ergot alkaloids.
- Describe the major clinical applications of the ergot drugs.

## CONCEPTS

Autacoids are endogenous substances that have important effects when studied as drugs but often have poorly defined physiologic roles. Histamine and serotonin (5-hydroxytryptamine [5-HT]) are 2 of the most important of these substances. Both are synthesized in the body from amino acid precursors and then eliminated by pathways very similar to those used for catecholamine synthesis and metabolism. The ergot alkaloids are a heterogeneous group of drugs that interact with serotonin receptors, dopamine receptors, and adrenoceptors.

### HISTAMINE

Histamine is formed from the amino acid histidine and is stored in high concentrations in mast cells. It is metabolized by amine oxidase enzymes and by methylation. Released from mast cells in response to immunoglobulin E (IgE)-mediated (immediate) allergic reactions, this autacoid plays an important pathophysiologic role in seasonal rhinitis (hay fever), urticaria, and angioneurotic edema. It may also play a physiologic role in the control of acid secretion in the stomach.

**A. Receptors & Effects:** Two receptors for histamine, $H_1$ and $H_2$, mediate most of the well-defined actions; a third ($H_3$) has recently been identified (Table 16–1).

1. **$H_1$ receptor.** This receptor is particularly important in smooth muscle effects; its biochemical mechanism is unclear. It causes bronchoconstriction, possibly by $IP_3$ release, and vasodilation, probably by release of EDRF. Local edema may form as a result of an action on capillary endothelium.
2. **$H_2$ receptor.** This receptor stimulates gastric acid secretion by parietal cells. It also has a

**Table 16–1.** Histamine and serotonin receptor subtypes.

| Receptor Subtype | Distribution | Postreceptor Mechanism | Antagonists |
|---|---|---|---|
| $H_1$ | Smooth muscle | Increases $IP_3$ | Diphenhydramine |
| $H_2$ | Stomach, heart, mast cells | Increases cAMP | Cimetidine |
| $H_3$ | CNS | Unknown | ? |
| $5\text{-}HT_{1a}$ | CNS | Decreases cAMP | Ipsapirone |
| $5\text{-}HT_{1b/1d}$[1] | CNS | Decreases cAMP | |
| $5\text{-}HT_{1c}$ | CNS | Increases $IP_3$ | Ritanserin |
| $5\text{-}HT_2$ | Platelets, smooth muscle, CNS | Increases $IP_3$ | Ritanserin |
| $5\text{-}HT_3$ | CNS | Opens Na/K ion channel | Ondansetron |
| $5\text{-}HT_4$ | Hippocampus, enteric nerves | Increases cAMP | |

[1]The $5\text{-}HT_{1b}$ receptor is thought to occur only in rodents.

cardiac stimulant effect. Both actions are caused by activation of adenylyl cyclase and increased levels of cAMP.

3. **$H_3$ receptor.** This receptor appears to be involved mainly in modulation of histaminergic neurotransmission in the CNS by presynaptic action.

**B. Clinical Use:** Histamine has no therapeutic applications, but the drugs that block its effects are important in clinical medicine.

## HISTAMINE $H_1$ ANTAGONISTS

**A. Classification & Prototypes:** A wide variety of antihistaminic $H_1$ blockers are available from several different chemical families. **Diphenhydramine** and **chlorpheniramine** may be considered prototypes. Because they have been developed for use in chronic conditions, they are all active by the oral route. Several newer agents (eg, **terfenadine**) have decreased CNS penetration.

**B. Mechanism of Action:** $H_1$ blockers are competitive pharmacologic antagonists at the $H_1$ receptor; they have no effect on histamine release from storage sites. Because their structure closely resembles that of some muscarinic blockers and alpha adrenoceptor blockers, many $H_1$ blockers also have significant effects at these autonomic receptors.

**C. Effects:** $H_1$-blocking drugs have sedative and anti-motion-sickness effects in the CNS. In the periphery, they competitively inhibit the effects of histamine (especially if given before histamine release). In addition, they may block muscarinic, alpha-adrenoceptor-mediated, and serotonin-mediated effects. Many $H_1$ blockers are potent local anesthetics.

**D. Clinical Use:** $H_1$ blockers have major applications in allergies of the immediate type (ie, those caused by antigen acting on IgE antibody-sensitized mast cells). These conditions include hay fever and urticaria. The drugs have a broad spectrum of adverse effects that limit their usefulness but can also be used to good effect (eg, the sedative effect is used in over-the-counter sleep aids). Dozens of $H_1$-blocking compounds are available.

**E. Toxicity:** Sedation is common, except with newer agents that do not enter the CNS readily (eg, terfenadine). Antimuscarinic effects such as dry mouth and blurred vision occur with some drugs in some patients. Alpha-blocking actions may cause orthostatic hypotension.

## HISTAMINE $H_2$ ANTAGONISTS

**A. Classification & Prototypes:** Four $H_2$ blockers are available; **cimetidine** is the prototype. They do not resemble $H_1$ blockers structurally. They are orally active, with half-lives of 1–3 hours.

**B. Mechanism of Action:** These drugs produce a surmountable pharmacologic blockade of histamine $H_2$ receptors.

**C. Effects:** The only therapeutic effect of importance is the reduction of gastric acid secretion. Blockade of cardiac $H_2$ receptor-mediated effects can be demonstrated, but has no clinical significance.

**D. Clinical Use:** In acid-peptic disease, especially duodenal ulcer, these drugs reduce symptoms, accelerate healing, and prevent recurrences. Acute ulcer is treated with several doses per day, whereas recurrence of the ulcer can often be prevented with a single bedtime dose. They are also effective in accelerating healing and preventing recurrences of gastric peptic ulcers. In Zollinger-Ellison syndrome, these drugs are very helpful in controlling symptoms (acid hypersecretion, severe ulceration, bleeding, and diarrhea) caused by a gastrinoma.

**E. Toxicity:** Cimetidine is a potent inhibitor of hepatic drug-metabolizing enzymes. It also has significant antiandrogen effects in many patients. Ranitidine has a weaker inhibitory effect on hepatic drug metabolism; neither it nor the newer $H_2$ blockers appear to have endocrine effects.

## SEROTONIN (5-HYDROXYTRYPTAMINE) & RELATED AGONISTS

Serotonin is produced from tryptophan and stored in the enterochromaffin cells of the gut and in the CNS. It appears to play a physiologic role as a neurotransmitter and possibly as a local hormone modulating gastrointestinal activity. Serotonin is also stored (but synthesized to only a minimal extent) in platelets.

**A. Receptors & Effects:**

1. **5-$HT_1$ receptors** make up a family of related cAMP- and $IP_3$-linked membrane receptors (Table 16–1). They are located primarily in the brain and mediate synaptic inhibition. The mechanism appears to involve increased potassium conductance. Peripheral 5-$HT_1$ receptors mediate both excitatory and inhibitory effects in various smooth muscle tissues.
2. **5-$HT_2$ receptors** are located in both brain and peripheral tissues. These receptors mediate synaptic excitation in the CNS. They mediate smooth muscle contraction (gut, bronchi, uterus, vessels) or dilation (vessels). The mechanism involves cyclic nucleotides or the phosphoinositide cascade (or both). In carcinoid tumor, this receptor probably mediates some of the vasodilation, diarrhea, and bronchoconstriction characteristic of the disease.
3. **5-$HT_3$ receptors** are located in the CNS. They open nonselective Na,K channels that mediate depolarization of neurons. Their role in brain function is not yet understood but includes some aspect of chemoreceptor-induced vomiting.

**B. Clinical Use:** Serotonin has no clinical applications.

**C. Sumatriptan:** Sumatriptan, a substituted indole, is a 5-$HT_{1d}$ agonist. It has recently been shown to be effective in the treatment of acute migraine and cluster headache attacks, strengthening the association of serotonin abnormalities with these headache syndromes.

## SEROTONIN ANTAGONISTS

**A. Classification & Prototypes:** **Ketanserin** is a 5-$HT_2$ and alpha-adrenoceptor blocker. **Phenoxybenzamine** (an alpha-adrenoceptor blocker) and **cyproheptadine** (an $H_1$ blocker) are also good 5-$HT_2$ blockers. **Ondansetron** is a 5-$HT_3$ blocker. The **ergot alkaloids** are partial agonists at 5-HT (and other) receptors (see below).

**B. Mechanism of Action:** Ketanserin and cyproheptadine are competitive pharmacologic antagonists. Phenoxybenzamine is an irreversible blocker. Ondansetron has a central antiemetic action. The mechanism is not understood.

**C. Effects:** In addition to inhibition of serotonin effects, these poorly selective agents have the effects of alpha blockers (ketanserin, phenoxybenzamine) or $H_1$ blockers (cyproheptadine).

**D. Clinical Use:** Ketanserin is under investigation as an antihypertension drug. Ketanserin, cyproheptadine, and phenoxybenzamine may all be of value in the treatment of carcinoid tumor, a neoplasm that secretes large amounts of serotonin (and peptides). Ondansetron is used to control emesis associated with cancer chemotherapy.

**E. Toxicity:** Adverse effects of ketanserin are those of alpha blockade and $H_1$ blockade. The toxicities of ondansetron include diarrhea and headache.

## ERGOT ALKALOIDS

These complex drugs are produced by a fungus found in spoiled grain. They are responsible for the epidemics of "St. Anthony's Fire" described during the Middle Ages. There are at least 20 naturally occurring members of the family, but only a few are used as therapeutic agents. The ergot alkaloids are *partial agonists* at alpha adrenoceptors and 5-$HT_2$ receptors. The balance of agonist versus antagonist effect varies from compound to compound. Some are also agonists at the dopamine receptor.

**A. Classification & Prototypes:**

1. **Vascular effects.** The prototype vasoconstrictor ergot is ergotamine.
2. **Uterine effects.** The prototype uterine stimulant (oxytocic drug) is ergonovine.
3. **CNS action. Bromocriptine** and **lysergic acid diethylamide (LSD)** are potent dopamine agonists in the CNS.

**B. Effects:** Receptor effects, summarized in Table 16–2, include the following:

1. **Vessels.** Ergot alkaloids can produce marked and prolonged alpha-receptor-mediated vasoconstriction. An overdose can cause ischemia and gangrene of the limbs.
2. **Uterus.** 5-$HT_2$ activation causes powerful contractions; near term, this is sufficient to cause abortion.
3. **Brain.** Hallucinations may be prominent with the naturally occurring ergots but are less common with therapeutic ergots; LSD is a semisynthetic ergot alkaloid. In the pituitary, some ergot alkaloids are potent dopaminelike inhibitors of prolactin secretion.

**C. Clinical Use:**

1. **Migraine.** Ergotamine is a mainstay of acute treatment. Methysergide and ergonovine are used prophylactically.
2. **Obstetric bleeding.** Ergonovine and ergotamine are effective agents for the reduction of postpartum bleeding.
3. **Hyperprolactinemia.** Bromocriptine has potent dopamine agonist effects. It is used to reduce prolactin secretion (dopamine is the physiologic prolactin release inhibitor). It also appears to reduce the size of pituitary tumors of the prolactin-secreting cells. Bromocriptine is also used in the treatment of Parkinson's disease.
4. **Other uses.** Methysergide has also been used in carcinoid tumor.

**D. Toxicity:** The toxic effects of ergot alkaloids are quite important, both from a public health standpoint (epidemics of ergotism from spoiled grain) and from the standpoint of overdose or abuse by individuals.

**Table 16–2.** Effects of ergot alkaloids at several receptors.[1,2]

| Ergot Alkaloid | Alpha Adrenoceptor | Dopamine Receptor | Serotonin Receptor (5-$HT_2$) | Uterine Smooth Muscle Stimulation |
|---|---|---|---|---|
| Bromocriptine | – | +++ | – | 0 |
| Ergonovine | + | + | –(PA) | +++ |
| Ergotamine | – –(PA) | 0 | +(PA) | +++ |
| Lysergic acid diethylamide (LSD) | 0 | +++ | – – – | ++ |
| Methysergide | +/0 | +/0 | – – –(PA) | 0 |

[1]Reproduced, with permission, from Katzung BG (editor): *Basic & Clinical Pharmacology,* 5th ed. Appleton & Lange, 1992.

[2]Agonist effects are indicated by +, antagonist by –, no effect by 0. Relative affinity for the receptor is indicated by the number of + or – signs. PA means partial agonist (both agonist and antagonist effects can be detected).

1. **Vascular effects.** Severe prolonged vasoconstriction can result in gangrene. The only effective antagonist is the physiologic antagonist, nitroprusside.
2. **Gastrointestinal effects.** Most ergot alkaloids cause gastrointestinal upset (nausea, vomiting, diarrhea) in many individuals.
3. **Genitourinary effects.** Marked uterine contractions may be produced. The uterus becomes progressively more sensitive to ergot alkaloids during pregnancy.
4. **CNS effects.** Hallucinations resembling psychosis are common with LSD but less common with the ergot alkaloids used in therapeutics.

## DRUG LIST

The following drugs are important members of the group discussed in this chapter. Prototype agents should be learned in detail; the major variants should be known well enough to list the factors that distinguish them from the prototypes and from each other; and the other significant agents should be recognized as belonging to a specific subclass.

| Subclass | Prototype | Major Variants | Other Significant Agents |
|---|---|---|---|
| Histamine agonists | Histamine | | |
| $H_1$ blockers | Chlorpheniramine | Terfenadine | Cyclizine, promethazine. |
| $H_2$ blockers | Cimetidine | | Ranitidine, famotidine, nizatidine. |
| 5-HT agonists | Serotonin | Sumatriptan | Ergot alkaloids (partial agonists). See Clinical Use. |
| 5-HT blockers | Ketanserin, ondansetron | Cyproheptadine | Ergot alkaloids (partial agonists). See Clinical Use. |

## QUESTIONS

**DIRECTIONS (items 1–4):** Each numbered item or incomplete statement in this section is followed by answers or by completions of the statement. Select the ONE lettered answer or completion that is BEST in each case.

1. Carcinoid tumor may be treated with
   **(A)** cyproheptadine
   **(B)** methysergide
   **(C)** phenoxybenzamine
   **(D)** ketanserin
   **(E)** all of the above

2. Drugs that can reverse one or more smooth muscle effects of circulating histamine in humans include all of the following EXCEPT
   **(A)** epinephrine
   **(B)** terbutaline
   **(C)** lysergic acid diethylamide
   **(D)** chlorpheniramine
   **(E)** phenylephrine

**3.** Many antihistamines ($H_1$ blockers) have additional effects; these are likely to include all of the following EXCEPT
(A) antimuscarinic reduction in bladder tone
(B) local anesthetic effects if injected
(C) anti-motion-sickness effect
(D) increase in total peripheral resistance
(E) sedation

**4.** All of the following are $H_2$-blocking drugs EXCEPT
(A) cimetidine
(B) nizatidine
(C) famotidine
(D) chlorpheniramine
(E) ranitidine

**DIRECTIONS (items 5–10):** Items 5–10 consist of lettered headings followed by a set of numbered phrases. For each numbered phrase, select the ONE lettered heading that is most closely associated with it. Each lettered heading may be selected once, more than once, or not at all.

(A) Ergotamine tartrate
(B) Ondansetron
(C) Bromocriptine
(D) Methysergide
(E) Cimetidine

**5.** Useful in the treatment of hyperprolactinemia

**6.** Effective in the treatment of peptic ulcer disease

**7.** Drug of choice in aborting an acute migraine headache

**8.** Used in management of chemotherapy-induced vomiting

**9.** Causes inhibition of hepatic metabolism of many drugs; some antiandrogenic effects

**10.** Partial agonist at serotonin receptors; used in prophylaxis of migraine

## ANSWERS

**1.** All of the drugs listed have been used in the treatment of carcinoid. Octreotide, a somatostatin analogue, has also been used in this condition. The answer is **(E).**

**2.** LSD is an ergot derivative, not a histamine antagonist. The answer is **(C).**

**3.** $H_1$ blockers do not activate receptors that mediate vasoconstriction, and some of them actually block alpha adrenoceptors. The answer is **(D).**

**4.** Chlorpheniramine is an $H_1$ blocker. The answer is **(D).**

**5.** The answer is **(C),** bromocriptine, a dopamine agonist.

**6.** Cimetidine is effective in reducing gastric acid secretion. The answer is **(E).**

**7.** Ergotamine is still the drug of choice in acute severe migraine. The answer is **(A).**

**8.** Ondansetron, a serotonin antagonist, is an antiemetic. The answer is **(B).**

**9.** Cimetidine, unlike the newer $H_2$ blockers, inhibits hepatic metabolism via the P-450 drug-oxidizing system. It also has weak antiandrogenic actions. The answer is **(E).**

**10.** Some ergot alkaloids are partial agonists at serotonin receptors. The answer is **(D).**

# Polypeptides 17

## OBJECTIVES

**Define the following terms:**

- Angiotensins I and II
- Atrial natriuretic factor
- Kallikrein
- Kininogen
- Renin

**You should be able to:**

- Name a partial agonist inhibitor of angiotensin and at least one drug that reduces the formation of angiotensin II.
- Outline the major effects of bradykinin and vasoactive intestinal polypeptide (VIP).
- Describe the function of angiotensin-converting enzyme (peptidyl dipeptidase, kininase II).
- Describe the effects of atrial natriuretic factor (ANF).

## CONCEPTS

**A. Classification & Prototypes:** Polypeptides comprise a large class of endogenous peptides that function as local and systemic hormones. Many are still poorly understood in terms of the physiologic or pathophysiologic roles they play and their possible clinical potential. They include angiotensin, bradykinin, vasoactive intestinal polypeptide (VIP), atrial natriuretic factor (ANF), substance P, vasopressin, insulin, glucagon, and several opioid peptides. Vasopressin is discussed in Chapters 15 and 36. Insulin and glucagon are discussed in Chapter 40 and the opioids in Chapter 30. The peptides discussed in this chapter and their effects are summarized in Table 17–1.

**B. Mechanisms:** These agents probably all act on cell surface receptors. Some appear to open ion channels; others cause release of intracellular second messengers.

### ANGIOTENSIN & ITS ANTAGONISTS

**A. Source & Disposition:** **Angiotensin I** is produced from angiotensinogen by renin, an enzyme released from the juxtaglomerular apparatus of the kidney. This inactive decapeptide is converted into **angiotensin II,** an octapeptide, by angiotensin-converting enzyme (ACE), also known as peptidyl dipeptidase or kininase II. Angiotensin II is the active form of the peptide. It is rapidly degraded by peptidases (angiotensinases).

**B. Effects:** Angiotensin II is a potent arteriolar vasoconstrictor and stimulant of aldosterone release. It increases vascular resistance and renal sodium retention.

**Table 17–1.** Some polypeptides and their effects.

| Polypeptide | Effects |
|---|---|
| Angiotensin II | Constricts arterioles; increases aldosterone secretion. |
| Bradykinin | Dilates arterioles; increases capillary permeability; stimulates sensory nerve endings. |
| Atrial natriuretic factor (ANF) | Dilates vessels; increases glomerular filtration; decreases sodium reabsorption; inhibits renin secretion; inhibits angiotensin II and aldosterone effects. |
| Vasoactive intestinal polypeptide (VIP) | Dilates vessels; relaxes bronchiolar and gastrointestinal smooth muscle. Probably a neurotransmitter. |
| Substance P | Dilates arterioles; contracts veins and smooth muscle of the intestines and bronchi. Probably a neurotransmitter. |

C. **Clinical Use:** In the past, angiotensin II was used via intra-arterial infusion to control bleeding in difficult-to-access sites. It no longer has any clinical applications.

D. **Antagonists:** As noted in Chapter 11, 2 types of antagonists are available. **Saralasin** is a partial agonist inhibitor at the angiotensin II receptor. ACE inhibitors (eg, captopril) are important agents for the treatment of hypertension. Block by either of these inhibitors is often accompanied by a compensatory increase in renin and angiotensin I levels.

## BRADYKININ

A. **Source & Disposition:** Bradykinin is one of several vasodilator kinins produced from kininogen by a family of enzymes, the kallikreins. It is rapidly degraded by various peptidases, including ACE.

B. **Effects:** Bradykinin is one of the most potent vasodilators known. It is thought to be involved in inflammation (as it causes edema and pain when released or injected into tissue). It can be released into salivary secretions, but its function there is unknown. It may play a role in the secretion of saliva.

C. **Clinical Use:** Bradykinin has no therapeutic application. However, it may play a role in the antihypertensive action of ACE inhibitors, as previously noted (Chapter 11).

D. **Antagonists:** There are no clinically important bradykinin antagonists.

## ATRIAL NATRIURETIC FACTOR

A. **Source & Disposition:** ANF is synthesized and stored in the cardiac atria of mammals. It is released from the atria in response to distension of the chambers.

B. **Effects:** ANF is a vasodilator as well as a natriuretic (sodium excretion-enhancing) agent. Its renal action includes increased glomerular filtration, decreased proximal tubular sodium reabsorption, and inhibitory effects on renin secretion. It also inhibits the actions of angiotensin II and aldosterone. Although it lacks positive inotropic action, it may play an important compensatory role in congestive heart failure by limiting sodium retention.

## VASOACTIVE INTESTINAL POLYPEPTIDE & SUBSTANCE P

VIP is a potent vasodilator but probably is physiologically more important as a neurotransmitter. It is found in the nervous system and in the gastrointestinal tract. Substance P is another neurotransmitter polypeptide with potent vasodilator action. It may also function as a local hormone in the gastrointestinal tract. Its highest concentrations are found in the parts of the nervous system that contain neurons subserving pain. There are no recognized clinical applications for these polypeptides or their antagonists.

## QUESTIONS

**DIRECTIONS (items 1–5):** Each numbered item or incomplete statement in this section is followed by answers or by completions of the statement. Select the ONE lettered answer or completion that is BEST in each case.

**1.** Regarding polypeptides,
**(A)** angiotensin I (a decapeptide) is the most potent of the series that includes angiotensinogen and angiotensin II (an octapeptide)
**(B)** bradykinin is a potent vasodilator with pain-inducing and edema-inducing effects
**(C)** atrial natriuretic factor increases cardiac contractility in congestive heart failure
**(D)** because they cannot cross the blood-brain barrier, polypeptides are not found in the brain
**(E)** bradykinin is inactivated by the enzyme kallikrein

**2.** Which of the following is frequently associated with increased gastrointestinal motility or diarrhea?
**(A)** Bethanechol
**(B)** Bradykinin
**(C)** Angiotensin
**(D)** Renin
**(E)** None of the above

**3.** A polypeptide that causes increased capillary permeability and edema is
**(A)** captopril
**(B)** angiotensin I
**(C)** bradykinin
**(D)** saralasin
**(E)** angiotensin II

**4.** Agents that produce vasoconstriction include all of the following EXCEPT
**(A)** angiotensin II
**(B)** epinephrine
**(C)** methysergide
**(D)** serotonin
**(E)** substance P

**5.** A vasodilator that can be inactivated by proteolytic enzymes is
**(A)** serotonin
**(B)** vasoactive intestinal polypeptide
**(C)** histamine
**(D)** angiotensin I
**(E)** isoproterenol

**DIRECTIONS (items 6–10):** Items 6–10 consist of lettered headings followed by a set of numbered phrases. For each numbered phrase, select the ONE lettered heading that is most closely associated with it. Each lettered heading may be selected once, more than once, or not at all.

**(A)** Angiotensin I
**(B)** Angiotensin II
**(C)** Bradykinin
**(D)** Substance P
**(E)** Vasoactive intestinal polypeptide

6. Produced in traumatized tissue; causes edema

7. Decapeptide precursor of a vasoconstrictor substance

8. Vasodilator found in peripheral and CNS sites; associated with sensory pain fibers

9. Octapeptide vasoconstrictor that increases in the blood of hypertensive patients treated with large doses of diuretics

10. Vasodilator that increases in the blood of patients treated with captopril

## ANSWERS

1. Angiotensin I is an inactive precursor. Atrial natriuretic factor has no effect on cardiac contractility. Polypeptides are found in high concentrations in parts of the brain because they are synthesized there. The answer is **(B)**.

2. The polypeptides listed here are not associated with marked increases in gastrointestinal motility. Bethanechol, a muscarinic cholinoceptor stimulant, is an effective stimulant of the gut. The answer is **(A)**.

3. Bradykinin causes a marked increase in permeability that is often associated with edema. The answer is **(C)**.

4. Substance P is a potent vasodilator. The answer is **(E)**.

5. Vasoactive intestinal polypeptide is the only polypeptide in the list that is a vasodilator. The answer is **(B)**.

6. Bradykinin is a mediator of tissue damage. The answer is **(C)**.

7. Angiotensin I is a decapeptide. The answer is **(A)**.

8. Substance P is a vasodilator. The answer is **(D)**.

9. Angiotensin II, an octapeptide, increases because the compensatory cardiovascular response causes an increase in renin secretion. The answer is **(B)**.

10. Bradykinin increases because the enzyme inhibited by captopril, ACE, normally degrades kinins as well as producing angiotensin II. The answer is **(C)**.

# Prostaglandins & Other Eicosanoids 18

## OBJECTIVES

**Define the following terms:**

- Abortifacient
- Cyclooxygenase
- Dysmenorrhea
- Endoperoxide
- Great vessel transposition
- Lipoxygenase
- Nonsteroidal anti-inflammatory drug (NSAID)
- Patent ductus arteriosus
- Phospholipase $A_2$
- Slow-reacting substance of anaphylaxis (SRS-A)

**You should be able to:**

- List the major effects of $PGE_2$ and $PGF_2$.
- List important sites of synthesis and the effects of thromboxane and prostacyclin in the vascular system.
- Explain the differing effects of aspirin on prostaglandin synthesis and on leukotriene synthesis.
- Explain the current concepts relating eicosanoids to anaphylactic shock.

## CONCEPTS

The eicosanoids are an important group of fatty acid derivatives that are produced from arachidonic acid derived from cell membrane lipids.

**A. Classification:** The principal eicosanoids are the **prostaglandins, prostacyclin, thromboxanes,** and **leukotrienes.** There are several series for most of the principal subgroups; these series are based on different substituents (indicated by A, B, C, etc) and different numbers of double bonds (indicated by subscript 2, 3, 4, etc) in the molecule.

**B. Synthesis:** Active eicosanoids are synthesized in response to various stimuli, eg, tissue injury. These stimuli activate phospholipases in the cell membrane, and arachidonic acid is produced from membrane lipid (Fig 18–1). Arachidonic acid can be metabolized to straight-chain products

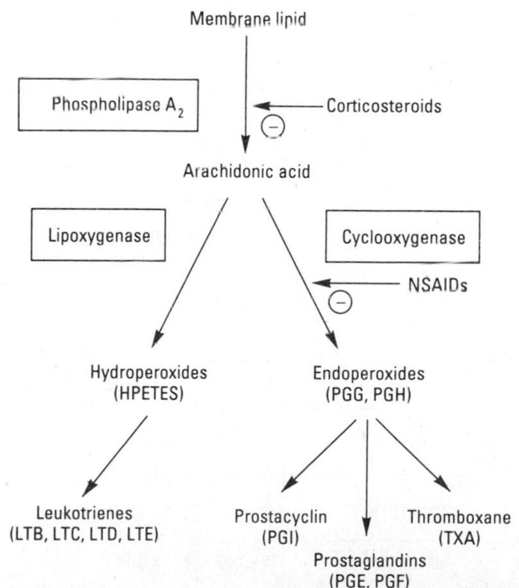


**Figure 18–1.** Synthesis of eicosanoids and sites of inhibitory effects of corticosteroids and nonsteroidal anti-inflammatory drugs (NSAIDs).

by lipoxygenase, finally producing leukotrienes. Alternatively, cyclization by the enzyme cyclooxygenase may occur, resulting in the production of prostacyclin, prostaglandins, or thromboxane. Note that thromboxane is preferentially synthesized in platelets, whereas prostacyclin is synthesized in the endothelial cells of vessels. All naturally occurring eicosanoids have very short half-lives and are inactive by the oral route.

**C. Mechanism of Action:** Most eicosanoid effects appear to be brought about by activation of cell surface receptors that couple to adenylyl cyclase (cAMP) or phosphatidylinositol ($IP_3$ and DAG) second messengers.

**D. Effects:** Various effects are produced on smooth muscle, platelets, the CNS, and other organs. Some of the most important effects are summarized in Table 18–1. Eicosanoids most directly involved in pathologic processes include thromboxane, a potent vasoconstrictor and platelet aggregation stimulant, and the leukotrienes $LTC_4$, $LTD_4$, and $LTE_4$, which together make up a bronchoconstriction mediator, slow-reacting substance of anaphylaxis (SRS-A). $LTB_4$ is a chemotactic factor important in inflammation. $PGE_2$ and prostacyclin may play important roles as naturally occurring vasodilators. PGE derivatives have a significant protective effect on the gastric mucosa. The mechanism may involve increased secretion of bicarbonate and mucus, decreased secretion of acid, or both. $PGE_2$ and $PGF_{2\alpha}$ are released in large amounts from the endometrium during menstruation and may play a physiologic role in labor. Dysmenorrhea is associated with uterine contractions induced by prostaglandins, specifically $PGF_{2\alpha}$. Therapeutic effects are described under Clinical Use.

**E. Clinical Use:**

1. **Obstetrics.** $PGE_2$ and $PGF_{2\alpha}$ produce strong contractions of the uterus. They are useful as abortifacients in the second trimester of pregnancy. Although effective in inducing labor at term, they produce more adverse effects (nausea, vomiting, diarrhea) than do other oxytocics used for this application. In Europe, the $PGE_1$ analogue misoprostol has been used with mifeprostone (RU486) as an abortifacient combination.
2. **Pediatrics.** $PGE_1$ is given as an infusion to maintain patency of the ductus arteriosus in infants with transposition of the great vessels until surgical correction can be undertaken.
3. **Dialysis.** Prostacyclin ($PGI_2$) is occasionally used to prevent platelet aggregation in dialysis machines.
4. **Gastroenterology.** Orally active synthetic PGE derivatives are in use or under investigation for treatment of peptic ulcer disease. They appear to act by increasing the secretion of protective mucus.
5. **Peptic ulcer associated with NSAID use.** Misoprostol is approved in the USA for the prevention of peptic ulcers in patients who must take high doses of nonsteroidal anti-inflammatory drugs for arthritis and have a history of ulcer associated with this use.

**F. Antagonists:**

1. **Corticosteroids.** As indicated in Fig 18–1, corticosteroids inhibit the production of arachidonic acid by phospholipases in the membrane. This effect is mediated by proteins that inhibit the action of phospholipase. This action is probably a major mechanism of the important anti-inflammatory action of corticosteroids.
2. **NSAIDs.** Aspirin and other nonsteroidal (ie, noncorticosteroid) anti-inflammatory drugs (NSAIDs) inhibit cyclooxygenase and the production of the thromboxane, prostaglandin, and

**Table 18–1.** Effects of some eicosanoids.[1]

| Effect | $PGE_2$ | $PGF_{2\alpha}$ | $PGI_2$ | $TXA_2$ | $LTB_4$ | $LTC_4$ | $LTD_4$ |
|---|---|---|---|---|---|---|---|
| Vascular tone | ↓ | ↑ or ↓ | ↓↓ | ↑↑↑ | ? | ↑, ↓ | ↑, ↓ |
| Bronchial tone | ↓↓ | ↑ | ↓ | ↑↑↑ | ? | ↑↑↑↑ | ↑↑↑↑ |
| Uterine tone | ↑↑ | ↑↑↑ | ↓ | ? | ? | ? | ? |
| Platelet aggregation | ↑ or ↓ | ? | ↓↓↓ | ↑↑↑ | ? | ? | ? |
| Leukocyte chemotaxis | ? | ? | ? | ? | ↑↑↑↑ | ? | ? |

[1]↑ = slight increase, ↑↑ = moderate, ↑↑↑ = high, and ↑↑↑↑ = very high; ↓ = slight decrease, ↓↓ = moderate, and ↓↓↓ = marked; ? = unknown effect.

prostacyclin branch of the synthetic path. Inhibition of cyclooxygenase by aspirin, unlike that by other NSAIDs, is irreversible. It is thought that some cases of aspirin allergy result from diversion of arachidonic acid to the leukotriene pathway when the cyclooxygenase-catalyzed prostaglandin pathway is blocked. The antiplatelet action of aspirin occurs because inhibition of thromboxane synthesis is essentially permanent in platelets; they lack the machinery for new protein synthesis. In contrast, inhibition of prostacyclin synthesis in the vascular endothelium is temporary because these nucleated cells can synthesize new enzyme. Inhibition of prostaglandin synthesis also results in important anti-inflammatory effects. Inhibition of synthesis of fever-inducing prostaglandins in the brain produces the antipyretic action of NSAIDs. Closure of a patent ductus arteriosus in an otherwise normal infant can be accelerated with potent NSAIDs such as indomethacin. ***Note:*** Although under intense investigation, no selective lipoxygenase inhibitors are available for clinical use at present.

## DRUG LIST

The following drugs are important members of the group discussed in this chapter. Prototype agents should be learned in detail; the major variants should be known well enough to list the factors that distinguish them from the prototypes and from each other; and the other significant agents should be recognized as belonging to a specific subclass.

| Subclass | Prototype | Major Variants | Other Significant Agents |
|---|---|---|---|
| Prostaglandins | $PGE_2$, $PGF_{2\alpha}$ | | $PGE_1$ |
| Prostacyclin | $PGI_2$ | | |
| Thromboxanes | $TXA_2$ | | |
| Leukotrienes | $LTC_4$ | LTB4 | $LTD_4$, $LTE_4$ |
| Phospholipase inhibitors | Prednisone and other corticosteroids | | |
| Cyclooxygenase inhibitors | Aspirin | Ibuprofen | Other NSAIDs |

## QUESTIONS

**DIRECTIONS (items 1–7):** Each numbered item or incomplete statement in this section is followed by answers or by completions of the statement. Select the ONE lettered answer or completion that is BEST in each case.

**1.** Which of the following is (are) frequently associated with increased gastrointestinal motility and diarrhea?
**(A)** Timolol
**(B)** Prostaglandins $E_1$ and $E_2$
**(C)** Corticosteroids
**(D)** Leukotriene $B_4$
**(E)** None of the above

**2.** Which of the following drugs inhibits cyclooxygenase irreversibly?
**(A)** Acetylsalicylic acid
**(B)** Hydrocortisone
**(C)** Ibuprofen
**(D)** Histamine
**(E)** Nitroprusside

**3.** Agents that cause vasoconstriction include all of the following EXCEPT
(A) angiotensin II
(B) prostacyclin
(C) methysergide
(D) cocaine
(E) thromboxane

**4.** A uterine stimulant derived from membrane lipid is
(A) serotonin
(B) bradykinin
(C) histamine
(D) prostaglandin $E_2$
(E) angiotensin

**5.** Agents that have been shown to protect the upper gastrointestinal tract from ulcer formation include all of the following EXCEPT
(A) certain prostaglandin E derivatives
(B) sucralfate
(C) atropine
(D) aspirin
(E) cimetidine

**6.** Recognized clinical indications for eicosanoids or their inhibitors include all of the following EXCEPT
(A) patent ductus arteriosus
(B) primary dysmenorrhea
(C) abortion
(D) hypertension
(E) transposition of the great arteries

**7.** All of the following have direct or indirect bronchoconstrictor action EXCEPT
(A) leukotriene $D_4$
(B) prostaglandin $E_2$
(C) prostaglandin $F_{2\alpha}$
(D) thromboxane $A_2$
(E) slow-reacting substance of anaphylaxis

**DIRECTIONS (items 8–12):** Items 8–12 consist of lettered headings followed by a set of numbered phrases. For each numbered phrase, select the ONE lettered heading that is most closely associated with it. Each lettered heading may be selected once, more than once, or not at all.

(A) Prednisone
(B) Ibuprofen
(C) Leukotriene $C_4$
(D) Acetylsalicylic acid
(E) Prostacyclin

**8.** Reversible inhibitor of platelet cyclo-oxygenase

**9.** Component of slow-reacting substance of anaphylaxis

**10.** Blocks phospholipase $A_2$ in the cell membrane

**11.** Increased levels may be responsible, in part, for some cases of aspirin hypersensitivity

**12.** Extremely potent vasodilator

## ANSWERS

1. Neither beta blockers (eg, timolol) nor corticosteroids increase gastrointestinal activity. Leukotriene $B_4$ is a chemotactic factor. The answer is **(B)**.

2. Hydrocortisone and other corticosteroids inhibit phospholipase, and histamine and nitroprusside have no recognized effect on the enzymes involved in eicosanoid synthesis. Ibuprofen inhibits cyclooxygenase reversibly. The answer is **(A)**, aspirin (acetylsalicylic acid).

3. Prostacyclin is a very effective vasodilator. The answer is **(B)**.

4. Although serotonin and, in some species, histamine may cause uterine stimulation, they are not derived from membrane lipid. The answer is **(D)**.

5. Aspirin has a direct irritant effect on the gastric mucosa and inhibits production of protective prostaglandins. The answer is **(D)**.

6. None of the vasodilator eicosanoids have a long enough duration of action or sufficient bioavailability to be useful in hypertension. The answer is **(D)**.

7. Prostaglandin $E_2$ is a very potent bronchodilator. Unfortunately, it is an irritant and causes coughing when inhaled. The answer is **(B)**.

8. NSAIDs other than aspirin are reversible inhibitors of cyclooxygenase. The answer is **(B)**.

9. The leukotriene C and D series are major components of slow-reacting substance of anaphylaxis. The answer is **(C)**.

10. Corticosteroids block phospholipase $A_2$, the enzyme that produces arachidonic acid. The answer is **(A)**.

11. It is thought that the leukotrienes are produced in increased amounts in patients with aspirin hypersensitivity when cyclooxygenase is blocked. The answer is **(C)**.

12. Prostacyclin is the only potent vasodilator in the list. The answer is **(E)**.

# 19 Bronchodilators & Other Agents Used in Asthma

## OBJECTIVES

**Define the following terms:**

- $Beta_2$-selective sympathomimetic
- Bronchial hyperreactivity
- Extrinsic asthma
- IgE-mediated disease
- Immunologic model for asthma
- Intrinsic asthma
- Leukotrienes
- Mast cell degranulation
- Mediators of bronchoconstriction
- Phosphodiesterase
- Tachyphylaxis

**You should be able to:**

- List the major classes of drugs used in asthma.
- Describe the mechanisms of action of these drug groups.
- List the major adverse effects of the most important asthma drugs.

## CONCEPTS

**A. Pathophysiology of Asthma:** Asthma is a disease characterized by airway inflammation and episodic, reversible bronchospasm. The immediate cause of the bronchial smooth muscle contraction is the release of several mediators from sensitized mast cells and other cells involved in immunologic responses. These mediators include the leukotrienes $LTC_4$, $LTD_4$, and $LTE_4$. In addition, chemoattractant mediators such as $LTB_4$ attract inflammatory cells to the airways. Asthma is often associated with marked bronchial hyperreactivity to various provocative inhaled substances including antigens, histamine, muscarinic agonists, $SO_2$, and cold air. This reactivity is partially mediated by vagal reflexes.

In extrinsic asthma, sensitized mast cells carry IgE antibodies. When these antibodies bind the appropriate antigens, they trigger calcium entry into the mast cell, which in turn causes synthesis and release of the leukotrienes listed above as well as stored mediators such as histamine. Intrinsic asthma is a form that is not associated with clear-cut provocation by external antigens.

**B. Mechanisms of Drug Action:** Drugs useful in asthma include bronchodilators (smooth muscle relaxants such as beta-adrenoceptor agonists and methylxanthines) and inhibitors of the synthesis or release of mediators from mast cells (Fig 19–1). The most important of the latter (with regard to asthma) are the corticosteroids and cromolyn.

## BETA-ADRENOCEPTOR AGONISTS

**A. Classification & Prototypes:** The most important sympathomimetics used in asthma are the $\beta_2$-selective agonists, although epinephrine and isoproterenol are still used occasionally. Of the selective agents, **albuterol, metaproterenol,** and **terbutaline** are the most important in the USA. They are given almost exclusively by inhalation, usually from pressurized aerosol canisters but occasionally by nebulizer. The inhalational route decreases the systemic dose (and adverse effects) while delivering a locally effective dose to the airway smooth muscle.

**B. Mechanism & Effects:** These agents act by increasing cAMP levels in smooth muscle cells, as described in Chapter 9.

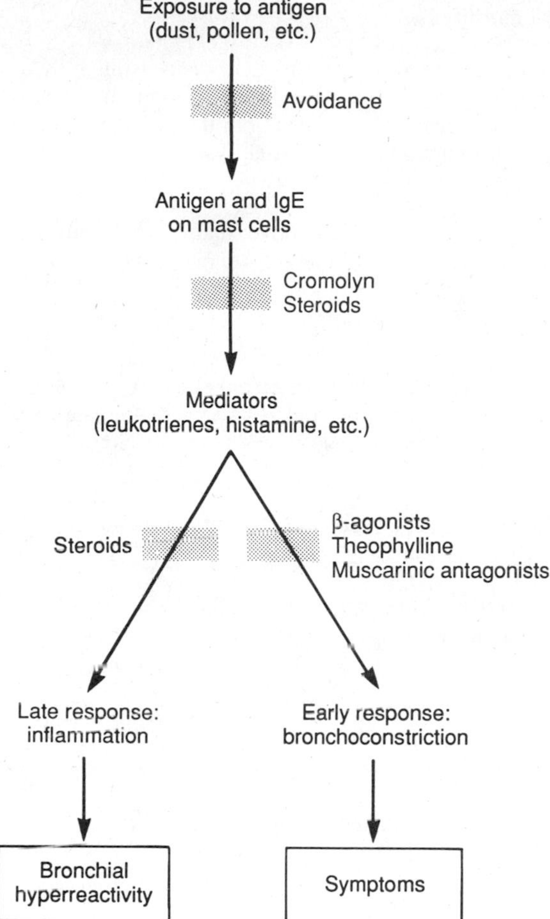


**Figure 19–1.** Summary of strategies for treatment of asthma. Therapeutic interventions are indicated by shaded bars. (Redrawn from Cockcroft DW: Ann Allergy 1985;*55*:857.)

**C. Clinical Use:** Sympathomimetics are used extensively in asthma. They are effective in almost all cases.

**D. Toxicity:** Skeletal muscle tremor is a common adverse $\beta_2$ effect. Beta$_2$ selectivity is relative. At high clinical dosage, these agents have significant $\beta_1$ effects. Even when they are given by inhalation, some cardiac effect (tachycardia) is common. Other adverse effects are rare. When the agents are used excessively, arrhythmias may occur.

## METHYLXANTHINES

**A. Classification & Prototypes:** The methylxanthines are purine derivatives. The 3 major groups of methylxanthines are found in plants and provide the stimulant agents in 3 common beverages: **caffeine** (coffee), **theophylline** (tea), and **theobromine** (cocoa). The theophylline group is the only one important in the treatment of asthma.

**B. Mechanism of Action:** The methylxanthines inhibit phosphodiesterase, the enzyme that degrades cAMP. However, this effect requires high concentrations of the drug. Methylxanthines also block adenosine receptors in the CNS and elsewhere, but a relationship between this action and the bronchodilating effect has not been clearly established. It is possible that bronchodilation is caused by a third, unrecognized, action.

**C. Effects:** When used to treat asthma, bronchodilation is the most important action. Increased strength of skeletal muscle (diaphragm) contraction has been demonstrated in some patients.

Other effects include CNS stimulation, cardiac stimulation, vasodilation, a slight increase in blood pressure, and increased gastrointestinal motility.

**D. Clinical Use:** The major clinical indication for the use of any methylxanthine is asthma; theophylline is the most important methylxanthine in clinical use. A newer methylxanthine derivative, pentoxifylline, is promoted as a remedy for intermittent claudication; this effect is said to result from decreased viscosity of the blood. Of course, the nonmedical use of the beverages listed above is far greater than the clinical uses of the methylxanthines.

**E. Toxicity:** The adverse effects are extensions of the effects listed above; nausea and vomiting, cardiac arrhythmias, tremor, insomnia, and convulsions may all result from overdosage.

## MUSCARINIC ANTAGONISTS

**A. Classification & Prototypes:** Atropine and other naturally occurring belladonna alkaloids were used for many years in the treatment of asthma, with only modest success. A quaternary antimuscarinic agent designed for aerosol use, **ipratropium,** has achieved greater success. It is delivered by pressurized aerosol and has little systemic action.

**B. Mechanism of Action:** Competitive block of muscarinic receptors prevents bronchoconstriction in some patients (especially children).

**C. Effects:** Because ipratropium is delivered directly to the airway and is poorly absorbed and distributed, systemic effects are small. However, large doses might be expected to produce typical peripheral atropinelike effects.

**D. Clinical Use:** Ipratropium is used in asthma. Muscarinic blockers are not useful in as large a fraction of the asthmatic population as are the $\beta_2$ agonists. However, in chronic obstructive pulmonary disease, the antimuscarinics may be more effective than $\beta$ agonists.

**E. Toxicity:** When given in excessive dosage, minor atropinelike toxic effects may occur.

## CROMOLYN

**A. Classification & Prototypes:** Cromolyn (disodium cromoglycate) is an unusual chemical and is the only member of its class available in the USA. It is extremely insoluble, so that even massive doses result in minimal systemic blood levels. It is given by aerosol for asthma.

**B. Mechanism of Action:** The mechanism of action of cromolyn is still poorly understood but appears to involve a decrease in the release of mediators (such as the leukotrienes and histamine) from mast cells. It is useful only for prophylaxis of asthma.

**C. Effects:** Because of its lack of absorption from the airway, cromolyn has only local effects.

**D. Clinical Use:** Asthma (especially in children) is by far the most important use. Nasal inhaler and eyedrop formulations are available for hay fever, and an oral formulation is used for food allergy.

**E. Toxicity:** Cough and irritation of the airway may occur, even at therapeutic dosage.

## CORTICOSTEROIDS

**A. Classification & Prototypes:** All of the corticosteroids (eg, **cortisol, prednisone;** see Chapter 38) are potentially beneficial in severe asthma. However, because of their toxicity, systemic (oral) corticosteroids are used only as a last resort. In contrast, local aerosol administration of surface-active corticosteroids (eg, **beclomethasone**) is relatively safe, and inhaled corticosteroids are becoming more common as first- or second-line therapy for individuals with moderate to severe asthma.

**B. Mechanism of Action:** The mechanism of action may be to block the synthesis of arachidonic acid by phospholipase $A_2$ (see Chapter 18). It has also been suggested that corticosteroids increase the responsiveness of beta adrenoceptors in the airway.

**C. Effects:** See Chapter 38.

**D. Clinical Use:** As well as asthma, corticosteroids have many other uses (see Chapter 38).

**E. Toxicity:** See Chapter 38. Local aerosol administration can result in adrenal suppression, but this is rarely significant. More commonly, changes in the oropharyngeal flora take place, resulting in candidiasis. If oral therapy is required, adrenal suppression can be reduced by using alternate-day therapy—ie, by giving the drug in slightly higher dosage every other day rather than smaller doses every day.

## DRUG LIST

The following drugs are important members of the group discussed in this chapter. Prototype agents should be learned in detail; the major variants should be known well enough to list the factors that distinguish them from the prototypes and from each other, and the other significant agents should be recognized as belonging to a specific subclass.

| Subclass | Prototype | Major Variants | Other Significant Agents |
|---|---|---|---|
| Beta agonists | Metaproterenol | | Terbutaline, albuterol |
| Methylxanthines | Theophylline | Aminophylline | Caffeine, theobromine |
| Muscarinic antagonist | Ipratropium | | |
| Cromolyn | Cromolyn | | |
| Corticosteroids | Beclomethasone | Prednisone | |

## QUESTIONS

**DIRECTIONS (items 1–4):** Each numbered item or incomplete statement in this section is followed by answers or by completions of the statement. Select the ONE lettered answer or completion that is BEST in each case.

**1.** One effect that theophylline, nitroglycerin, isoproterenol, and histamine have in common is
**(A)** direct stimulation of cardiac contractile force
**(B)** tachycardia
**(C)** increased gastric acid secretion
**(D)** postural hypotension
**(E)** throbbing headache

**2.** Which of the following is NOT a recognized action of terbutaline?
**(A)** Diuretic effect
**(B)** Positive inotropic effect
**(C)** Skeletal muscle tremor
**(D)** Smooth muscle relaxation
**(E)** Tachycardia

**3.** Of the following, the most likely to have adverse effects when used for severe asthma in a 10-year-old child is
(A) daily administration of albuterol by aerosol
(B) daily administration of prednisone by mouth
(C) daily administration of beclomethasone by aerosol
(D) daily administration of cromolyn by inhaler
(E) daily administration of theophylline in long-acting oral form

**4.** The major action of cromolyn is
(A) smooth muscle relaxation in the bronchi
(B) stimulation of cortisol release by the adrenals
(C) block of calcium channels in lymphocytes
(D) block of mediator release from mast cells
(E) block of cAMP synthesis in basophils

**DIRECTIONS (items 5–10):** Items 5–10 consist of lettered headings followed by a set of numbered phrases. For each numbered phrase, select the ONE lettered heading that is most closely associated with it. Each lettered heading may be selected once, more than once, or not at all.

(A) Aminophylline
(B) Ipratropium
(C) Corticosteroids
(D) Epinephrine
(E) Cromolyn

**5.** Bronchodilator; useful in chronic obstructive pulmonary disease; very unlikely to cause cardiac arrhythmia

**6.** Nonselective but very potent and efficacious bronchodilator; not active by the oral route

**7.** Prophylactic agent that stabilizes mast cells

**8.** Direct bronchodilator useful in asthma by the oral route

**9.** Parenteral form is life-saving in severe status asthmaticus; inhibits phospholipase $A_2$

**10.** Methylxanthine salt used mainly in asthma

## ANSWERS

**1.** Aminophylline does not cause headache. Nitroglycerin does not increase gastric acid secretion. Isoproterenol does not cause either. Histamine may cause all of the effects listed. The answer is **(B).**

**2.** Terbutaline is a "selective" $\beta_2$-receptor agonist, but in moderate to high doses it induces $\beta_1$ cardiac effects as well as $\beta_2$-mediated smooth and skeletal muscle effects. The answer is **(A).**

**3.** If oral corticosteroids must be used, alternate-day therapy is preferred because it interferes less with normal growth in children. The answer is **(B).**

**4.** The answer is **(D),** inhibition of mediator release from mast cells.

**5.** Ipratropium is the bronchodilator that is most likely to be useful in chronic obstructive pulmonary disease without causing arrhythmias. The answer is **(B).**

**6.** Epinephrine is still one of the most potent and efficacious agents available for asthma. However, because it is nonselective, $\beta_2$-selective agents are preferred. The answer is **(D).**

7. Cromolyn is useful only for prophylaxis. It stabilizes mast cells. The answer is **(E)**.

8. Aminophylline, a salt of theophylline, is active by the oral route; it is a bronchodilator. The answer is **(A)**.

9. Parenteral corticosteroids are life-saving in status asthmaticus. They probably act by reducing production of leukotrienes (see Chapter 18). The answer is **(C)**.

10. As noted in the answer to question 8, aminophylline is a salt of theophylline. The answer is **(A)**.

# Part V. Drugs That Act in the Central Nervous System

# Introduction to CNS Pharmacology 20

## OBJECTIVES

**Define the following terms:**

- Diffuse neuronal system
- Hierarchic neuronal system
- Voltage-gated channels
- Receptor-operated channels
- EPSP
- IPSP
- Synaptic mimicry

**You should be able to:**

- List the criteria for accepting a chemical as a neurotransmitter.
- Describe the mechanisms by which drugs cause presynaptic and postsynaptic modulation of synaptic transmission.
- List the major excitatory central neurotransmitters.
- List the major inhibitory central neurotransmitters.
- Describe the mechanism of strychnine's convulsant action.

## CONCEPTS

**A. Targets of CNS Drug Action:** Drugs that act on the CNS appear to do so by changing ion flow through transmembrane channels.

1. **Types of receptor-channel coupling.** The effect may be (1) a receptor-mediated effect directly on the channel protein, (2) receptor-mediated and coupled through second messengers, or (3) a perturbation of the channel that results from changes in the lipid environment caused by the solubility of the drug in the lipid.
2. **Types of channels.** Channels can be divided into voltage-sensitive (electrically gated) and transmitter-sensitive (chemically gated or receptor-operated) groups. Some electrically gated channels (eg, calcium channels) are closely regulated by chemical transmitters. Electrically gated channels are concentrated on the axons of nerve cells, whereas chemically gated ones are found on cell bodies and on both sides of synapses.
3. **Role of ion current carried by the channel.** In general, excitatory postsynaptic potentials (EPSPs) are generated by opening channels that conduct sodium or calcium. In some instances these depolarizing potentials result from *closing* potassium channels. Inhibitory postsynaptic potentials (IPSPs) are generated by opening potassium or chloride channels.

**B. Sites & Mechanisms of Drug Action:** Most therapeutically important CNS drugs act on chemically gated channels. Their sites of action are therefore in synapses. Possible mechanisms are indicated in Figure 20–1. Drugs may act presynaptically by altering the production, storage, release, reuptake, or metabolism of transmitter chemicals. Other agents activate or block postsyn-

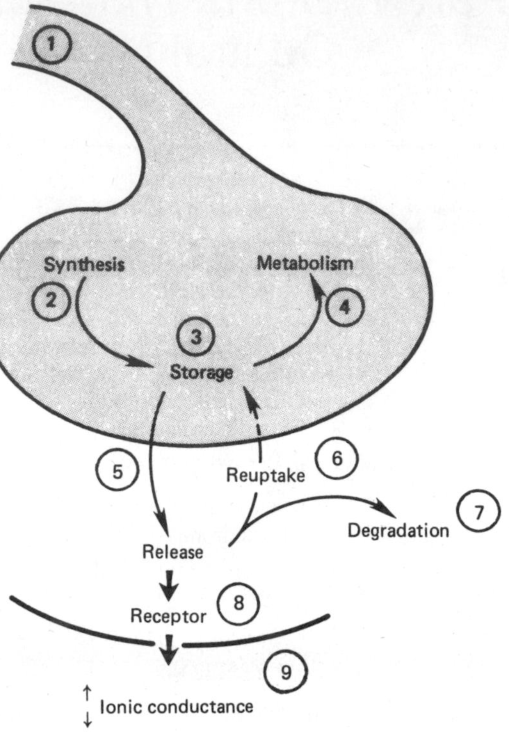

**Figure 20–1.** Sites of drug action. Schematic drawing of steps at which drugs can alter synaptic transmission. (1) Action potential in presynaptic fiber; (2) synthesis of transmitter; (3) storage; (4) metabolism; (5) release; (6) reuptake; (7) degradation; (8) receptor for the transmitter; (9) receptor-induced increase or decrease in ionic conductance. (Reproduced, with permission, from Katzung BG [editor]: *Basic & Clinical Pharmacology,* 5th ed. Appleton & Lange, 1992.)

aptic receptors for specific transmitters. A few toxic substances damage or kill the nerve cell (eg, kainic acid; 6-hydroxydopamine; 1-methyl-4-phenyl-1,2,3,6-tetrahydropyridine [MPTP]).

**C. Role of CNS Organization:** The CNS contains 2 types of neuronal systems, hierarchic and nonspecific (or diffuse).

1. **Hierarchic systems.** These systems are clearly delimited in their anatomic distribution and generally contain large, myelinated, rapidly conducting fibers. They control major sensory and motor functions. The transmitters include aspartate and glutamate. These systems also include numerous small inhibitory interneurons, which utilize gamma-aminobutyric acid (GABA) or glycine as transmitters. Drugs that affect these systems tend to have well-defined effects.
2. **Diffuse systems.** Diffuse systems are broadly distributed, with a single cell frequently sending processes to many different areas. The axons are fine and form synapses with many cells. The transmitters are often amines (norepinephrine, dopamine, serotonin) or peptides. Drugs that affect these systems will often have very general effects (eg, on sleep or mood).

**D. Transmitters at Central Synapses:**

1. **Criteria for transmitter status.** To be accepted as a neurotransmitter, a candidate chemical must be present in higher concentration in the synaptic area than in other areas (localization), must be released by electrical or chemical stimulation, and must produce the same sort of postsynaptic response that is seen with physiologic activation of the synapse (mimicry).
2. **Recognized transmitters**
   a. **Nonpeptide transmitters.** A list of these is given in Table 20–1.
   b. **Peptide transmitters.** Many peptides that have been identified in the CNS appear to meet most or all of the criteria for acceptance as neurotransmitters. The best defined of this group are the opioid peptides (beta-endorphin, met- and leu-enkephalin, and dynorphin). Peptide transmitters differ from nonpeptide transmitters in that (1) the peptides are synthesized in the cell body and transported to the nerve ending via axonal transport and (2) no reuptake or specific enzyme mechanisms have been identified for terminating their action.

**Table 20–1.** Summary of nonpeptide neurotransmitter pharmacology in the central nervous system.[1]

| Transmitter | Anatomy | Receptor Subtypes and Preferred Agonists[2] | Antagonists[2] | Receptor Mechanisms |
|---|---|---|---|---|
| Acetylcholine | Cell bodies at all levels; long and short connections. | Muscarinic ($M_1$): muscarine, McN-A-343 | Pirenzepine, atropine | Excitatory: decrease in $K^+$ conductance. |
| | | Muscarinic ($M_2$): muscarine, bethanechol | Atropine | Inhibitory: increase in $K^+$ conductance. |
| | Motoneuron-Renshaw cell synapse. | Nicotinic: nicotine | Dihydro-β-erythroidine | Excitatory: increase in cation conductance. |
| Dopamine | Cell bodies at all levels; short, medium, and long connections. | $D_1$: SKF 38393 | Phenothiazines, SCH 23390 | Inhibitory: (?) increases cAMP. |
| | | $D_2$: apomorphine | Phenothiazines, butyrophenones | Inhibitory: increase in $K^+$ conductance. |
| GABA | Supraspinal interneurons; spinal interneurons involved in presynaptic inhibition. | $GABA_A$: muscimol | Bicuculline, picrotoxin | Inhibitory: increase in $Cl^-$ conductance. |
| | | $GABA_B$: baclofen | 2-OH saclofen, CGP 35348 | Inhibitory (presynaptic): decrease in $Ca^{2+}$ conductance.<br>Inhibitory (postsynaptic): increase in $K^+$ conductance. |
| Glutamate; aspartate | Relay neurons at all levels. | N-Methyl-D-aspartate (NMDA) | 2-Amino-5-phosphonovalerate, CPP | Excitatory: increase in cation conductance, particularly $Ca^{2+}$. |
| | | AMPA, quisqualate, kainate | CNQX | Excitatory: increase in cation conductance but not $Ca^{2+}$. |
| | | ACPD, quisqualate | . . . | Excitatory: decrease in $K^+$ conductance. |
| Glycine | Spinal interneurons and some brain stem interneurons. | Taurine, β-alanine | Strychnine | Inhibitory: increase in $Cl^-$ conductance. |
| 5-Hydroxytryptamine (serotonin) | Cell bodies in midbrain and pons project to all levels. | $5\text{-}HT_{1A}$: LSD, 8-OH DPAT | Metergoline, spiperone | Inhibitory: increase in $Cl^-$ conductance. |
| | | $5\text{-}HT_{1C}$ | Mesulergine | ? |
| | | $5\text{-}HT_2$: LSD, DOB | Ketanserin | Excitatory: decrease in $K^+$ conductance. |
| | | $5\text{-}HT_3$: 2-methyl-5-HT | ICS 205930 | Excitatory: increase in cation conductance. |
| Norepinephrine | Cell bodies in pons and brain stem project to all levels. | $Alpha_1$: phenylephrine | Prazosin | Excitatory: decrease in $K^+$ conductance. |
| | | $Alpha_2$: clonidine | Yohimbine | Inhibitory: increase in $K^+$ conductance. |
| | | $Beta_1$: isoproterenol, dobutamine | Atenolol, practolol | Excitatory: decrease in $K^+$ conductance; mediated by cAMP. |
| | | $Beta_2$: salbutamol | Butoxamine | Inhibitory: may involve increase in electrogenic sodium pump. |

[1]Reproduced, with permission, from Katzung BG (editor): *Basic & Clinical Pharmacology,* 5th ed. Appleton & Lange, 1992.
[2]Abbreviations: ACPD = *trans*-1-amino-cyclopentyl-1,3-dicarboxylate; AMPA = DL-α-amino-3-hydroxy-5-methylisoxazole-4-proprionate; CGP 35348 = 3-aminopropyl(diethoxymethyl)phosphinic acid; CNQX = 6-cyano-7-nitroquinoxaline-2,3-dione; CPP = 3-(2-carboxypiperazin-4-yl)propyl-1-phosphonic acid; DOB = 5-bromo-2,5-dimethoxyamphetamine; 8-OH DPAT = 8-hydroxy-2(di-n-propylamino)tetralin.

## QUESTIONS

**DIRECTIONS (items 1–3):** Each numbered item or incomplete statement in this section is followed by answers or by completions of the statement. Select the ONE lettered answer or completion that is BEST in each case.

**1.** Each of the following is recognized as a central neurotransmitter EXCEPT
**(A)** serotonin (5-hydroxytryptamine, 5-HT)
**(B)** norepinephrine
**(C)** dopamine
**(D)** cAMP
**(E)** acetylcholine

**2.** Possible mechanisms of action of CNS drugs include all of the following EXCEPT
**(A)** reduced uptake of peptide transmitters into the nerve terminal
**(B)** increased chloride conductance in the postsynaptic cell
**(C)** increased release of transmitter from the terminal
**(D)** increased sodium conductance in the postsynaptic cell
**(E)** all of the above

**3.** Neurotransmitters may
**(A)** increase chloride conductance, resulting in an IPSP
**(B)** increase potassium conductance, resulting in an EPSP
**(C)** increase sodium conductance, resulting in an IPSP
**(D)** increase calcium conductance, resulting in an IPSP
**(E)** all of the above

**DIRECTIONS (items 4–7):** Items 4–7 consist of lettered headings followed by a set of numbered phrases. For each numbered phrase, select the ONE lettered heading that is most closely associated with it. Each lettered heading may be selected only once.

**(A)** Norepinephrine
**(B)** GABA
**(C)** Acetylcholine
**(D)** Glutamate
**(E)** Dopamine

**4.** Increases chloride conductance

**5.** Stimulates production of cAMP; little effect on alpha receptors

**6.** Increases potassium conductance; an ester

**7.** Increases sodium and calcium conductance; an amino acid

## ANSWERS

**1.** Cyclic AMP is undoubtedly important as a second messenger in the CNS, but there is no evidence that it acts as a neurotransmitter. The answer is **(D).**

**2.** No uptake of peptides has been demonstrated. All of the other effects listed have been identified in the brain. The answer is **(A).**

3. Chloride and potassium currents result in IPSPs. Sodium and calcium currents cause EPSPs. The answer is **(A)**.

4. Increased chloride conductance is the major effect of GABA. The answer is **(B)**.

5. Dopamine increases adenylyl cyclase activity and increases cAMP levels by activating $D_1$ receptors. (Dopamine inhibits cAMP production via $D_2$ receptors.) The answer is **(E)**.

6. Increased potassium conductance via $M_2$ receptor activation is a major mechanism of acetylcholine-induced IPSPs. The answer is **(C)**.

7. Glutamate is an excitatory amino acid transmitter that increases both sodium and calcium conductance. The answer is **(D)**.

# Sedative-Hypnotic Drugs 21

## OBJECTIVES

**Define the following terms:**

- Sedation
- Hypnosis
- REM sleep
- Tolerance
- Physical dependence
- Anxiolytic
- Anesthesia
- Coma
- Psychologic dependence

**You should be able to:**

- Identify the major chemical classes of sedative-hypnotics.
- Describe the sequence of CNS effects of a typical sedative-hypnotic over the entire dose range.
- Describe the pharmacodynamics of benzodiazepines, including interactions with neuronal membrane receptors.
- Compare the pharmacokinetics of commonly used benzodiazepines and barbiturates and understand how differences between them apply to clinical use.
- Describe the clinical uses of sedative-hypnotics.

## CONCEPTS

### A. Classification & Pharmacokinetics

1. **Description.** The sedative-hypnotics belong to a chemically heterogeneous class of drugs that produce dose-dependent CNS depressant effects. These range from sedation and relief of anxiety (anxiolysis), through hypnosis (facilitation of sleep), to anesthesia and coma (Fig 21–1). The most important subgroup is made up of the **benzodiazepines,** but representatives of other subgroups, including **barbiturates, carbamates, alcohols,** and **cyclic ethers,** are still used. The steepness of the dose-response curve varies among drug groups; those with flatter curves, such as benzodiazepines, are safer for clinical use (Fig 21–1).
2. **Absorption and distribution.** Most of these drugs are lipid-soluble and are absorbed well

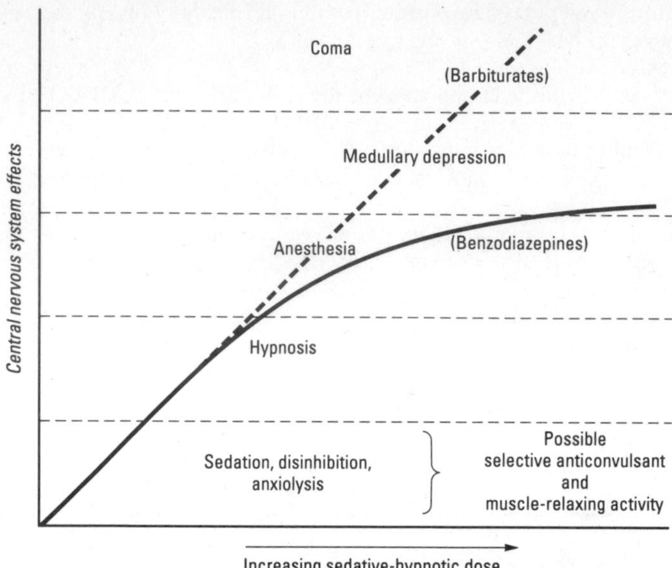


**Figure 21–1.** Relationships between sedative-hypnotic dose and CNS effects.

from the gastrointestinal tract, with good distribution to the brain. Drugs with the highest lipid solubility (eg, **thiopental**) enter the CNS rapidly and can be used as induction agents in anesthesia. The CNS effects of thiopental are terminated by rapid **redistribution** of the drug from the brain to other tissues.

3. **Metabolism and excretion.** Sedative-hypnotics are metabolized prior to elimination from the body, mainly by hepatic enzymes. Metabolic rates and pathways vary among different drugs. Plasma half-lives range from a few hours (eg, for triazolam) to over 36 hours (eg, for chlordiazepoxide). Most benzodiazepines are converted initially to active metabolites with long plasma half-lives. After several days of therapy with such drugs (eg, diazepam, flurazepam), accumulation of **active metabolites** can lead to excessive sedation. With the exception of phenobarbital, of which a part is excreted unchanged in the urine, the barbiturates are extensively metabolized via oxidation at the C5 position. Chloral hydrate is oxidized to trichloroethanol, an active metabolite.

**B. Mechanism of Action:** No single mechanism of action for sedative-hypnotics has been identified, and the different chemical subgroups may have different actions. Certain drugs (eg, benzodiazepines) facilitate neuronal membrane inhibition by acting at specific receptors.

1. **Benzodiazepine receptors** are present in many brain regions, including the thalamus, limbic structures, and the cerebral cortex. They form part of a $GABA_A$ receptor-chloride ion channel macromolecular complex. Binding of benzodiazepines to these receptors appears to facilitate the inhibitory actions of GABA, which are exerted through increased chloride ion conductance. Flumazenil, an antagonist at benzodiazepine receptors, reverses the central nervous system effects of benzodiazepines. Certain beta-carbolines have a high affinity for benzodiazepine receptors and can elicit anxiogenic and convulsant effects. They are classified as **inverse agonists.**
2. **Barbiturates** depress neuronal activity in the midbrain reticular formation, facilitating and prolonging the inhibitory effects of GABA and glycine. They do not bind to benzodiazepine receptors, but appear to interact with chloride ion channels. They may also block the excitatory transmitter glutamic acid.
3. The newer drug **buspirone** interacts with the $5\text{-}HT_{1A}$ subclass of brain serotonin receptors as a partial agonist, but the precise mechanism of its anxiolytic effect is unknown.

**C. Effects:** CNS effects of the sedative-hypnotics depend on the dose, as shown in Fig 21–1. Depressant effects are additive when 2 or more drugs are given together.

1. **Sedation,** with relief of anxiety and disinhibition, may occur; in animals, punishment-suppressed behavior is released.
2. **Hypnosis** (promotion of sleep onset and increase of duration of sleep) occurs. Rapid eye movement (REM) sleep stages are usually decreased, and, upon withdrawal from chronic drug use, a rebound increase in REM sleep may occur.
3. **Anesthesia,** with amnesia, loss of consciousness, and suppression of reflexes, can be produced by most barbiturates (eg, thiopental) and certain benzodiazepines (eg, midazolam).
4. **Anticonvulsant effects** are associated only with particular drugs (eg, phenobarbital, diazepam) that reduce the spread of epileptiform activity without excessive CNS depression.
5. **Muscle relaxation** occurs at high dosage for most sedative-hypnotics, but diazepam is effective in treating specific spasticity states, including cerebral palsy, at sedative dose levels.
6. **Medullary depression** occurs at very high doses and leads to respiratory arrest, hypotension, and cardiovascular collapse. These effects are the cause of death in overdose.
7. **Tolerance** and **dependence** occur when sedative-hypnotics are used continuously or in high dosage. Tolerance involves a decrease in responsiveness. There may be cross-tolerance between different chemical subgroups. Psychologic dependence occurs frequently and involves the compulsive use of these drugs to reduce anxiety. Physical dependence constitutes an altered state that leads to an abstinence syndrome (withdrawal state) when the drug is discontinued. Withdrawal signs may include anxiety and tremors, as well as seizures that may be life-threatening.

**D. Clinical Use:** Most of these uses can be predicted from the pharmacodynamic effects outlined above. Major uses include the treatment of anxiety states (chlordiazepoxide, diazepam, oxazepam) and sleep disorders (flurazepam, triazolam, secobarbital, chloral hydrate). Selective uses include the management of grand mal seizures (phenobarbital), status epilepticus (diazepam), muscle spasticity (diazepam), phobic anxiety states (alprazolam); induction of anesthesia (thiopental); and in general anesthesia (midazolam). Longer-acting sedative-hypnotics are used in the detoxification of physically dependent patients. The anxiolytic effects of buspirone occur without marked sedation, but take several days to develop.

**E. Toxicity:** Important toxic effects include the following:

1. **Excess CNS depression.** This includes decreased psychomotor functioning and unwanted daytime sedation following use as hypnotics. These adverse effects occur most often with benzodiazepines that have active metabolites with long half-lives (flurazepam); therefore, short-acting drugs that do not form active metabolites (oxazepam, lorazepam) may be preferred. The dose of the sedative-hypnotic should be reduced in the elderly patient.
   a. **Additive CNS depression,** which occurs with other drugs in this class as well as with antihistamines, antipsychotic drugs, and ethanol, is the most common result of drug interactions involving sedative-hypnotics. Ethanol is less likely to cause additive CNS depression with buspirone than with other sedative-hypnotics.
   b. **Overdosage,** with severe respiratory and cardiovascular depression, is more likely to occur with barbiturates than with benzodiazepines and is managed symptomatically.
2. **Other effects.** Short-acting hypnotics (eg, triazolam) may cause daytime rebound anxiety and amnesia. Barbiturates and carbamates (but not benzodiazepines) induce the formation of liver microsomal enzymes that metabolize drugs and hormones. This enzyme induction has led to multiple drug interactions. Barbiturates may also precipitate porphyria in susceptible patients. Chloral hydrate may displace coumarins from plasma protein-binding sites and increase anticoagulant effects.

## DRUG LIST

The following drugs are important members of the group discussed in this chapter. Prototype agents should be learned in detail; the major variants should be known well enough to list the factors that distinguish them from the prototypes and from each other; and the other significant agents should be recognized as belonging to a specific subclass.

| Subclass | Prototype | Major Variants | Other Significant Agents |
|---|---|---|---|
| Benzodiazepines | Chlordiazepoxide, diazepam, temazepam | Alprazolam | Flurazepam, lorazepam, nitrazepam, oxazepam, triazolam |
| Barbiturates | Phenobarbital, pentobarbital, thiopental | | Secobarbital, methohexital |
| Carbamates | Meprobamate | | |
| Alcohols | Ethanol | Chloral hydrate | |
| Azospirodecanediones | Buspirone | | |

## QUESTIONS

**DIRECTIONS (items 1–5):** Each numbered item or incomplete statement in this section is followed by answers or by completions of the statement. Select the ONE lettered answer or completion that is BEST.

**1.** All of the following may be caused by treatment with moderate to large doses of a benzodiazepine EXCEPT
**(A)** decreased performance on tests of psychomotor function
**(B)** loss of effectiveness with continued use as hypnotic agents
**(C)** seizures with abrupt discontinuance after chronic use
**(D)** increase in the activity of $\alpha$-aminolevulinic acid (ALA) synthetase with continued use
**(E)** additive depression of the central nervous system with alcoholic beverages

**2.** All of the following statements concerning the barbiturates are accurate EXCEPT:
**(A)** With physical dependence, the symptoms of the abstinence syndrome are most severe during withdrawal from use of shorter-acting barbiturates
**(B)** Renal elimination of phenobarbital is increased by urinary acidification
**(C)** Barbiturates are contraindicated in patients with acute intermittent porphyria
**(D)** In terms of CNS depressant effects, barbiturates exhibit a steeper dose-response relationship than benzodiazepines

**3.** Concerning the clinical uses of sedative-hypnotics, all of the following are recognized indications EXCEPT:
**(A)** Diazepam is used for muscle spasticity in patients with cerebral palsy
**(B)** Grand mal epilepsy in children can be treated with phenobarbital
**(C)** Alprazolam appears to have selective anxiolytic effects in patients who suffer from panic attacks
**(D)** Chlordiazepoxide is useful in the detoxification of alcoholic patients
**(E)** Secobarbital is effective in the management of patients with bipolar affective disorders

**4.** Characteristic properties of sedative-hypnotic drugs include all of the following EXCEPT:
**(A)** Cross-tolerance occurs between the barbiturates and the benzodiazepines
**(B)** Administration to a pregnant patient during the immediate predelivery period will result in depression of neonatal vital functions
**(C)** High doses lead to increases in the time spent in REM sleep
**(D)** May cause respiratory depression in patients with chronic obstructive pulmonary disease
**(E)** Toxic levels depress myocardial contractility and reduce vascular tone

**5.** Which ONE of the following best describes the mechanism of action of benzodiazepines?
**(A)** Blockade of the excitatory actions of glutamic acid
**(B)** Inhibition of GABA transaminase leading to increased levels of GABA
**(C)** Activation of glycine receptors in the spinal cord
**(D)** Facilitation of GABA-mediated increases in chloride ion conductance
**(E)** Increase in dopamine-stimulated adenylyl cyclase activity

**DIRECTIONS (items 6–10):** Items 6–10 consist of lettered headings followed by a set of numbered statements. For each numbered statement, select the ONE lettered heading that is most closely associated with it. Each lettered heading may be selected once, more than once, or not at all.

**(A)** Buspirone
**(B)** Triazolam
**(C)** Flumazenil
**(D)** Chloral hydrate
**(E)** Phenobarbital

**6.** This drug has a shorter half-life than others in its chemical class. It is widely used as a hypnotic and may cause daytime anxiety and amnestic effects.

**7.** This drug reverses some of the effects of benzodiazepines by acting as an antagonist at brain benzodiazepine receptors.

**8.** This pro-drug is biotransformed to an active metabolite. It may increase anticoagulant effects by displacement of warfarin from plasma protein-binding sites.

**9.** The anxiolytic actions of this drug may take several days to develop. It acts as a partial agonist on brain serotonin receptors.

**10.** The chronic use of this drug may lead to an increase in the rates of metabolism of warfarin, phenytoin, and digitalis compounds.

## ANSWERS

**1.** In contrast to the barbiturates and carbamates, chronic therapy with benzodiazepines does not lead to increased activity of liver drug-metabolizing enzymes (eg, P-450 family) or of enzymes involved in porphyrin synthesis (eg, ALA synthetase). However, the benzodiazepines are CNS depressants that exert additive effects with ethanol. With chronic use, tolerance and both psychologic and physical dependence occur. The answer is **(D)**.

**2.** As a weak acid ($pK_a$ 7), phenobarbital will exist mainly in the protonated (nonionized) form in the urine at acid pH and will therefore be reabsorbed in the renal tubule. Increase in renal elimination is facilitated by urinary alkalinization, so that a larger proportion of the drug is in the ionized (polar) state. The answer is **(B)**.

**3.** Sedative-hypnotic drugs have no long-term benefit in the management of bipolar affective disorders. The answer is **(E)**.

**4.** A characteristic effect of sedative-hypnotics, especially when used as hypnotics, is a decrease in the time spent in REM sleep. Increases in REM sleep (rebound) may occur during withdrawal from chronic use of sedative-hypnotics. Note that all drugs in this class cross the placental barrier. The answer is **(C)**.

**5.** Benzodiazepines are thought to exert most of their CNS effects through the mediation of the inhibitory neurotransmitter GABA, which causes membrane hyperpolarization through an increase in chloride ion conductance. Benzodiazepines interact with specific receptors that are components of the GABA receptor-chloride ion channel macromolecular complex. The answer is **(D)**.

**6.** Triazolam is currently widely prescribed as a hypnotic drug. Oversedation is less common with triazolam than with flurazepam, presumably because of its short plasma half-life. However, side effects of triazolam include disinhibition, hyperexcitability, daytime rebound anxiety, and effects on memory. The answer is **(B)**.

7. Flumazenil is a benzodiazepine congener that acts as an antagonist at benzodiazepine receptors. It reverses some of the CNS depressant effects of benzodiazepines and appears to be useful in treating benzodiazepine overdosage. The answer is **(C)**.

8. Chloral hydrate is metabolized to trichloroethanol, the active moiety. It displaces certain drugs from plasma protein-binding sites and may cause bleeding when administered to patients given warfarin. The chronic use of chloral hydrate has been associated with an increased incidence of neoplastic disease. The answer is **(D)**.

9. Buspirone is a novel anxiolytic drug that appears to interact with a subclass of brain serotonin receptors. Its effects develop slowly, and although it is less likely than conventional sedative-hypnotics to exert additive CNS depressant effects, caution is advised. The answer is **(A)**.

10. With chronic administration, phenobarbital increases the activity of hepatic drug-metabolizing enzymes, including cytochrome P-450. This may lead to increases in the rate of metabolism of many drugs administered concomitantly, with decreases in the intensity and duration of their effects. The answer is **(E)**.

# 22 Alcohols

## OBJECTIVES

**Define the following terms:**

- Alcoholism
- Psychologic and physical dependence
- Tolerance, cross-tolerance
- Wernicke-Korsakoff syndrome
- Acute ethanol intoxication
- Alcohol withdrawal syndrome
- Fetal alcohol syndrome

**You should be able to:**

- Describe the pharmacodynamics and pharmacokinetics of acute ethanol ingestion.
- List the toxic effects of chronic ethanol ingestion.
- Outline the treatment of (a) ethanol overdosage and (b) the alcohol withdrawal syndrome.
- Describe the toxicity and treatment of acute poisoning with (a) methanol and (b) ethylene glycol.

## CONCEPTS

Ethanol is the most important alcohol of pharmacologic interest. It has few medical applications, but its abuse is responsible for major medical and socioeconomic problems. Other alcohols of toxicologic importance are methanol and ethylene glycol.

### ETHANOL

A. **Pharmacokinetics:** Ethanol is rapidly and completely absorbed after ingestion and distributed to all body tissues; its volume of distribution is equivalent to that of total body water. Two enzyme systems metabolize ethanol to acetaldehyde:

1. **Alcohol dehydrogenase.** This is a cytosolic, NAD-dependent enzyme found mainly in the liver and gut. It accounts for the metabolism of low to moderate doses of ethanol. Because of the limited supply of the coenzyme NAD, the reaction has zero-order kinetics that result in a fixed capacity for ethanol metabolism of about 7–10 g/h. In chronic ethanol use, the use of NAD for its metabolism leads to a deficiency of the coenzyme for its normal metabolic functions. Gut metabolism of ethanol is reported to be lower in women than in men.
2. **Microsomal ethanol-oxidizing system (MEOS).** This is a liver microsomal mixed-function oxidase system whose activity increases with chronic exposure to ethanol or inducing agents such as barbiturates. This may be partially responsible for the increased tolerance to ethanol that occurs with chronic use.

   Acetaldehyde formed from the oxidation of ethanol is rapidly metabolized to acetic acid by aldehyde dehydrogenase, a mitochondrial enzyme found in the liver and many other tissues. Aldehyde dehydrogenase is inhibited by **disulfiram** and by other drugs including **metronidazole, oral hypoglycemics,** and some **cephalosporin antibiotics.**

## B. Acute Effects:

The major acute effects of ethanol on the CNS include sedation, loss of inhibition, impaired judgment, slurred speech, and ataxia. Higher doses lead to loss of consciousness, anesthesia, and coma with fatal respiratory and cardiovascular depression. The mechanisms underlying these actions are not understood but may involve effects on neuronal membrane fluidity and synaptic transmission. Additive CNS depression occurs with concomitant administration of sedative-hypnotics, phenothiazines, and tricyclic antidepressants. Ethanol, even at relatively low concentrations in the blood, significantly depresses the heart. Vascular smooth muscle is relaxed, which leads to vasodilation, sometimes with marked hypothermia. Ethanol also relaxes uterine smooth muscle.

## C. Chronic Effects:

1. **Tolerance and dependence.** Tolerance occurs mainly as a result of CNS adaptation but may be partly caused by an increased rate of ethanol metabolism. There is cross-tolerance to other sedative-hypnotic drugs. Both psychologic dependence and physical dependence are marked, the latter demonstrated by an abstinence syndrome upon abrupt discontinuance of ethanol intake by the chronic user.
2. **Liver.** Gluconeogenesis is reduced and hypoglycemia and fat accumulation may occur through NAD depletion; nutritional deficiencies may contribute to this process. Progressive loss of liver function occurs with hepatitis and cirrhosis. Hepatic dysfunction is often more severe in females, perhaps because higher concentrations of alcohol reach the liver in women.
3. **Gastrointestinal system.** Irritation, inflammation, bleeding, and scarring of the gut wall occur and may cause absorption defects and exacerbate nutritional deficiencies
4. **CNS.** Thiamine deficiency associated with ethanol use leads to the Wernicke-Korsakoff syndrome, which is characterized by ataxia, confusion, and paralysis of the extraocular muscles. Prompt treatment with parenteral thiamine is essential to prevent permanent brain damage.
5. **Endocrine system.** Gynecomastia, testicular atrophy, and salt retention occur, partly because of altered steroid metabolism in the cirrhotic liver.
6. **Cardiovascular system.** Chronic ethanol use is associated with an increased incidence of hypertension, anemia, and myocardial infarction.
7. **Fetal alcohol syndrome.** Ethanol use in pregnancy is associated with teratogenic effects, including mental retardation, growth deficiencies, and characteristic malformations of the face and head.

## D. Treatment of Acute & Chronic Alcoholism:

1. **Excessive CNS depression** due to acute ingestion of ethanol is managed by maintenance of vital signs and prevention of aspiration after vomiting.
2. **Alcohol withdrawal syndromes** are characterized by insomnia, tremor, anxiety, and, in severe cases, delirium tremens (DTs) and life-threatening convulsions. Peripheral effects include nausea, vomiting, diarrhea, and arrhythmias. The abstinence syndrome is usually managed by treatment with a long-acting sedative-hypnotic (eg, diazepam), but the intensity may also be reduced by clonidine or propranolol.
3. Treatment of alcoholism is a complex sociomedical problem, and the disease is characterized by a high relapse rate. The aldehyde dehydrogenase inhibitor disulfiram is used adjunctively

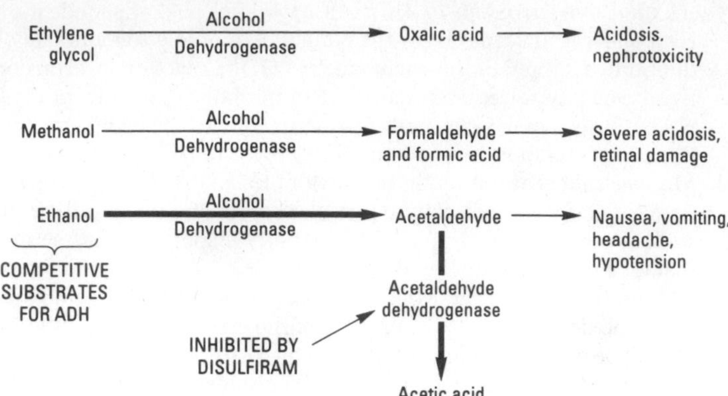


**Figure 22–1.** Toxic metabolites of alcohols. The oxidation of alcohols by alcohol dehydrogenase (ADH) results in the formation of metabolites that cause serious toxicities. Ethanol, a preferred substrate for ADH, is used in methanol or ethylene glycol poisoning to slow the rate of formation of the toxic metabolites of these alcohols. Acetaldehyde formed from ethanol is oxidized rapidly by aldehyde dehydrogenase except in the presence of disulfiram.

in some treatment programs. If ethanol is consumed by a patient who has taken disulfiram, acetaldehyde accumulation leads to nausea, headache, flushing, and hypotension (Fig 22–1).

## OTHER ALCOHOLS

**A. Methanol:** Methanol is sometimes used by alcoholics when they are unable to obtain ethanol. Intoxication from methanol (alone) may include visual dysfunction, gastrointestinal distress, shortness of breath, loss of consciousness, and coma. Methanol is metabolized to formaldehyde, which can cause severe acidosis, retinal damage, and blindness. The formation of this toxic metabolite is retarded by prompt intravenous administration of ethanol, which acts as a preferred substrate for alcohol dehydrogenase and competitively inhibits the oxidation of methanol (Fig 22–1).

**B. Ethylene Glycol:** Industrial exposure to ethylene glycol (by inhalation or skin absorption) or self-administration (eg, by drinking antifreeze products) leads to severe acidosis and renal damage from the metabolism of ethylene glycol to oxalic acid. Initial treatment with ethanol may slow or prevent formation of this toxic metabolite via competition for oxidation by alcohol dehydrogenase. Alcohol dehydrogenase is inhibited by **4-methylpyrazole,** an "orphan drug," also used as an antidote in methanol and ethylene glycol toxicity.

## QUESTIONS

**DIRECTIONS (items 1–5):** Each numbered item or incomplete statement in this section is followed by answers or by completions of the statement. Select the ONE lettered answer or completion that is BEST in each case.

**1.** All of the following may occur after acute administration of ethanol EXCEPT
**(A)** myocardial depression
**(B)** additive CNS depression with phenothiazines
**(C)** contraction of uterine smooth muscle
**(D)** inhibition of liver microsomal drug-metabolizing enzymes
**(E)** hypothermia

**2.** All of the following are signs or symptoms of chronic ethanol use EXCEPT
**(A)** distal paresthesias
**(B)** gynecomastia and testicular atrophy
**(C)** fatty liver and hepatitis
**(D)** gastric irritation and bleeding
**(E)** decreased liver alcohol dehydrogenase levels

**3.** All of the following statements about the biodisposition of ethanol are accurate EXCEPT:
**(A)** Ethanol is absorbed at all levels of the gastrointestinal tract
**(B)** Acetaldehyde is the initial product of ethanol metabolism
**(C)** After an oral dose, plasma levels of ethanol are higher in women than in men
**(D)** Metabolism of ethanol follows first-order kinetics
**(E)** Ethanol is a more effective substrate for alcohol dehydrogenase than methanol is

**4.** All of the following statements about ethanol are correct EXCEPT:
**(A)** Flushing, headache, nausea and vomiting are likely effects of drinking alcoholic beverages in patients who have consumed disulfiram
**(B)** The Wernicke-Korsakoff syndrome occurs following withdrawal from chronic use of ethanol
**(C)** The main objective of drug therapy in ethanol withdrawal is to prevent seizures, delirium, and arrhythmias
**(D)** Long-acting benzodiazepines are preferred in ethanol detoxification
**(E)** intravenous phenytoin may be used during ethanol withdrawal in patients with a history of seizures

**5.** All of the following statements about methanol or ethylene glycol are accurate EXCEPT:
**(A)** The presence of flickering white spots before the eyes is an initial sign of methanol poisoning
**(B)** Administration of bicarbonate may be required to counteract metabolic acidosis in methanol toxicity
**(C)** Disulfiram is used in the management of poisoning from methanol or ethylene glycol to decrease their metabolism to toxic products
**(D)** Oxalate crystals are usually present in the urine following ingestion of ethylene glycol
**(E)** Initiation of dialysis procedures is an important step in the management of methanol or ethylene glycol toxicity

**DIRECTIONS (items 6–8):** Items 6–8 consist of lettered headings followed by a set of numbered statements. For each numbered statement, select the ONE lettered heading that is most closely associated with it. Each lettered heading may be selected once, more than once, or not at all.

**(A)** Aldehyde dehydrogenase
**(B)** Microsomal ethanol-oxidizing system (MEOS)
**(C)** Alcohol dehydrogenase
**(D)** Monoamine oxidase

**6.** A cytoplasmic zinc-containing enzyme that is primarily responsible for the oxidation of low to moderate doses of ethanol

**7.** The activity of this enzyme is induced by chronic exposure to ethanol or barbiturates

**8.** Fomepizole (4-methylpyrazole) is a potent inhibitor of this enzyme

## ANSWERS

**1.** Ethanol relaxes both uterine and vascular smooth muscle. Its effect on the uterus is to prolong labor. Vasodilation occurs and at high doses may lead to hypothermia. The answer is **(C)**.

2. Chronic ingestion of ethanol is not associated with a decrease in the activity of liver alcohol dehydrogenase, although the activities of other hepatic enzymes may be changed. The answer is **(E).**

3. A characteristic feature of ethanol biodisposition is that its elimination via metabolism follows zero-order kinetics. This results from the limited availability of NAD, the cofactor in alcohol dehydrogenase-mediated ethanol oxidation. The higher plasma levels in women after oral ingestion may occur because the activity of gastric alcohol dehydrogenase is lower in women than men. The answer is **(D).**

4. The Wernicke-Korsakoff syndrome occurs with ethanol use, not withdrawal, but it may be difficult to distinguish from the acute confusional state that often accompanies alcohol withdrawal. It is characterized by paralysis of the external eye muscles, ataxia, and altered mentation. The syndrome is associated with thiamine deficiency but is rarely seen in the absence of alcoholism. The answer is **(B).**

5. Disulfiram is an inhibitor of aldehyde dehydrogenase, the enzyme that converts acetaldehyde (formed from ethanol) to acetic acid. It is sometimes used adjunctively in alcoholic rehabilitation programs, since ethanol ingestion leads to toxic accumulation of acetaldehyde in the presence of the drug. Disulfiram does not inhibit alcohol dehydrogenase (ADH) and thus does not block the metabolism of methanol or ethylene glycol. However, ethanol—as a preferred substrate for alcohol dehydrogenase—competitively decreases the metabolism of the other alcohols and is used clinically in the management of methanol and ethylene glycol toxicity. The answer is **(C).**

6. Alcohol dehydrogenase, a cytosolic enzyme that contains zinc, is the main enzyme involved in the oxidation of low to moderate doses of ethanol. NAD is required as a cofactor, and its concentration is rate-limiting. The enzyme also oxidizes methanol to formaldehyde and oxidizes ethylene glycol to oxalic acid. The answer is **(C).**

7. MEOS is a mixed function oxidase enzyme requiring NADPH as a cofactor. It plays a significant role in ethanol oxidation to acetaldehyde only when blood alcohol levels are high. With chronic exposure to ethanol, the activity of MEOS may increase via enzyme induction, and this may play a role in "metabolic tolerance." The answer is **(B).**

8. A potent inhibitor of alcohol dehydrogenase, 4-methylpyrazole blocks the conversion of methanol and ethylene glycol to their toxic metabolites. The answer is **(C).**

# Antiepileptic Drugs 23

## OBJECTIVES

**Define the following terms:**

- Absence (petit mal) seizures
- Generalized tonic-clonic (grand mal) seizures
- Infantile spasms
- Myoclonic jerking
- Partial and generalized seizures
- Status epilepticus

**You should be able to:**

- List the major drugs used for partial and generalized tonic-clonic seizures and describe their main adverse effects.
- List the major drugs used for absence seizures and describe their main toxic effects.
- Describe the pharmacokinetic factors that must be considered in designing a dosage regimen for antiepileptic drugs.

## CONCEPTS

**A. Classification:** Epilepsy comprises a group of chronic syndromes that involve the recurrence of seizures (a **seizure** is a limited period of abnormal discharge of cerebral neurons). Subgroups of antiepileptic drugs are selective in their therapeutic effects for specific types of seizures. Several chemical subgroups of antiepileptic drugs are structurally related to each other; these include hydantoins (eg, **phenytoin**), barbiturates (eg, **phenobarbital**), and succinimides (eg, **ethosuximide**). There are also 3 unrelated subgroups, benzodiazepines (eg, **diazepam, clonazepam**), tricyclics (eg, **carbamazepine**), and **valproic acid.**

**B. Pharmacokinetics:** Antiepileptic drugs are commonly used for long periods and can cause adverse effects. Consideration of their pharmacokinetic properties is important for avoiding toxicity and drug interactions. Determination of plasma levels and clearance rates of some drugs in individual patients may be necessary for optimum therapy. This is particularly important with phenytoin, which undergoes first-pass metabolism that is saturable at high dosages. In general, antiepileptic drugs are well absorbed orally and have good bioavailability. They are usually metabolized via hepatic enzymes, and active metabolites are formed in some cases (see below). Plasma concentrations may reach toxic levels in the presence of other drugs that inhibit antiepileptic drug metabolism.

Specific pharmacokinetic features of interest include (a) nonlinear rates of hepatic metabolism of phenytoin; (b) induction of liver enzymes by barbiturates and carbamazepine; (c) competition for plasma protein-binding sites between phenytoin and other drugs (anticoagulants, sulfonamides), leading to **drug interactions;** and the formation of active metabolites from primidone (phenobarbital and phenylethylmalonamide) and from trimethadione (dimethadione).

**C. Mechanisms of Action:** The general action of antiepileptic drugs is to inhibit the generation of repetitive action potentials in epileptic foci. The mechanisms by which this occurs are not identical for all antiepileptic drugs.

1. **Phenytoin and carbamazepine.** At therapeutic concentrations, phenytoin and carbamazepine appear to act at similar sites in neuronal membranes to block sodium channels. This action is use-dependent and results in prolongation of the inactivated state of the $Na^+$ channel that follows an action potential. Valproic acid may exert similar effects.
2. **Benzodiazepines and barbiturates.** Benzodiazepines interact with specific receptors that are components of the $GABA_A$ receptor-chloride ion channel macromolecular complex to facilitate the inhibitory effects of GABA. Phenobarbital and other barbiturates interact with

**Table 23–1.** Toxic effects and complications of the use of antiepileptic drugs.

| Antiepileptic Drug | Toxic Effects & Complications |
|---|---|
| Benzodiazepines | Sedation, tolerance, dependence |
| Carbamazepine | Diplopia, ataxia, enzyme induction, blood dyscrasias |
| Ethosuximide | Gastrointestinal distress, lethargy, headache |
| Phenobarbital | Sedation, enzyme induction, tolerance, dependence |
| Phenytoin | Nystagmus, diplopia, ataxia, sedation, gingival hyperplasia, hirsutism, anemias |
| Valproic acid | Gastrointestinal distress, hepatotoxicity (rare but possibly fatal) |

chloride ion channels to enhance the inhibitory actions of GABA, and they also block the quisqualate receptor subclass of the excitatory neurotransmitter glutamic acid.

3. **Succinimides.** Ethosuximide inhibits low-threshold (T-type) $Ca^{2+}$ currents, especially in thalamic neurons that act as pacemakers to generate rhythmic cortical discharge.
4. **Other mechanisms.** GABA transaminase, which is inhibited by valproic acid at high concentrations, is irreversibly inactivated by the new drug **vigabatrin** at therapeutic levels. This action may lead to enhanced inhibitory effects of GABA at synaptic sites.

**D. Clinical Use:** A seizure diagnosis is important for prescribing an appropriate drug (or combination of drugs). The appropriate therapy is chosen on the basis of anticipated toxicity or complications and the prior responsivity pattern.

1. **Generalized tonic-clonic (grand mal) and partial seizures.** Carbamazepine, phenytoin, phenobarbital (for children), and valproic acid.
2. **Absence (petit mal) seizures.** Ethosuximide, valproic acid, or clonazepam.
3. **Infantile spasms.** Clonazepam or nitrazepam (also corticotropin).
4. **Status epilepticus.** Diazepam or lorazepam.
5. **Myoclonic syndromes.** Valproic acid or clonazepam.

**E. Toxicity:** Chronic outpatient therapy with antiepileptic drugs may cause specific toxic effects, as shown for the major agents in Table 23–1.

1. **Teratogenic potential** with phenytoin (fetal hydantoin syndrome) and valproic acid (spina bifida) is of particular concern.
2. **Overdoses** of antiepileptics may lead to respiratory depression, which should be treated supportively.
3. **Withdrawal** from antiepileptic drugs should be accomplished gradually to prevent increased seizure frequency and severity.

## DRUG LIST

The following drugs are important members of the group discussed in this chapter. Prototype agents should be learned in detail; the major variants should be known well enough to list the factors that distinguish them from the prototypes and from each other; and the other significant agents should be recognized as belonging to a specific subclass.

| Subclass | Prototype | Major Variants | Other Significant Agents |
|---|---|---|---|
| Barbiturates | Phenobarbital, primidone | | Mepharbital |
| Benzodiazepines | Diazepam | Lorazepam, clorazepate | Clonazepam, nitrazepam |
| Carboxylic acids | Valproic acid | | Sodium valproate |
| Hydantoins | Phenytoin | | Mephenytoin |
| Succinimides | Ethosuximide | | Phensuximide |
| Tricyclics | Carbamazepine | | |

## QUESTIONS

**DIRECTIONS (items 1–4):** Each numbered item or incomplete statement in this section is followed by answers or by completions of the statement. Select the ONE lettered answer or completion that is BEST in each case.

**1.** Drugs used in the treatment of partial seizures include all of the following EXCEPT
**(A)** valproic acid
**(B)** phenytoin
**(C)** ethosuximide
**(D)** carbamazepine
**(E)** primidone

**2.** Which of the following drugs is most likely to be effective in myoclonic syndromes?
**(A)** Valproic acid
**(B)** Phenobarbital
**(C)** Phenytoin
**(D)** Ethosuximide
**(E)** Carbamazepine

**3.** All of the following statements concerning antiepileptic drugs are correct EXCEPT.
**(A)** At high plasma levels phenytoin elimination follows zero-order kinetics
**(B)** Phenobarbital increases the activity of hepatic α-aminolevulinic acid (ALA) synthetase
**(C)** The mechanism of action of carbamazepine involves block of sodium ion channels in neuronal membranes
**(D)** Gastrointestinal distress is a common adverse effect of valproic acid
**(E)** Sedation and development of physical dependence are serious problems with the chronic use of ethosuximide in the treatment of seizure states

**4.** All of the following drugs are effective in the treatment of absence (petit mal) seizures EXCEPT
**(A)** clonazepam
**(B)** ethosuximide
**(C)** phenytoin
**(D)** valproic acid

**DIRECTIONS (items 5–10):** Items 5–10 consist of lettered headings followed by a set of numbered statements. For each numbered statement, select the ONE lettered heading that is most closely associated with it. Each answer may be selected once, more than once, or not at all.

**(A)** Diazepam
**(B)** Carbamazepine
**(C)** Phenytoin
**(D)** Valproic acid
**(E)** Ethosuximide

**5.** This drug is used for both partial and generalized tonic-clonic seizures. It should be avoided in the management of pregnant women because it is teratogenic. It may cause hirsutism and gingival hyperplasia.

**6.** Chronic use of this drug leads to the induction of hepatic drug-metabolizing enzymes. Other clinical applications include the management of trigeminal neuralgia.

**7.** Hepatic metabolism of this drug leads to the formation of a toxic metabolite that has been implicated in the development of severe hepatotoxicity, especially in young children.

**8.** In the blood, this drug is approximately 90% protein-bound. Displacement of the drug from plasma protein-binding sites by anticoagulants increases its adverse effects, which include nystagmus, diplopia, and ataxia.

**9.** This drug is used by the intravenous route in status epilepticus. It interacts with specific receptors that are components of the $GABA_A$ receptor-chloride ion channel macromolecular complex.

**10.** There is concern about idiosyncratic blood dyscrasias, including aplastic anemia and agranulocytosis, with the use of this drug.

## ANSWERS

**1.** Phenytoin, carbamazepine, and barbiturates are used for both generalized tonic-clonic and partial seizures. Valproic acid is also useful in partial seizures. Succinimides (ethosuximide, phensuximide) are not effective in grand mal or in partial seizures. The answer is **(C).**

**2.** Specific myoclonic syndromes are usually treated with valproic acid, although some patients may respond to clonazepam or other benzodiazepines. The answer is **(A).**

**3.** Ethosuximide causes few behavioral toxicities, and patients are unlikely to develop psychologic or physical dependence. Gastric distress is its most common toxicity. Note the dose-dependent variations in the rate of metabolism of phenytoin, which contribute to patient variability in the relationship between dose and plasma levels. In addition to induction of liver drug-metabolizing enzymes, phenobarbital increases porphyrin synthesis. The answer is **(E).**

**4.** Of the 4 drugs listed for absence seizures, ethosuximide and valproic acid are usually preferred because they are nonsedating. Clonazepam has the disadvantage of dose-related sedation and the development of tolerance. Phenytoin is not effective in absence seizures. The answer is **(C).**

**5.** Both phenytoin and valproic acid are teratogenic, but hirsutism and gingival hyperplasia are characteristic of phenytoin, and should allow you to distinguish between the 2 drugs. Note that spina bifida is a characteristic teratogenic effect of valproic acid. The answer is **(C).**

**6.** Carbamazepine, like phenobarbital, it is an effective inducer of liver microsomal drug-metabolizing enzymes. It is also effective in treating trigeminal neuralgia, and—possibly—manic states. The answer is **(B).**

**7.** Valproic acid is very effective in treating petit mal seizures and has also been used for myoclonic syndromes. Its most common adverse effect is gastrointestinal distress. A much more serious toxicity of valproic acid is hepatotoxicity, an effect thought to be caused by formation of a reactive metabolite. This adverse effect has resulted in a number of fatalities. The answer is **(D).**

**8.** Phenytoin-binding sites on plasma proteins are shared by other drugs, including anticoagulants, sulfonamides, salicylates, and phenylbutazone. These drugs may displace phenytoin and, by increasing the concentration of free phenytoin in the blood, will magnify its adverse effects. The answer is **(C).**

**9.** Of the drugs listed, both diazepam and phenytoin may be administered intravenously in status epilepticus. The actions of diazepam result from binding to benzodiazepine receptors, leading to the facilitation of the inhibitory effects of GABA. The answer is **(A).**

**10.** Idiosyncratic blood dyscrasias have occurred with carbamazepine, mostly in elderly patients treated for trigeminal neuralgia. Several fatalities have occurred. The answer is **(B).**

# General Anesthetics 24

## OBJECTIVES

**Define the following terms:**

- Amnesia
- Balanced anesthesia
- Inhalation anesthesia
- Minimal alveolar anesthetic concentration (MAC)
- Analgesia
- General anesthesia
- Intravenous anesthesia
- Stages of anesthesia

**You should be able to:**

- Identify the main inhalational and intravenous anesthetic agents and describe their pharmacodynamic properties.
- Describe the relationship between the blood:gas partition coefficient of an inhalational anesthetic and the speed of onset (and offset) of anesthesia with it.
- Describe how changes in pulmonary ventilation and blood flow can influence the speed of onset (and offset) of inhalation anesthesia.
- Describe the pharamcodynamics and pharmacokinetics of the commonly used intravenous anesthetics

## CONCEPTS

**A. General Anesthesia:** General anesthesia is characterized by a state of unconsciousness, analgesia, and amnesia, with skeletal muscle relaxation and loss of reflexes. General anesthetics are CNS depressants with actions that can be induced and terminated more rapidly than can those of sedative-hypnotics. Although not seen clearly with modern agents, which act rapidly, the progressively greater depth of central depression associated with increasing the dose or time of exposure is reflected by the traditional **stages of anesthesia:**

1. **Analgesia.** Initially, the patient has a decreased awareness of pain but is still conscious.
2. **Disinhibition.** The patient next experiences a loss of consciousness and amnesia, but reflexes are enhanced and respiration is typically irregular.
3. **Surgical anesthesia.** The patient is unconscious and has no pain reflexes; respiration is regular, and blood pressure is maintained.
4. **Medullary depression.** Finally, the patient experiences severe respiratory and cardiovascular depression that requires mechanical and pharmacologic support.

**B. Balanced Anesthesia:** In practice, the state of general anesthesia is usually achieved by the use of several pharmacologic agents, including certain intravenous drugs to induce the anesthetic state, gaseous anesthetics to maintain anesthesia, and neuromuscular blocking agents to effect muscle relaxation. Such drug protocols are called **combination** or **balanced anesthesia.**

**C. Mechanism of Action:** The mechanisms of action of general anesthetics are unclear, but these drugs usually increase the threshold for firing of CNS neurons. The potency of most inhaled anesthetics correlates positively with their lipid solubility. Possible mechanisms of action include block of ion channels by interactions with membrane lipids or proteins, as well as effects on central neurotransmitter mechanisms. CNS neurons have different sensitivities to general anesthetics; inhibition of neurons involved in pain pathways occurs before inhibition of neurons in the midbrain reticular formation.

## INHALED ANESTHETICS

**A. Classification & Pharmacokinetics of Onset of Action:** The agents currently used in inhalation anesthesia are nitrous oxide and the halogenated hydrocarbons including halothane, enflurane, isoflurane, and methoxyflurane. Desflurane is investigational. They are administered as gases, and the **partial pressure,** or "tension," of a particular anesthetic is a measure of its concentration in the body. The speed of induction of anesthetic effects depends on several factors:

1. **Inspired gas concentration.** A high partial pressure of the gas in the lungs results in more rapid attainment of anesthetic levels in the blood.
2. **Blood:gas partition coefficient.** The more rapidly a drug equilibrates with the blood, the more quickly it passes into the brain to produce anesthetic effects. Drugs with low blood solubility (eg, nitrous oxide) equilibrate more rapidly than do drugs with a higher partition coefficient (eg, halothane), as illustrated in Fig 24–1.
3. **Ventilation rate.** The greater the ventilation, the more rapid the rise in alveolar and blood concentrations of the agent and the more rapid the onset of anesthesia (Fig 24–1).
4. **Pulmonary blood flow.** This inversely modifies the rate at which the gas partial pressure rises and thus affects the speed of onset of anesthesia.

**B. Elimination:** Anesthesia is terminated by redistribution of the drug from the brain to the blood and elimination of the drug through the lungs. Halothane and methoxyflurane are also metabolized to a significant extent by liver enzymes.

**C. Minimum Alveolar Anesthetic Concentration (MAC):** The potency of inhaled anesthetics is best measured by the minimum alveolar anesthetic concentration (MAC). This is defined as the alveolar concentration required to eliminate the response to a standardized painful stimulus in 50% of patients. Each anesthetic has a defined MAC, but this concentration may vary among patients depending on age, cardiovascular status, use of adjuvant drugs, etc. The range of MACs for different agents is illustrated by a comparison of nitrous oxide (MAC > 100%) and methoxyflurane (MAC = 0.16%). Isoflurane, enflurane, and halothane have MACs between 0.75 and 1.5%.

**D. Effects:**

1. **CNS effects.** Inhaled anesthetics reduce the metabolic rate in the brain but reduce vascular resistance and thus increase cerebral blood flow. This may lead to an increase in intracranial pressure. High concentrations of enflurane may cause spike-and-wave activity and muscle twitching.

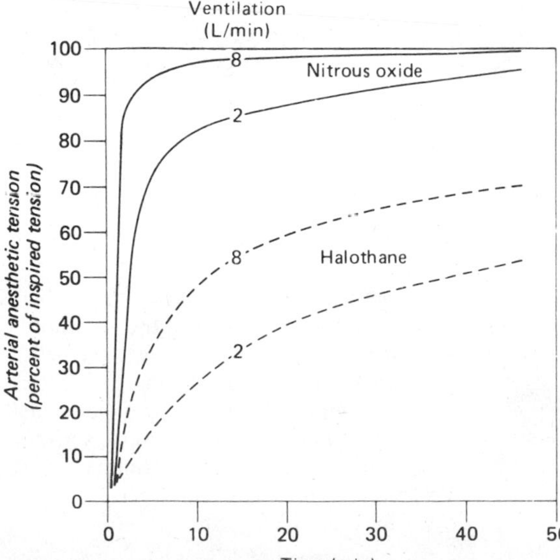


**Figure 24–1.** Ventilation rate and arterial anesthetic tensions. (Reproduced, with permission, from Katzung BG [editor]: *Basic & Clinical Pharmacology,* 5th ed. Appleton & Lange, 1992.)

2. **Cardiovascular effects.** Most inhaled anesthetics decrease arterial blood pressure moderately. Enflurane and halothane are myocardial depressants that decrease cardiac output, whereas isoflurane causes peripheral vasodilation. Nitrous oxide is less likely to lower blood pressure than are other gaseous anesthetics.
3. **Respiratory effects.** The rate of respiration may be increased by inhaled anesthetics, but the tidal volume is decreased, leading to an increase in arterial $CO_2$ tension. Inhaled anesthetics decrease the ventilatory response to hypoxia even at subanesthetic concentrations (eg, during recovery). Nitrous oxide has the smallest effect on respiration.
4. **Toxicity.** Postoperative hepatitis has occurred (rarely) following halothane anesthesia in patients experiencing hypovolemic shock or other severe stress. Fluoride released by metabolism of methoxyflurane may cause renal insufficiency after prolonged anesthesia. Prolonged exposure to nitrous oxide decreases methionine synthetase activity and may lead to megaloblastic anemia.

## INTRAVENOUS ANESTHETICS

**A. Classification, Pharmacokinetics, & Pharmacodynamics:** Several different chemical classes of drugs are used as intravenous agents in anesthesia.

1. **Barbiturates. Thiopental, thiamylal,** and **methohexital** have high lipid solubility, which promotes rapid entry into the brain and results in surgical anesthesia in one circulation time. They are used for induction of anesthesia and for short surgical procedures. Their anesthetic effects are terminated by redistribution from the brain to other tissues, but hepatic metabolism is required for their elimination from the body (Fig 24–2). They are respiratory and circulatory depressants, and because they depress cerebral blood flow, they can decrease intracranial pressure.
2. **Benzodiazepines. Midazolam** has been used adjunctively with gaseous anesthetics and narcotics. The onset of its CNS effects is slower than that of thiopental, and it has a longer duration of action. Cases of severe postoperative respiratory depression have occurred. The antagonist flumazenil accelerates recovery from midazolam and other benzodiazepines.
3. **Arylcyclohexylamines. Ketamine** produces a state called "dissociative anesthesia," in which the patient remains conscious but has marked catatonia, analgesia, and amnesia. It is an antagonist of glutamic acid, blocking the actions of this excitatory transmitter at its NMDA receptor. Ketamine is a cardiovascular stimulant and increases intracranial pressure. It causes disorientation and hallucinations during recovery, attenuated by diazepam.
4. **Narcotic-analgesics. Morphine** and **fentanyl** are used with other CNS depressants (nitrous oxide, benzodiazepines) in certain high-risk patients who may not survive a full general anesthetic. Respiratory depression with these drugs may be reversed postoperatively with narcotic antagonists.

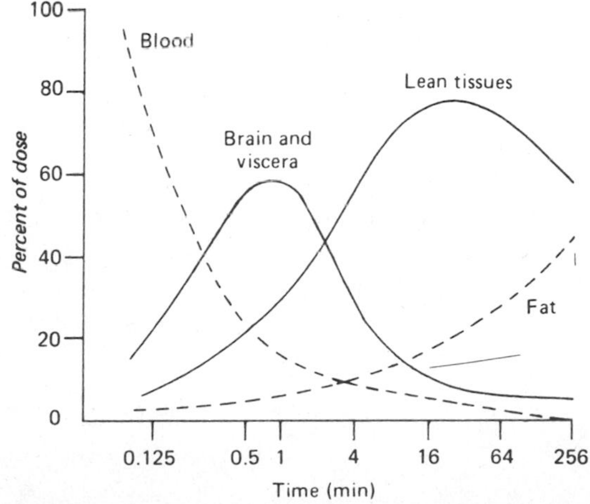


**Figure 24–2.** Redistribution of thiopental after an intravenous bolus administration. (Reproduced, with permission, from Katzung BG [editor]: *Basic & Clinical Pharmacology*, 5th ed. Appleton & Lange, 1992.)

5. **Propofol. Propofol** is similar to the intravenous barbiturates in its rate of onset and duration of anesthesia. It is used as an induction agent and for short anesthetic procedures. However, it may cause hypotension as a result of cardiac depression and vasodilation.

## DRUG LIST

The following drugs are important members of the group discussed in this chapter. Prototype agents should be learned in detail; the major variants should be known well enough to list the factors that distinguish them from the prototypes and from each other.

| Subclass | Prototype | Major Variants |
|---|---|---|
| Inhalation anesthetics | Halothane | Enflurane, isoflurane, methoxyflurane |
| | Nitrous oxide | |
| Intravenous anesthetics | Thiopental | Thiamylal, methohexital |
| | Midazolam | |
| | Ketamine | |
| | Morphine, fentanyl, and similar narcotics | |

## QUESTIONS

**DIRECTIONS (items 1–5):** Each numbered item or incomplete statement in this section is followed by answers or by completions of the statement. Select the ONE lettered answer or completion that is BEST in each case.

**1.** All of the following statements about the onset of anesthesia using inhalation agents are accurate EXCEPT:
**(A)** Onset of anesthesia is very slow with agents that have a low blood:gas coefficient
**(B)** Onset of anesthesia is accelerated by increasing inspired anesthetic gas concentration
**(C)** The effects of nitrous oxide occur very rapidly
**(D)** Decreasing the ventilation rate during gas inhalation will slow the onset of anesthesia
**(E)** Anesthetic effects develop slowly with methoxyflurane

**2.** All of the following statements about the halogenated hydrocarbon gaseous anesthetics are accurate EXCEPT:
**(A)** Isoflurane decreases the systemic vascular resistance and has minimal effects on cardiac output
**(B)** All cause decreased mean arterial pressure
**(C)** During recovery from anesthesia, compensatory ventilatory responses to anoxia are reduced
**(D)** These agents facilitate contraction of uterine smooth muscle
**(E)** All cause decreased hepatic and renal blood flow

3. All of the following are adverse effects that may occur with the use of inhalational agents EXCEPT:
   (A) Halothane may increase intracranial pressure in patients with head injury
   (B) Mild, generalized muscle twitching occurs with high doses of enflurane
   (C) Postoperative hepatitis is associated mostly with the use of isoflurane
   (D) Vasopressin-resistant polyuric renal insufficiency may occur with the use of methoxyflurane
   (E) Since it may cause megaloblastic anemia, nitrous oxide is an occupational hazard for staff working in poorly ventilated dental operating rooms

4. All of the following statements concerning MAC are accurate EXCEPT:
   (A) At a given level of anesthesia, measurement of alveolar concentrations of different anesthetics allows potency comparisons
   (B) MACs give information about the slope of the dose-response curve
   (C) The MAC value for nitrous oxide in humans is greater than 100%
   (D) MACs decrease in elderly patients
   (E) The simultaneous use of opioid analgesics lowers the MAC for gas anesthetics

5. All of the following statements concerning the intravenous anesthetics are accurate EXCEPT:
   (A) Intravenous barbiturates decrease cerebral blood flow
   (B) Redistribution of the drug from the brain to other body tissues is responsible for termination of the anesthetic effects of thiopental
   (C) Ketamine is a cardiovascular depressant
   (D) High doses of opioid analgesics can be used in cardiac surgery with minimal circulatory deterioration
   (E) Intraoperative use of benzodiazepines prolongs the postanesthetic recovery period and may cause amnesia

**DIRECTIONS (items 6–10):** Items 6–10 consist of lettered headings followed by a set of numbered sentences. For each numbered sentence, select the ONE lettered heading that is most closely associated with it. Each lettered heading may be selected once, more than once, or not at all.

(A) Midazolam
(B) Methoxyflurane
(C) Propofol
(D) Halothane
(E) Ketamine

6. This drug is a high-potency gas anesthetic (low MAC) that is metabolized—at a higher rate than other inhaled anesthetics—with release of fluoride ions

7. This drug interacts with the NMDA subclass of brain glutamate receptors

8. Postanesthetic CNS depression following the use of this agent may be reversed by administration of flumazenil

9. This agent is a phenol derivative that causes rapid anesthesia and marked decrease in systemic blood pressure

10. This halogenated inhalational agent is associated with a low incidence of postoperative hepatitis, especially in patients who have had periods of anoxia during surgery

## ANSWERS

1. Arterial gas tension increases slowly following inhalation of anesthetics with high blood solubility (eg, methoxyflurane). This results in a slow equilibration with the brain and slower induc-

tion of anesthesia than occurs with agents of low blood solubility (eg, nitrous oxide). The answer is **(A)**.

2. The halogenated hydrocarbon anesthetics are potent uterine muscle relaxants. This action may be useful for intrauterine manipulation during delivery, but may increase bleeding during dilation and curettage. Nitrous oxide has little effect on uterine musculature. The answer is **(D)**.

3. Hepatitis following general anesthesia has been linked to the use of halothane, although the incidence of severe hepatic necrosis is only about one of 35,000 halothane administrations. The results of animal experiments suggest that halothane hepatotoxicity may be due to the formation of a toxic metabolite produced under anoxic conditions. Hepatotoxicity has not been reported following isoflurane administration, and it may be relevant that this agent is the most slowly metabolized of the fluorinated hydrocarbons. The answer is **(C)**.

4. Dose-response characteristics of gas anesthetics are difficult to measure, since is not possible to estimate brain concentrations of such drugs at different stages of CNS depression. On the basis of alveolar gas concentration measurements we can conclude that dose-response relationships are steep. Whereas a dose of 1 MAC of any agent may prevent movement in response to surgical stimulation in 50% of patients, individual patients may require from 0.5 to 1.5 MACs. MACs give no information about the **slope** of the dose-response curve. The answer is **(B)**.

5. Ketamine routinely produces cardiac stimulation, with increases in heart rate, cardiac output, and arterial blood pressure. This is a distinctive property of ketamine, as is the high incidence of postanesthetic emergence reactions including disorientation, vivid dreams, and hallucinations. The answer is **(C)**.

6. Methoxyflurane is the most potent halogenated gas anesthetic. Its MAC is 0.16%, compared with 0.75% for halothane and 1.4% for isoflurane. Its hepatic metabolism is more extensive than that of the other agents, releasing fluoride ions at levels that can be nephrotoxic. The answer is **(B)**.

7. Ketamine is an antagonist at NMDA glutamate receptors in the brain. It is not clear whether such actions contribute to its anesthetic effects. There is some evidence that ketamine and other drugs that block NMDA receptors may have neuronal protective value in the management of cerebral ischemic states. The answer is **(E)**.

8. Flumazenil is a benzodiazepine receptor antagonist. It accelerates recovery from postoperative CNS depression due to midazolam or other benzodiazepines used in anesthesia, such as diazepam and lorazepam. The short duration of action of flumazenil may necessitate multiple doses. The answer is **(A)**.

9. Propofol (2,6-diisopropylphenol) is a newer intravenous anesthetic that has properties and uses similar to those of thiopental. However, it is more cardiodepressant than intravenous barbiturates, causing a marked decrease in systemic blood pressure on induction. The answer is **(C)**.

10. Use of halothane is associated with a very low (1 in 35,000 cases) incidence of postoperative hepatitis. This toxicity may result from a reactive metabolite produced under hypoxic conditions. The answer is **(D)**.

# Local Anesthetics 25

## OBJECTIVES

**You should be able to:**

- Describe the mechanism of blockade of the nerve impulse by local anesthetics.
- Discuss the relation between pH, $pK_a$, and the onset or intensity of blockade.
- List the factors that determine the susceptibility of nerve fibers to blockade.
- List the major toxic effects of the local anesthetics.
- Explain use-dependent blockade.

## CONCEPTS

Local anesthesia is the condition that results when sensory input from a local area to the CNS is blocked. The local anesthetics constitute a group of chemically similar agents that block the sodium channels of excitable membranes. Because they can be administered locally by topical application or by injection in the target area, their anesthetic effect can be restricted to a localized area. When given intravenously, these drugs have effects on other tissues.

**A. Chemistry:** Most local anesthetic drugs are esters or amides of simple benzene derivatives. They carry an amine function and are therefore ionizable through the gain of a proton ($H^+$). As discussed in Chapter 1, the degree of ionization is a function of the $pK_a$ of the drug and the pH of the medium. Because the pH of tissue may differ from the usual 7.4 (for example, it may be as low as 6.4 in infected tissue), the degree of ionization of the drug will vary. Because the $pK_a$ of most local anesthetics is between 8.0 and 9.0 (benzocaine is an exception), infection-associated variations in pH can have significant effects on the proportion of ionized to nonionized drug. The question of the active form of the drug (ionized versus nonionized) is discussed below.

**B. Pharmacokinetics:** Local anesthetics are readily absorbed from the injection site after subcutaneous administration. The duration of local action is therefore limited unless blood flow to the area is reduced. This can be accomplished by administration of a vasoconstrictor (usually an alpha-agonist sympathomimetic) with the local anesthetic agent. Cocaine is an exception to this rule since it has intrinsic sympathomimetic action (because it inhibits norepinephrine reuptake into nerve terminals); it does not require any additional vasoconstrictor. Surface activity (ability to reach superficial nerves when applied to the surface of mucous membranes) is a property of only a few local anesthetics, including cocaine and benzocaine. Ester local anesthetics are metabolized by plasma cholinesterases; this metabolism may be rapid. Procaine and chloroprocaine have half-lives of only 1–2 minutes. The amides are hydrolyzed in the liver and have half-lives from 1.8 to 6 hours. Bupivacaine is a very lipid-soluble and long-acting local anesthetic. Liver dysfunction may increase the half-life of amide local anesthetics.

**C. Mechanism of Action:** Local anesthetics block voltage-dependent sodium channels and reduce the influx of ions, thereby preventing normal depolarization of the membrane and blocking conduction of the action potential. This effect occurs from the cytoplasmic side of the membrane. Since the drug molecule must cross the lipid membrane to reach the cytoplasm, the more lipid-soluble (nonionized) form would be expected to reach effective intracellular concentrations more rapidly than would the ionized form. On the other hand, once inside the membrane, the ionized form of the drug appears to be the more effective blocking entity. Thus both ionized and nonionized forms of the drug play a part in reaching the receptor site and causing the effect. The affinity of the receptor site within the sodium channel for the local anesthetic is a function of the state of the channel—whether it is resting, open, or inactivated—and therefore follows the same rules of use dependence and potential dependence that were described for the sodium channel-blocking antiarrhythmic drugs (see Chapter 14).

**D. Effects:** Differential sensitivity of different types of nerve fibers to local anesthetics is associated with several factors, including fiber diameter, myelination, physiologic firing rate, and anatomic location. In general, smaller fibers are blocked more easily than larger ones and myelinated fibers are blocked more easily than unmyelinated ones. Because of the use-dependent character of the blockade, rapidly firing fibers are blocked more quickly than slowly firing fibers. Fibers located in the periphery of a nerve bundle are blocked sooner than those in the core because they are exposed earlier to higher concentrations of the anesthetic. The effects of these drugs on the heart as group I antiarrhythmic agents are discussed in Chapter 14. They also have weak blocking effects on skeletal muscle neuromuscular transmission.

**E. Clinical Use:** The local anesthetics are most commonly used for minor surgical procedures. Their injection in carbonated solutions may accelerate their onset of action. High concentrations of extracellular $K^+$ may enhance local anesthetic activity, whereas elevated extracellular $Ca^{2+}$ concentrations may antagonize it. Local anesthetics are also used in spinal anesthesia and for producing autonomic blockade in ischemic conditions of the limbs. Repeated epidural injection may lead to tachyphylaxis.

**F. Toxicity:**

1. **CNS effects.** The most important toxic effects of the local anesthetics are those in the CNS. These actions include the mood elevation induced by cocaine. The other local anesthetics produce a spectrum of effects, including light-headedness or sedation, restlessness, nystagmus, and tonic-clonic convulsions. Severe convulsions may be followed by coma with respiratory and cardiovascular depression.
2. **Cardiovascular effects.** With the exception of cocaine, all local anesthetics are vasodilators. Patients with preexisting cardiovascular disease may show heart block and other disturbances of cardiac electrical function at high plasma levels of local anesthetics. Bupivacaine causes severe cardiovascular toxicity, including arrhythmias and hypotension, if given intravenously. The ability of cocaine to block norepinephrine reuptake at sympathetic neuroeffector junctions, plus its vasoconstricting actions, may contribute to its cardiotoxicity.
3. **Other toxic effects.** Prilocaine is metabolized to products that include an agent capable of causing methemoglobinemia. The ester-type local anesthetics are metabolized to products that cause antibody formation in some patients. Allergic responses to local anesthetics can usually be avoided by using an agent from the amide class.
4. **Treatment of toxicity.** Severe toxicity is best treated symptomatically. Convulsions are often treated with a short-acting sedative-hypnotic such as thiopental or diazepam. Hyperventilation with oxygenation is helpful. Occasionally, a neuromuscular blocking drug may be indicated to control violent convulsive activity. The cardiovascular toxicity of bupivacaine overdose is difficult to treat and has caused fatalities.

## DRUG LIST

The following drugs are important members of the group discussed in this chapter. Prototype agents should be learned in detail; the major variants should be known well enough to list the factors that distinguish them from the prototypes and from each other; and the other significant agents should be recognized as belonging to a specific subclass.

| Subclass | Prototype | Major Variants | Other Significant Agents |
|---|---|---|---|
| Ester anesthetics | Procaine | Cocaine, benzocaine | Tetracaine |
| Amide anesthetics | Lidocaine | Bupivacaine | Etidocaine, prilocaine |

## QUESTIONS

**DIRECTIONS (items 1–7):** Each numbered item or incomplete statement in this section is followed by answers or by completions of the statement. Select the ONE lettered answer or completion that is BEST in each case.

**1.** Actions of local anesthetics include all of the following EXCEPT
**(A)** blockade of voltage-dependent sodium channels
**(B)** preferential binding to resting channels
**(C)** slowing of axonal impulse conduction
**(D)** an increase in membrane refractory period

**2.** The $pK_a$ of lidocaine is 7.9. At pH 6.9, the fraction in the ionized form will be
**(A)** 1%
**(B)** 10%
**(C)** 50%
**(D)** 90%
**(E)** 99%

**3.** All of the following statements about nerve blockade with local anesthetics are accurate EXCEPT:
**(A)** Activity may be reduced when the anesthetic is injected into infected tissues
**(B)** Block is faster in onset with smaller-diameter fibers
**(C)** Activity is use-dependent
**(D)** Smaller-diameter fibers recover faster

**4.** The most important effect of local anesthetic overdosage is
**(A)** skin rash
**(B)** renal failure
**(C)** seizures
**(D)** gangrene
**(E)** bronchoconstriction

**5.** Factors that influence the duration or intensity of action of local anesthetics include all of the following EXCEPT
**(A)** blood flow through the tissue
**(B)** activity of acetylcholinesterase
**(C)** use of vasoconstrictors
**(D)** amount of local anesthetic injected
**(E)** tissue pH

**6.** You have a vial containing 4 mL of a 2% solution of lidocaine. How much lidocaine is present in 1 mL?
**(A)** 2 mg
**(B)** 8 mg
**(C)** 20 mg
**(D)** 80 mg

**7.** All of the following statements about the toxicity of local anesthetics are accurate EXCEPT:
**(A)** Allergic reactions are more likely to occur with mepivacaine than procaine
**(B)** Cyanosis may occur following injection of large doses of prilocaine, especially in patients with pulmonary disease
**(C)** Intravenous injection of local anesthetics may depress cardiac pacemaker activity
**(D)** In overdosage, hyperventilation (with oxygen) is helpful in preventing seizures and arrhythmias

**DIRECTIONS (items 8–10):** Items 8–10 consist of lettered headings followed by a set of numbered statements. For each numbered statement, select the ONE lettered heading that is most clearly associated with it. Each lettered heading may be selected once, more than once, or not at all.

**(A)** Lidocaine
**(B)** Cocaine
**(C)** Bupivacaine
**(D)** Benzocaine
**(E)** Procaine

**8.** This drug is an ester and has high surface activity. It has vasoconstrictive actions that may be useful clinically.

**9.** This drug has a slow onset and the longest duration of action of any local anesthetic. Its cardiac actions occur at normal heart rates.

**10.** Poorly soluble in aqueous fluids, this drug remains at the site of its application and is not absorbed into the systemic circulation. It has low toxic potential.

## ANSWERS

**1.** Local anesthetics bind preferentially to sodium channels in the open and inactivated states. Recovery from drug-induced block is 10–1000 times slower than recovery of channels from normal inactivation. Resting channels have a low affinity for local anesthetics. The answer is **(B)**.

**2.** Since the drug is a weak base, it will be more ionized (protonated) at pH values lower than its $pK_a$. Since the pH given is 1 log unit lower (more acid) than the $pK_a$, the ratio of ionized to nonionized drug will be 90:10. The answer is **(D)**. (Recall from Chapter 1 that at $pH = pK_a$, the ratio is 1:1; at 1 log unit difference, the ratio is 90:10; at 2 units difference, it is 99:1; etc.)

**3.** Smaller-diameter nerve fibers are more sensitive to local anesthetics and are blocked more rapidly than those of larger size. As the local concentration of drug declines during recovery from local anesthesia, smaller fibers continue to be blocked and are the last to recover. The answer is **(D)**.

**4.** Of the effects listed, the most important in local anesthetic overdose concerns the CNS. Such effects can include sedation or restlessness, nystagmus, convulsions, coma, and respiratory depression. Diazepam suppresses seizures caused by local anesthetics without effects on ventilation or circulation. Note that gangrene may occur when local anesthetics with high concentrations of sympathomimetics are injected into the extremities, as a result of the vasoconstrictor actions of the latter drugs. This effect is rare and is most likely to occur after inadvertent intra-arterial injection. The answer is **(C)**.

**5.** The ester group of local anesthetics is metabolized by plasma (and tissue) pseudocholinesterases. They are poor substrates for acetylcholinesterase, and the activity of this enzyme does not play a part in terminating the actions of local anesthetics. Individuals with genetically based defects in pseudocholinesterase activity are unusually sensitive to procaine and other esters. The answer is **(B)**.

**6.** The fact that you have 4 mL of a solution of lidocaine is irrelevant. A 2% solution of any drug contains 2 g/100 mL. The amount of lidocaine in 1 mL of a 2% solution is 0.02 grams, or 20 mg. The answer is **(C)**.

**7.** Allergic reactions to local anesthetics are infrequent, even though many persons provide medical histories of presumptive hypersensitivity to this class of drugs. When they occur, an ester derivative (eg, procaine) is usually involved and there is no cross-reactivity with amide local anesthetics. The answer is **(A).**

8. Cocaine is an ester anesthetic with high surface activity. It is the only local anesthetic that inhibits the reuptake of catecholamines at adrenergic terminals. It may cause pupillary mydriasis, as well as other sympathomimetic effects including vasoconstriction. The latter effect has been of value in topical anesthesia for surgery of the nasal mucosa. The answer is **(B).**

9. You may be able to identify this drug as bupivacaine from its long duration of action. Unlike lidocaine, the actions of bupivicaine on cardiac cells occur at normal heart rates. Accidental intravenous administration of bupivicaine may lead to cardiovascular collapse. The answer is **(C).**

10. Benzocaine is an ester that is used for topical anesthesia. Because of its low toxic potential, it has been used for anesthesia of large surface areas, including those within the oral cavity. Despite its limited absorption, methemoglobinemia has occurred when large doses are used in small children. The answer is **(D).**

# Skeletal Muscle Relaxants 26

## OBJECTIVES

**Define the following terms:**

- Depolarizing blockade
- Desensitization
- Malignant hyperthermia
- Nondepolarizing blockade
- Spasmolytic
- Stabilizing blockade

**You should be able to:**

- Describe the transmission process at the neuromuscular end-plate and the points at which drugs can modify this process.
- List 3 nondepolarizing neuromuscular blockers and one depolarizing neuromuscular blocker and compare their pharmacokinetics.
- Describe the differences between depolarizing and nondepolarizing blockers from the standpoint of tetanic and posttetanic twitch strength.
- Describe the method of reversal of nondepolarizing blockade.
- List the major drugs used in the treatment of skeletal muscle spasticity and describe their mechanisms.

## CONCEPTS

### NEUROMUSCULAR BLOCKERS

A. **Classification & Prototypes:** Skeletal muscle contraction is evoked by a nicotinic cholinergic transmission process. It is therefore subject to the same types of pharmacologic modification as autonomic ganglionic transmission. Blockade of transmission at the end-plate (the postsynaptic structure bearing the nicotinic receptors) is clinically useful in producing relaxation of muscle, a requirement for surgery. The neuromuscular blockers are structurally related to acetylcholine and are either antagonists (nondepolarizing type) or agonists (depolarizing type) at the nicotinic end-plate receptor. The prototype nondepolarizing agent is **tubocurarine;** the prototype depolarizing drug is **succinylcholine.**

**B. Nondepolarizing Neuromuscular Blocking Drugs:**

1. **Pharmacokinetics.** Most nondepolarizing agents have relatively long half-lives, ranging from 30 minutes to several hours. They are given parenterally. All except vecuronium and atracurium depend on the kidneys for elimination, and their half-lives are extended in patients with impaired renal function (Table 26–1).
2. **Mechanism of action.** These drugs act as surmountable blockers, meaning that the blockade can be overcome by increasing the amount of agonist (acetylcholine) in the synaptic cleft. Therefore the drugs in this group behave as though they compete with acetylcholine at the receptor, and their effect is reversed by cholinesterase inhibitors. However, there is evidence that some of them may also act directly to plug the ion channel operated by the acetylcholine receptor. Posttetanic potentiation is preserved in the presence of these agents, but tension during the tetanus fades rapidly. See Table 26–2 for additional details.

**C. Depolarizing Neuromuscular Blocking Drugs:**

1. **Pharmacokinetics.** Succinylcholine is an ester that strongly resembles acetylcholine: It is composed of 2 acetylcholine molecules linked end to end. Succinylcholine is metabolized by plasma cholinesterase (butyryl-cholinesterase or pseudocholinesterase) and has a duration of action of only a few minutes if given as a single dose. It is given by continuous infusion if prolonged paralysis is to be produced with this drug. (More often, paralysis is initiated with succinylcholine and then continued with a nondepolarizing agent.) Succinylcholine is not rapidly hydrolyzed by acetylcholinesterase.
2. **Mechanism of action.** Depolarizing blockers act like nicotinic agonists and depolarize the neuromuscular end-plate. The initial depolarization is often accompanied by twitching and fasciculations. Because tension cannot be maintained in skeletal muscle without periodic repolarization and depolarization of the end-plate, continuous depolarization results in muscle relaxation and paralysis. As with the nondepolarizing blockers, some evidence suggests that these drugs can also plug the end-plate channel. When succinylcholine is given over a long period, its effect changes from continuous depolarization (phase I) to one of gradual repolarization with resistance to depolarization (phase II), ie, a curarelike blockade.

**D. Reversal of Blockade:** The action of nondepolarizing blockers is readily reversed by increasing the concentration of normal transmitter at the receptors. This is best accomplished by administration of cholinesterase inhibitors such as neostigmine or edrophonium. In contrast, the paralysis produced by depolarizing blockers is facilitated by cholinesterase inhibitors in phase I. The block is reversed by cholinesterase inhibitors in phase II.

**E. Toxicity:**

1. **Respiratory paralysis.** The action of full doses of neuromuscular blockers leads directly to respiratory paralysis. If mechanical ventilation is not provided, the patient will asphyxiate.
2. **Autonomic effects and histamine release.** Some of these agents have autonomic effects or cause release of histamine, either of which can result in cardiovascular disturbances. These actions are summarized in Table 26–3.
3. **Interactions.** Aminoglycoside antibiotics and antiarrhythmic drugs potentiate and prolong the relaxant action of neuromuscular blockers.

**Table 26–1.** Pharmacokinetic characteristics of neuromuscular blocking drugs.

| Drug | Duration of Maximal Effect | Half-Life | Route or Mechanism of Elimination |
|---|---|---|---|
| Tubocurarine | 60 min | 120 min | Kidney, excreted in urine |
| Pancuronium | 60 min | 90–150 min | Kidney, excreted in urine |
| Vecuronium | 30 min | 70 min | Liver, excreted in bile |
| Atracurium | 20–30 min | 20 min | Spontaneous breakdown in plasma |
| Succinylcholine | 5–10 min | 1–2 min | Hydrolysis by plasma cholinesterase |

**Table 26–2.** Comparison of a typical nondepolarizing muscle relaxant (tubocurarine) and a depolarizing muscle relaxant (succinylcholine).[1]

| | | Succinylcholine | |
|---|---|---|---|
| | **Tubocurarine** | **Phase I** | **Phase II** |
| Administration of tubocurarine | Additive | Antagonistic | Augmented[2] |
| Administration of succinylcholine | Antagonistic | Additive | Augmented[2] |
| Effect of neostigmine | Antagonistic | Augmented[2] | Antagonistic |
| Initial excitatory effect on skeletal muscle | None | Fasciculations | None |
| Response to a tetanic stimulus | Unsustained | Sustained[3] | Unsustained |
| Posttetanic facilitation | Yes | No | Yes |
| Rate of recovery | 30–60 min[4] | 4–8 min | >20 min4 |

[1]Reproduced, with permission, from Katzung BG (editor): *Basic & Clinical Pharmacology,* 5th ed. Appleton & Lange, 1992.
[2]It is not known whether this interaction is additive or synergistic (superadditive).
[3]The amplitude is decreased, but the response is sustained.
[4]The rate depends on the dose and on the completeness of neuromuscular blockade.

## SPASMOLYTIC DRUGS

Certain diseases of the CNS (eg, cerebral palsy, multiple sclerosis, stroke) are associated with abnormally high reflex activity in the neuronal pathways controlling skeletal muscle, with resulting painful spasm. (Bladder and anal sphincter control is also affected in most cases and may require autonomic drugs for management.) The goal of spasmolytic therapy is reduction of excessive skeletal muscle tone without reduction of strength.

**A. Classification & Prototypes:** The spasmolytic drugs do not resemble acetylcholine in structure or effect. They act in the CNS or in the skeletal muscle cell rather than at the neuromuscular end-plate. Three drugs are used: **diazepam,** a benzodiazepine (see Chapter 21); **baclofen,** a GABA agonist; and **dantrolene,** an agent that acts on the sarcoplasmic reticulum of skeletal muscle. All 3 agents are usually used by the oral route. Recent clinical studies suggest that refractory cases may respond to chronic intrathecal administration of baclofen.

**B. Mechanism of Action:** The 3 spasmolytic drugs act by 3 different mechanisms. Two act in the spinal cord: Diazepam facilitates GABA-mediated presynaptic inhibition, and baclofen acts as a $GABA_B$ agonist, causing a reduction in the tonic output of the primary spinal motoneurons. Dantrolene acts in the skeletal muscle cell to reduce the release of activator calcium from the sarcoplasmic reticulum. Dantrolene is also effective in the treatment of malignant hyperthermia, a

**Table 26–3.** Autonomic effects of neuromuscular blocking drugs.[1]

| Drug | Effect on Autonomic Ganglia | Effect on Cardiac Muscarinic Receptors | Effect on Histamine Release |
|---|---|---|---|
| Succinylcholine | Stimulates | Stimulates | Slight |
| Tubocurarine | Blocks | None | Moderate |
| Metocurine | Blocks weakly | None | Slight |
| Pancuronium | None | Blocks moderately | None |
| Vecuronium | None | None | None |
| Atracurium | None | None | Slight |

[1]Modified and reproduced, with permission, from Katzung BG (editor): *Basic & Clinical Pharmacology,* 5th ed. Appleton & Lange, 1992.

genetically determined disorder characterized by massive calcium release from skeletal muscle sarcoplasmic reticulum. Malignant hyperthermia is most often triggered by general anesthesia or neuromuscular blocking drugs. In this emergency condition, dantrolene is given intravenously.

C. **Toxicity:** The sedation produced by diazepam is significant but milder than that produced by other sedative-hypnotic drugs at doses that induce equivalent muscle relaxation. Baclofen produces less sedation than diazepam. Dantrolene causes significant muscle weakness but less sedation than either diazepam or baclofen.

## DRUG LIST

The following drugs are important members of the group discussed in this chapter. Prototype agents should be learned in detail; the major variant and the other significant agents should be known well enough to list the factors that distinguish them from the prototypes and from each other.

| Subclass | Prototype | Major Variants | Other Significant Agents |
|---|---|---|---|
| Nondepolarizing neuromuscular blockers | Tubocurarine | Atracurium | Vecuronium, pancuronium, pipecuronium |
| Depolarizing blockers | Succinylcholine | | Decamethonium |
| Spasmolytic drugs | Diazepam, baclofen, dantrolene | | |

## QUESTIONS

**DIRECTIONS (items 1–6):** Each numbered item or incomplete statement in this section is followed by answers or by completions of the statement. Select the ONE lettered answer or completion that is BEST in each case.

**1.** Edrophonium facilitates the initial relaxant effect of
(**A**) tubocurarine
(**B**) pancuronium
(**C**) atracurium
(**D**) succinylcholine
(**E**) vecuronium

**2.** Which of the following is most often associated with histamine release in some patients?
(**A**) Tubocurarine
(**B**) Pancuronium
(**C**) Atracurium
(**D**) Succinylcholine
(**E**) Vecuronium

**3.** Characteristics of phase I depolarizing neuromuscular blockade include
(**A**) well-sustained tetanic tension
(**B**) marked muscarinic blockade
(**C**) muscle fasciculations in the later stages of block
(**D**) reversible by pyridostigmine
(**E**) all of the above

**4.** Characteristics of nondepolarizing neuromuscular blockade include
(A) stimulation of autonomic ganglia
(B) poorly sustained tetanic tension
(C) block of posttetanic potentiation
(D) significant muscle fasciculations during onset of block
(E) histamine-blocking action

**5.** Which of the following will NOT cause skeletal muscle contractions or twitching?
(A) Nicotine
(B) Vecuronium
(C) Succinylcholine
(D) Acetylcholine

**6.** Which of the following has a duration of action shorter than 15 minutes when given as a single injection?
(A) Atracurium
(B) Vecuronium
(C) Pancuronium
(D) Succinylcholine
(E) Tubocurarine

**DIRECTIONS (items 7–10):** Items 7–10 consist of lettered headings followed by a set of numbered phrases. For each numbered phrase, select the ONE lettered heading that is most closely associated with it. Each lettered heading may be selected once, more than once, or not at all.

(A) Tubocurarine
(B) Dantrolene
(C) Succinylcholine
(D) Diazepam
(E) Baclofen

**7.** Prevents release of calcium from the sarcoplasmic reticulum

**8.** Depolarizes the neuromuscular end-plate

**9.** Reversed by neostigmine, even at the start of its effect

**10.** GABA analog (agonist at $GABA_B$ receptors) that reduces motor neuron outflow.

## ANSWERS

**1.** Only depolarizing blockers are facilitated by cholinesterase inhibitors. The answer is **(D)**.

**2.** The answer is **(A)**, tubocurarine.

**3.** Phase I depolarizing blockade is not associated with muscarinic blockade, nor is it reversible with cholinesterase inhibitors. Muscle fasciculations occur at the start of the action of succinylcholine. The answer is **(A)**.

**4.** Nondepolarizing blockers result in poorly sustained tetanus and do not cause fasciculations at any time during their action (Table 26–2). The answer is **(B)**.

**5.** Nicotine, succinylcholine, and acetylcholine cause end-plate depolarization and skeletal muscle contractions (they are nicotinic receptor agonists). Vecuronium is a nondepolarizing blocker and does not cause contraction at any dose. The answer is **(B)**.

**6.** Of the listed drugs, only succinylcholine has a duration of action shorter than 15 minutes. The answer is **(D).**

**7.** Dantrolene is the only commonly used spasmolytic that acts inside the skeletal muscle cell. It interferes with calcium release. The answer is **(B).**

**8.** Succinylcholine is the only nicotinic agonist in the answer list. The answer is **(C).**

**9.** Only nondepolarizing blockade can be reversed by cholinesterase inhibitors. The answer is **(A).**

**10.** Baclofen is a $GABA_B$ agonist. The answer is **(E).**

# 27 Drug Therapy of Parkinson's Disease & Other Movement Disorders

## OBJECTIVES

**Define the following terms:**

- Dopaminergic-cholinergic balance
- Dyskinesia
- Levodopa adjunct
- Movement disorder
- On-off phenomena

**You should be able to:**

- Describe the mechanisms by which levodopa, bromocriptine, amantadine, selegiline, and muscarinic blockers alleviate parkinsonism.
- Describe the therapeutic and toxic effects of the antiparkinsonism agents.
- List the chemical agents and drugs that cause parkinsonism symptoms.
- Identify the drugs used in management of tremor, Huntington's disease, drug-induced dyskinesias, and Wilson's disease.

## CONCEPTS

### ANTIPARKINSONISM AGENTS

Parkinsonism is a common neurologic movement disorder that develops in diseases which involve dysfunction in the basal ganglia and associated brain structures. Its symptoms (mnemonic *raft*) include muscle *r*igidity, *a*kinesia, *f*lat facies, and *t*remor (at rest). The disease, of uncertain etiology, occurs with increasing frequency during aging, from the fifth or sixth decade of life. Its pathologic characteristics include a decrease in the levels of dopamine and degeneration of dopaminergic neurons in the nigrostriatal tract. The reduction of normal dopaminergic neurotransmission is accompanied by a reciprocal increase in cholinergic neurotransmission; thus, dopamine and acetylcholine activities appear to be out of balance in Parkinson's disease. Many drugs can cause parkinsonian symptoms, which are usually reversible. The most important of these are the butyrophenone and phenothiazine **antipsychotic drugs,** which block brain dopamine receptors. **Reserpine,** at high doses, causes similar symptoms, presumably via the depletion of brain dopamine. **MPTP** (1-methyl-4-phenyl-1,2,3,6-tetrahydropyridine), a by-product of the attempted illicit synthesis of a meperidine analog, causes irreversible parkinsonism through destruction of dopaminergic neurons in the nigrostriatal tract. Treatment with inhibitors of monoamine oxidase (MAO) type B protects against MPTP neurotoxicity in animals.

Drug treatment of Parkinson's disease involves increasing brain dopamine functional activity or decreasing brain cholinergic (muscarinic) functional activity (or both).

## A. Levodopa:

1. **Mechanism of action.** Because dopamine has low bioavailability and does not readily cross the blood-brain barrier, its precursor, L-dopa (levodopa), is used. This amino acid is converted to dopamine by the enzyme aromatic L-amino acid decarboxylase, which is present in many body tissues, including the brain. Lower doses of levodopa can be used if given with **carbidopa,** an inhibitor of the decarboxylase that does not cross the blood-brain barrier.
2. **Pharmacologic effects.** Levodopa ameliorates many parkinsonism symptoms, particularly bradykinesia, and there is a decreased mortality rate among patients who take it. However, the drug does not cure parkinsonism, and responsiveness decreases with time, which may reflect disease progression. Clinical responses may fluctuate quite rapidly, changing from akinesia to dyskinesia over a few hours. These so-called **on-off phenomena** may be related partly to changes in levodopa levels in plasma. **"Drug holidays,"** periods of a few weeks during which the drug is not taken, are sometimes used to reduce response fluctuations and toxic effects.
3. **Toxicity.** Most adverse effects are dose-dependent. Peripheral toxicity is less common when levodopa is used with carbidopa.
   a. **Gastrointestinal disturbances** include anorexia, nausea, and vomiting.
   b. **Cardiovascular effects** include tachycardia, postural hypotension, and cardiac arrhythmias.
   c. **Dyskinesias** include choreoathetosis of the face and extremities.
   d. **Behavioral effects** include anxiety, agitation, confusion, delusions, hallucinations, and depression.

## B. Bromocriptine:

1. **Mechanism of action.** Bromocriptine is an ergot alkaloid that acts as a partial agonist at certain dopamine receptors in the brain, increasing the functional activity of dopamine neurotransmitter pathways, including those involved in extrapyramidal functions. **Pergolide** is a dopamine agonist at both $D_1$ and $D_2$ receptors, recently approved for use in parkinsonism. It acts similarly to bromocriptine and may decrease response fluctuations and prolong the effectiveness of levodopa. Pergolide loses efficacy with time.
2. **Clinical indications.** Bromocriptine may be used in conjunction with levodopa (and with anticholinergic drugs) and in patients who are refractory to or cannot tolerate levodopa.
3. **Toxicity**
   a. Gastrointestinal effects include nausea and vomiting.
   b. Postural hypotension is common, especially at the start of therapy.
   c. Dyskinesias occur, which are similar to those induced by levodopa.
   d. Mental disturbances include confusion and hallucinations.
   e. Miscellaneous effects, including pulmonary infiltrates and erythromelalgia, are occasionally reported; these usually clear promptly after the drug is stopped.

## C. Amantadine:

1. **Mechanism of action.** This drug enhances dopaminergic neurotransmission by mechanisms that may involve increasing the synthesis or release of dopamine or inhibiting the reuptake of dopamine.
2. **Pharmacologic effects.** The drug may improve bradykinesia, rigidity, and tremor but is usually effective for only a few weeks. It also has antiviral effects.
3. **Toxicity**
   a. **Mental disturbances** include restlessness, agitation, insomnia, confusion, hallucinations, and acute toxic psychosis.
   b. **Dermatologic reactions** include livedo reticularis.
   c. **Peripheral edema.**

**D. Selegiline (deprenyl):** This drug is a selective inhibitor of MAO type B, the enzyme form that metabolizes dopamine in preference to norepinephrine and serotonin. It may increase brain dopamine levels and act as an adjunctive agent to levodopa in Parkinson's disease.

**E. Acetylcholine-Blocking Drugs:** Antimuscarinic drugs may improve the tremor and rigidity of parkinsonism but have little effect on bradykinesia. The agents differ in potency and in their efficacy in different patients. CNS toxic effects include drowsiness, inattention, confusion, delusions, and hallucinations. Peripheral adverse effects are typical of atropinelike drugs.

## DRUG THERAPY OF OTHER MOVEMENT DISORDERS

**A. Tremor:** Physiologic and essential tremors are clinically similar conditions characterized by postural tremor. They may be alleviated by beta-adrenoceptor-blocking drugs such as **propranolol.** Such agents should be used with caution in patients with congestive heart failure, asthma, or hypoglycemia.

**B. Huntington's Disease:** This inherited disorder appears to result from a brain neurotransmitter imbalance such that GABA functions are diminished and dopaminergic functions are enhanced. There may also be a cholinergic deficit, since the choline acetyltransferase level is decreased in the basal ganglia. Drug therapy involves the use of amine-depleting drugs such as **tetrabenazine** or antipsychotic agents (such as **haloperidol** or a **phenothiazine**) that block dopamine receptors. Attempts to enhance brain GABA and acetylcholine activities by using drugs have not been successful in this disease.

**C. Drug-Induced Dyskinesias:** Parkinsonian symptoms caused by antipsychotic agents are usually reversible by lowering the drug dosage, changing the therapy to a drug that is less toxic to extrapyramidal function, or using muscarinic blockers. Levodopa and bromocriptine are not useful, because dopamine receptors are blocked by the antipsychotic drugs. **Tardive dyskinesias** that develop from neuroleptic therapy are possibly a form of denervation supersensitivity. They are not readily reversed, and no specific drug therapy is available.

**D. Wilson's Disease:** This recessively inherited disorder of copper metabolism results in hepatic and neurologic dysfunction. Treatment involves use of the chelating agent **penicillamine** (dimethylcysteine), which removes excess copper. Toxic effects of penicillamine include gastrointestinal distress, myasthenia, optic neuropathy, and blood dyscrasias.

# DRUG LIST

The following drugs are important members of the group discussed in this chapter. Prototype agents should be learned in detail; the other significant agents should be recognized as belonging to a specific subclass.

| Subclass | Prototype | Other Significant Agents |
|---|---|---|
| Dopamine agonists | Levodopa, bromocriptine | Pergolide |
| Indirect dopamine agonists | Amantadine, selegiline | |
| Levodopa adjuncts | Carbidopa | |
| Anticholinergic drugs | Benztropine | Biperiden, orphenadrine, trihexyphenidyl |

## QUESTIONS

**DIRECTIONS (items 1–4):** Each numbered item or incomplete statement in this section is followed by answers or by completions of the statement. Select the ONE lettered answer or completion that is BEST in each case.

**1.** All of the following statements concerning levodopa are accurate EXCEPT:
**(A)** Choreoathetosis of the face and distal extremities is an important unwanted effect
**(B)** Fluctuations in clinical response occur with increasing frequency as treatment continues
**(C)** It effectively antagonizes akinesia and tremor caused by antipsychotic drugs
**(D)** It should be avoided in patients with a history of melanoma

**2.** Which of the following statements about carbidopa is accurate?
**(A)** It crosses the blood-brain barrier
**(B)** It inhibits monoamine oxidase type A
**(C)** It is converted to the false transmitter, carbidopamine
**(D)** It inhibits aromatic L-amino acid decarboxylase
**(E)** It inhibits monoamine oxidase type B

**3.** All of the following statements about bromocriptine are accurate EXCEPT:
**(A)** It should not be administered to patients on antimuscarinic drugs
**(B)** It may cause pulmonary infiltrates
**(C)** It is contraindicated in patients with a history of psychosis
**(D)** It is a direct-acting dopamine receptor agonist

**4.** Concerning drugs and parkinsonism, all of the following statements are accurate EXCEPT:
**(A)** Useful therapeutic effects of amantadine may disappear after only a few weeks of treatment
**(B)** The toxic effects of MPTP on nigrostriatal dopaminerfic neurons depend on its prior metablolism via monoamine oxidase type B.
**(C)** The primary therapeutic benefit of antimuscarinic drugs in parkinsonism is their ability to relieve bradykinesia (akinesia)
**(D)** The limited efficacy of pergolide may be due to down-regulation of dopamine receptors
**(E)** Selegiline (deprenyl) may increase the adverse effects of levodopa

**DIRECTIONS (items 5–9):** Items 5–9 consist of lettered headings followed by a set of numbered statements. For each numbered statement, select the ONE lettered heading that is most closely associated with it. Each lettered heading may be selected once, more than once, or not at all.

**(A)** Amantadine
**(B)** Selegiline (deprenyl)
**(C)** Levodopa
**(D)** Trihexyphenidyl
**(E)** Pergolide

**5.** Contraindicated in prostatic hypertrophy and obstructive gastrointestinal disease.

**6.** Potentiates dopaminergic function possibly by increasing the release or blocking the reuptake of dopamine. Livedo reticularis may occur during treatment.

**7.** A drug recently approved for the treatment of parkinsonism. It directly stimulates both $D_1$ and $D_2$ dopamine receptors.

**8.** A selective inhibitor of monoamine oxidase type B.

**9.** This drug may cause hypertensive crisis if given with an inhibitor of monoamine oxidase type A, since it is a precursor of norepinephrine.

## ANSWERS

1. Levodopa, the mainstay of drug treatment of idiopathic parkinsonism, is not effective in antagonizing the akinesia, rigidity, and tremor caused by treatment with antipsychotic agents. The primary reason is that such drugs are potent blockers of dopamine receptors. Parkinsonlike side effects of neuroleptics are reversible when the dose is decreased and are attenuated by antimuscarinic agents. The answer is **(C)**.

2. Carbidopa is an inhibitor of aromatic L-amino acid decarboxylase, the enzyme that converts levodopa to dopamine. It acts only on the enzyme present in peripheral tissues (eg, liver), since it does not enter the CNS. Its use in combination with levodopa decreases the dose requirement and reduces peripheral side effects of levodopa. The answer is **(D)**.

3. The use of agents that promote dopaminergic transmission in combination with antimuscarinic drugs is common in the treatment of parkinsonism. Bromocriptine does not complicate treatment with antimuscarinic drugs or amantadine. It should be used at reduced doses if combined with levodopa to avoid intolerable side effects. The answer is **(A)**.

4. The drug most effective in relieving the bradykinesia of parkinsonism, and the disabilities arising from it, is levodopa. Antimuscarinic drugs may improve the tremor and rigidity of parkinsonism, but have little effect on bradykinesia. The answer is **(C)**.

5. Recall from autonomic pharmacology that the contraindications listed are typical for drugs that block acetylcholine at muscarinic receptors. Add to this list angle-closure glaucoma. The answer is **(D)**.

6. The antiviral agent amantadine has antiparkinsonism activity, possibly promoting dopaminergic neurotransmission by the mechanism listed. Its benefits may be short-lived, disappearing after only a few weeks of treatment. Its adverse effects include CNS excitation, peripheral edema, and dermatologic reactions. The answer is **(A)**.

7. Pergolide is approved for use in the treatment of parkinsonism. It is a dopamine receptor agonist similar to bromocriptine in its actions. The drug loses its efficacy with time, possibly owing to down-regulation of dopamine receptors. The answer is **(E)**.

8. Selegiline (deprenyl) inhibits monoamine oxidase type B, the enzyme that metabolizes dopamine. It may prove useful as an adjunctive agent to levodopa in parkinsonism. When used early in parkinsonism, selegiline can delay the requirement for levodopa. Its selective inhibitory action precludes untoward reactions with tyramine, which is metabolized by monoamine oxidase type A. The answer is **(B)**.

9. The only selection that is a catecholamine precursor is levodopa. Remember that the drug is a precursor of norepinephrine and epinephrine as well as dopamine, and that they are metabolized primarily by monoamine oxidase type A. The answer is **(C)**.

# Antipsychotic Drugs & Lithium

# 28

## OBJECTIVES

**Define the following terms:**

- Bipolar disorder
- Extrapyramidal reaction
- Neuroleptic
- Tardive dyskinesia
- Neuroleptic malignant syndrome

**You should be able to:**

- Describe the dopamine hypothesis of schizophrenia.
- List the major dopaminergic tracts in the CNS. mesocortical, mesolimbic, nigrostriatal
- Describe the behavioral effects of antipsychotic drugs on normal and schizophrenic individuals.
- List the adverse effects of the major antipsychotic drugs.
- Describe the pharmacokinetics and pharmacodynamics of lithium.

## CONCEPTS

### ANTIPSYCHOTIC DRUGS

The antipsychotic drugs (**neuroleptics**) are effective in controlling many of the symptoms of psychotic illness. Although not cured by drug therapy, the symptoms of schizophrenia (thought disorder, emotional withdrawal, and hallucinations or delusions) may be ameliorated by antipsychotic drugs. Chronic therapy, which is often needed, can result in severe toxicity in some patients.

**A. Classification:** The major chemical subgroups of antipsychotic drugs are the **phenothiazines** (chlorpromazine, thioridazine, fluphenazine); the **thioxanthenes** (thiothixene); and the **butyrophenones** (haloperidol). Several newer heterocyclic drugs (clozapine, loxapine, molindone) appear to be effective in schizophrenia and may have fewer extrapyramidal adverse effects than standard drugs.

**B. Pharmacokinetics:** The antipsychotic drugs are well absorbed when given orally and, because they are lipid-soluble, readily enter the CNS and most other body tissues. Many are bound extensively to plasma proteins. These agents require metabolism by liver enzymes prior to their elimination, and they have long plasma half-lives that permit once-daily dosage. Parenteral forms of fluphenazine, thioridazine, and haloperidol are used for rapid initiation of therapy. In the past, parenteral chlorpromazine was used for this purpose.

**C. Mechanism of Action:** The **dopamine hypothesis of schizophrenia** proposes that this psychotic disorder is caused by a *relative excess* of functional activity of the neurotransmitter dopamine in the brain. It is based on the following observations: (1) Most antipsychotic drugs block brain dopamine receptors. (2) Dopamine receptor-agonist drugs (eg, amphetamine, levodopa) exacerbate schizophrenia. (3) An increased density of dopamine receptors has been detected in certain brain regions of untreated schizophrenics.

**Blockade of dopamine receptors** in the mesocortical and mesolimbic pathways of the CNS is generally considered to be the mechanism of action of conventional antipsychotics. Binding affinity to the $D_2$ subclass of dopamine receptors correlates well with clinical antipsychotic potency. Some of these agents exert blocking actions on other brain neurotransmitter receptors including serotonin receptors and alpha adrenoceptors, but such actions do not correlate well with antipsychotic effects. The atypical drug clozapine has a higher affinity for $D_4$ and 5-$HT_2$ receptors than for $D_1$ or $D_2$ receptors.

**D. Effects:** The effects of antipsychotic drugs result from their interactions with receptors in the brain and in peripheral tissues.

1. **Dopamine receptor blockade.** Dopaminergic tracts in the brain include the mesocortical-mesolimbic pathways (mentation, mood), the nigrostriatal tract (extrapyramidal function), the tuberoinfundibular pathways (control of prolactin release), and the chemoreceptor trigger zone (emesis). Mesocortical-mesolimbic dopamine receptor blockade presumably underlies antipsychotic effects, and a similar action on the chemoreceptor trigger zone leads to useful antiemetic properties of some antipsychotic drugs. Adverse effects resulting from dopamine receptor blockade include extrapyramidal dysfunction and hyperprolactinemia.
2. **Muscarinic receptor blockade.** Atropinelike effects (dry mouth, constipation, urinary retention, and visual problems) are often pronounced during use of thioridazine and phenothiazines with aliphatic side-chains (chlorpromazine). Tolerance to some of these side effects may develop. Antimuscarinic CNS effects may include a toxic confusional state.
3. **Alpha-receptor blockade.** Postural hypotension, impotence, and failure to ejaculate occur; these effects are most likely with phenothiazines.
4. **$H_1$-receptor blockade.** Most often seen with short-side-chain phenothiazines, $H_1$-receptor blockade provides the basis for their use as antipruritics and may contribute to sedative effects.
5. **Sedation.** More marked with phenothiazines than with other antipsychotics, this sedation is normally perceived as unpleasant by nonpsychotic individuals.

## E. Clinical Use:

1. Treatment of schizophrenia. These drugs reduce hyperactivity, bizarre ideation, hallucinations, and delusions and thus facilitate the patient's functioning in an outpatient environment. There is no evidence that the different drugs have differing efficacies as antischizophrenic agents, but individual patients may respond more favorably to a particular drug. Clozapine is reported to be effective in some patients refractory to standard antipsychotic drugs.
2. Initial treatment of mania.
3. Management of psychotic aspects of schizoaffective disorders.
4. Treatment of Tourette's syndrome (especially haloperidol).
5. Use as antiemetics (eg, prochlorperazine), particularly in chemical or radiation-induced emesis.
6. Use as antipruritics in patients with intractable itching, and for preoperative sedation (eg, promethazine).

## F. Toxicity:

1. **Extrapyramidal adverse effects** that are dose-dependent include a **parkinsonismlike syndrome** (with akinesia, rigidity, and tremor), which is reversible with decrease in dose and antagonized by atropinelike drugs. This syndrome occurs more frequently with haloperidol and the more potent piperazine side-chain phenothiazines (eg, fluphenazine, trifluoperazine). Other extrapyramidal dysfunctions include akathisia and dystonias. Choreoathetoid movements of the face and tongue **(tardive dyskinesia)** may develop late in therapy and may be difficult to reverse upon drug discontinuance. Tardive dyskinesia may be attenuated by increasing neuroleptic dosage, which has led to the suggestion that this condition is caused by dopamine receptor sensitization.
2. **Autonomic adverse effects** include those due to blockade of peripheral muscarinic and alpha adrenoceptors. They may be more difficult to manage in elderly patients.
3. **Endocrine and metabolic effects** include weight gain, gynecomastia, the galactorrhea-amenorrhea syndrome, and infertility.
4. **The neuroleptic malignant syndrome** may occur in patients who are particularly sensitive to the extrapyramidal effects of antipsychotic drugs. Muscle rigidity, impairment of sweating, hyperpyrexia, and autonomic instability occur and may be life-threatening. Treatment involves the use of dopamine agonists and dantrolene.
5. **Miscellaneous toxicities.** Visual impairment caused by retinal deposits has occurred with thioridazine; this drug may also cause severe conduction defects in the heart. Clozapine causes a small but important (1–3%) incidence of agranulocytosis.
6. **Overdosage** with antipsychotics other than thioridazine is not usually fatal. Hypotension often responds to fluid replacement. Neuroleptics lower the convulsive threshold and may cause seizures, which are usually managed with diazepam or phenytoin. Thioridazine overdose, because of the drug's effect on cardiac conduction, is more difficult to treat.

## LITHIUM & TREATMENT OF BIPOLAR (MANIC-DEPRESSIVE) DISORDER

**A. Pharmacokinetics:** Lithium is absorbed rapidly and completely from the gut. It is distributed through body water and excreted by the kidneys with a half-life of about 20 hours. Plasma levels should be monitored from the start of therapy to establish an effective and safe dosage regimen. Thiazides interfere with the renal clearance of lithium and may increase plasma concentrations to toxic levels.

**B. Mechanism of Action:** The mechanism of action is not well defined. Lithium inhibits the recycling of neuronal membrane phosphoinositides involved in the generation of inositol trisphosphate ($IP_3$) and diacylglycerol (DAG), which act as second messengers in both alpha-adrenoceptor and muscarinic neurotransmission.

**C. Clinical Use:** Lithium is used in the treatment of bipolar affective disorder (manic-depressive disease). Maintenance therapy with lithium decreases manic behavior and modulates both the frequency and the magnitude of mood swings. Antipsychotic and sedative drug therapy may also be required, especially at the initiation of lithium treatment. The tricyclic antiepileptic drug carbamazepine has been used to treat mania in patients who respond inadequately to lithium.

**D. Toxicity:** Undesirable effects include tremor, sedation, leukocytosis, thyroid dysfunction, and reversible nephrogenic diabetes insipidus. Lithium may cause teratogenic effects.

## DRUG LIST

The following drugs are important members of the drug groups discussed in this chapter. Prototype agents should be learned in detail; the other significant agents should be recognized as belonging to a specific subclass. ***Note:*** Some authorities consider chlorpromazine obsolete because of its associated high incidence of toxic effects.

| Subclass | Prototype | Other Significant Agents |
|---|---|---|
| Phenothiazines | | |
| Aliphatic | Chlorpromazine | |
| Piperidine | Thioridazine | Mesoridazine |
| Piperazine | Trifluoperazine | Perphenazine, fluphenazine |
| Thioxanthenes | Thiothixene | |
| Butyrophenones | Haloperidol | |
| Dibenzoxapines | Loxapine, clozapine | |
| Dihydroindolones | Molindone | |
| Lithium | Lithium | |

## QUESTIONS

**DIRECTIONS (items 1–6):** Each numbered item or incomplete statement in this section is followed by answers or by completions of the statement. Select the ONE lettered answer or completion that is BEST in each case.

**1.** Concerning the dopamine hypothesis of schizophrenia, all of the following statements are accurate EXCEPT:
**(A)** Positron emission tomography has shown increased dopamine receptors in the brains of both untreated and drug-treated schizophrenics
**(B)** Psychotic effects may occur during treatment of a Parkinson's disease patient with dopamine receptor agonists
**(C)** Clinical potency of most antipsychotic drugs correlates well with their affinities for dopamine $D_1$ receptors
**(D)** Drug treatment of schizophrenics sometimes results in changes in the cerebrospinal fluid levels of the dopamine metabolite homovanillic acid

**2.** Pharmacodynamic properties of phenothiazines include all of the following EXCEPT
**(A)** antagonism at central and peripheral muscarinic receptors
**(B)** selective blockade of histamine $H_2$ receptors
**(C)** lowered seizure threshold
**(D)** alpha-adrenoceptor-blocking actions
**(E)** decreased psychomotor activity

**3.** The following statements concerning adverse effects of antipsychotic drugs are all accurate EXCEPT:
**(A)** Mydriasis and postural hypotension are likely side effects of chlorpromazine
**(B)** Retinal deposits occur with high doses of thioridazine
**(C)** Anticholinergic drugs usually reverse tardive dyskinesias
**(D)** Acute dystonic reactions usually respond to diphenhydramine
**(E)** Blood counts are mandatory during use of clozapine to detect agranulocytosis

**4.** Clinical uses of antipsychotic drugs include all of the following EXCEPT
**(A)** management of emesis during radiation therapy
**(B)** treatment of schizoaffective disorders
**(C)** management of Tourette's syndrome
**(D)** treatment of the amenorrhea-galactorrhea syndrome
**(E)** acute management of the manic phase of bipolar disorder

**5.** Akinesia, rigidity, and tremor occur more frequently during treatment with haloperidol than with thioridazine. The most likely explanation is that
**(A)** haloperidol has a low affinity for dopamine receptors
**(B)** thioridazine interacts specifically with serotonin receptors
**(C)** thioridazine has greater blocking actions on brain muscarinic receptors
**(D)** haloperidol acts presynaptically to stimulate dopamine release

**6.** All of the following statements concerning drug treatment of manic-depressive (bipolar) affective disorders are accurate EXCEPT:
**(A)** During pregnancy, lithium dosage must be lowered because its renal clearance is decreased
**(B)** Propranolol usually relieves the tremor that may occur at therapeutic dose levels of lithium
**(C)** Lithium dosage may have to be lowered in patients taking oral diuretics
**(D)** Patients unable to tolerate lithium may respond favorably to carbamazepine

**DIRECTIONS (items 7–11):** Items 7–11 consist of lettered headings followed by a set of numbered sentences. For each numbered sentence, select the ONE lettered heading that is most clearly associated with it. Each lettered heading may be selected once, more than once, or not at all.

**(A)** Bromocriptine
**(B)** Promethazine
**(C)** Lithium
**(D)** Trifluoperazine
**(E)** Thioridazine

**7.** The calming and antiemetic properties of this drug, together with its atropinelike and antihistaminic properties, form the basis for its nonpsychiatric use in preoperative sedation

**8.** This phenothiazine is a "high-potency" drug that, compared with chlorpromazine, is less sedating and causes less severe autonomic adverse effects

**9.** This drug may cause abnormal electrocardiograms, and cardiotoxicity is enhanced if it is administered with agents that have quinidinelike actions

**10.** This drug may be used to counteract the excessive dopamine receptor blockade characteristic of the neuroleptic malignant syndrome

**11.** Typical adverse effects of this drug include tremor, edema, and nephrogenic diabetes insipidus

---

## ANSWERS

**1.** Antipsychotic drugs block brain dopamine receptors, but they bind weakly to the $D_1$ receptor, and there is no correlation between their affinities for this receptor subtype and their clinical potency (in contrast to the strong correlation between $D_2$ receptor binding and clinical potency). All of the other statements are accurate. The answer is **(C).**

**2.** The phenothiazine antipsychotics block both muscarinic and alpha adrenoceptors. Sedative actions contribute to psychomotor depression, and they may lower the threshold to seizures. Although they antagonize histamine $H_1$ receptors, they have minimal effects on $H_2$ receptors and are not indicated for the management of peptic ulcers. The answer is **(B).**

**3.** Late-occurring choreoathetoid movements (tardive dyskinesias) are the most important adverse effect of antipsychotic drugs. They may be caused by a relative cholinergic deficiency, secondary to supersensitivity of striatal dopamine receptors. Anticholinergic drugs are not effective, and improvement may occur when antipsychotic drugs are discontinued. The answer is **(C).**

**4.** Hyperprolactinemia and the amenorrhea-galactorrhea syndrome may occur as an adverse effect during treatment with antipsychotic drugs because they block dopamine receptors in the tuberoinfundibular tract. The answer is **(D).**

**5.** Adverse effects resembling Parkinson's disease are more common with haloperidol than with thioridazine. The most likely explanation is that thioridazine exerts more pronounced blocking actions at brain muscarinic receptors. This action partly compensates for dopamine receptor blockade in the nigrostriatal tract such that extrapyramidal function is more effectively balanced. The answer is **(C).**

**6.** Reliance is placed on measurements of serum lithium concentrations for optimum dosage regimens. Lithium clearance is influenced by many factors including renal function, serum sodium concentration, hydration state, and the presence of other drugs. By increasing renal elimination of sodium, diuretics may decrease lithium clearance. In pregnancy lithium clearance is increased, necessitating a corresponding increase in lithium dose for effective maintenance. Note that lithium crosses the placental barrier and is excreted in breast milk. The answer is **(A).**

**7.** With the exception of thioridazine, phenothiazines exert strong antiemetic effects. Phenothiazines with short side-chains have marked histamine $H_1$ receptor-blocking action and are used for relief of pruritus, or, in the case of promethazine, as preoperative sedatives. The answer is **(B).**

**8.** Chlorpromazine is no more effective in the treatment of schizophrenia than are other drugs that have fewer adverse effects. The piperazine subclass of phenothiazines, which includes fluphenazine and trifluoperazine, are more potent than chlorpromazine and more specific in their pharmacologic effects. The answer is **(D).**

**9.** Thioridazine has several distinctive properties. At high doses it causes retinal deposits that, in advanced cases, resemble retinitis pigmentosa. It also has quinidinelike actions on the heart, and in overdose it may cause cardiac conduction block. The answer is **(E).**

**10.** The neuroleptic malignant syndrome is characterized by muscle rigidity, high fever, and autonomic instability. It may result from rapid block of dopamine receptors in patients who are highly sensitive to the extrapyramidal effects of antipsychotic drugs. Treatment involves the physical control of fever, the use of muscle relaxants (eg, dantrolene or diazepam), and the administration of the dopamine receptor agonist bromocriptine. The answer is **(A).**

**11.** The adverse effects described are typical of lithium. The answer is **(C).**

# 29 Antidepressants

## OBJECTIVES

**Define the following terms:**

- Endogenous depression
- Tricyclic antidepressant
- Bipolar affective disorder
- Amine hypothesis of mood
- Second-generation antidepressant

**You should be able to:**

- Describe the probable mechanisms and the major pharmacodynamic properties of tricyclic antidepressants.
- List the toxic effects that occur during chronic therapy with tricyclic antidepressants.
- Describe the therapeutic use and toxic effects of MAO inhibitors.
- Identify second-generation antidepressants and their distinctive properties.
- Identify the major drug interactions associated with the use of antidepressant drugs.

## CONCEPTS

Depression is a common medical condition with both psychologic and physical symptoms. The 3 major types are (1) **reactive depression,** which is a response to external events; (2) **bipolar affective (manic-depressive) disorder,** which is discussed in Chapter 28; and (3) **endogenous depression,** which is a depression of mood without any obvious medical or situational causes. Three groups of drugs are used to treat endogenous depression: the **tricyclic antidepressants;** the **second-generation**

**agents,** which are related to the tricyclic agents; and the **monoamine oxidase inhibitors.** The **amine hypothesis of mood** postulates that brain amines, particularly norepinephrine and serotonin, are neurotransmitters in pathways that function in the expression of mood states. According to the amine hypothesis, a functional decrease in the activity of such amines would result in depression; a functional increase of activity would result in mood elevation. Difficulties with this hypothesis include the facts that (1) antidepressant drugs cause an immediate change in amine activity but require weeks to achieve clinical effects; and (2) these drugs cause a slow *down*-regulation of amine receptors.

### A. Classification & Pharmacokinetics:

1. The tricyclic drugs (eg, **imipramine, amitriptyline**) are structurally related to the phenothiazine antipsychotics and share some of their pharmacologic effects. They are well absorbed orally but may undergo first-pass metabolism. Extensive hepatic metabolism is required prior to their elimination, and they may form active metabolites. Their plasma half-lives usually permit once-daily dosing.
2. The second-generation drugs **(amoxapine, fluoxetine, maprotiline, trazodone)** have varied chemical structures. Their pharmacokinetics are similar to those of the tricyclic drugs.
3. The MAO inhibitors (eg, **phenelzine, tranylcypromine**) are structurally related to amphetamines. Tranylcypromine is faster in onset but has a shorter duration of action than do other MAO inhibitors. They are all inhibitors of hepatic drug-metabolizing enzymes and cause many drug interactions.

### B. Mechanism of Action:

1. **Acute effect.** The acute effect of tricyclic drugs is to inhibit the uptake mechanisms responsible for the termination of the synaptic actions of both norepinephrine and serotonin in the brain. This is thought to result in potentiation of their neurotransmitter actions. The MAO inhibitors increase brain amine levels by interfering with their metabolism; this is presumed to enhance their actions as neurotransmitters. The acute actions of certain second-generation drugs appear to result from the selective block of reuptake of norepinephrine (eg, with maprotiline) or serotonin (eg, with fluoxetine). The potential sites of action of antidepressants are shown in Fig 29–1.
2. **Chronic effect.** Our understanding of mechanisms of these drugs is complicated by the fact that chronic treatment of animals with antidepressant drugs causes a down-regulation of brain

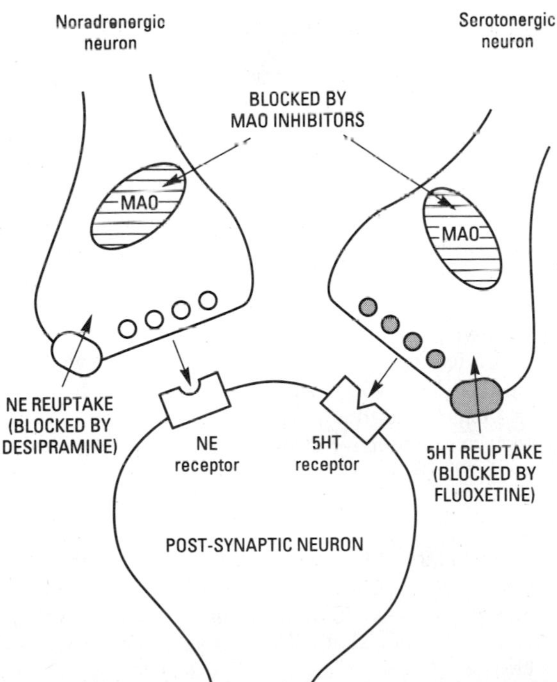


**Figure 29–1.** Possible sites of action of antidepressant drugs. Blockade of the reuptake of brain norepinephrine and serotonin increases the synaptic activities of the neurotransmitters. Inhibition of MAO increases the presynaptic levels of both norepinephrine and serotonin, which leads to increased neurotransmitter effects. These are acute actions of antidepressants; chronic therapy may lead to down-regulation of brain beta receptors.

**Table 29–1. Pharmacodynamics of common tricyclic antidepressants and newer "second-generation" agents.[1]**

| Drug | Sedation | Muscarinic Receptor Blockade | Inhibition of Reuptake of | |
|---|---|---|---|---|
| | | | Norepinephrine | Serotonin |
| Amitriptyline | +++ | +++ | ++ | +++ |
| Amoxapine | ++ | + | ++ | + |
| Desipramine | + | + | +++ | – |
| Doxepin | +++ | +++ | + | ++ |
| Fluoxetine | + | + | – | +++ |
| Imipramine | ++ | + | + | ++ |
| Maprotiline | ++ | + | +++ | - |
| Nortriptyline | ++ | + | + | + |
| Protriptyline | – | ++ | +++ | – |
| Trazodone | +++ | – | - | + |

[1] – = none; + = slight; ++ = moderate; +++ = marked

norepinephrine receptors, especially beta adrenoceptors. This change in adrenoceptors may result in a decrease in the neurotransmitter actions of norepinephrine, an action that is not in simple accord with the amine hypothesis of mood. Down-regulation of beta receptors also occurs during treatment with MAO inhibitors or selective blockers of serotonin reuptake.

### C. Effects:

1. **Amine uptake blockade** is a major property of tricyclics and most second-generation drugs. Inhibition of the norepinephrine and serotonin uptake mechanisms varies (Table 29–1). Norepinephrine reuptake is blocked in the autonomic nervous system (as well as the CNS), which may lead to sympathomimetic effects.
2. **Sedation** is a common CNS effect of tricyclic drugs (least with protriptyline and desipramine) and of second-generation drugs (Table 29–1). In contrast, MAO inhibitors may be mildly stimulating.
3. **Muscarinic receptor blockade** occurs with all tricyclics but is particularly marked with amitriptyline and doxepin (Table 29–1). The newer agents appear to be less potent antimuscarinics, and atropinelike effects are minimal with trazodone.
4. **Cardiovascular effects** include hypotension from alpha-adrenoceptor blockade (tricyclics) and depression of cardiac conduction. The latter effect may lead to arrhythmias.
5. **Convulsive threshold** is lowered by tricyclic drugs, and MAO inhibitors may also cause seizures if they are taken in overdosage.

### D. Clinical Use:

1. The management of endogenous depression is the major use of this class of drugs. A variable therapeutic response of patients to individual drugs is characteristic. Tricyclic drugs are thought to be most useful in patients with psychomotor retardation, sleep disturbances, poor appetite, weight loss, and decreased libido. MAO inhibitors may be most useful in patients with significant anxiety, phobic features, and hypochondriasis.
2. Second-generation drugs may prove to be as effective as tricyclics, possibly with fewer adverse effects. Their use is rapidly increasing, particularly in refractory cases of depression.
3. Additional clinical uses of tricyclic drugs include the treatment of enuresis, chronic pain states, acute panic attacks, phobias and obsessive-compulsive disorders (clomipramine).
4. *Tricyclic antidepressants are not recommended for use as anxiolytics.*

### E. Toxicity:

1. The adverse effects of tricyclic antidepressants, in large part predictable from their pharmacodynamics, include the following: (1) excessive sedation, lassitude, fatigue, and, sometimes, confusion; (2) sympathomimetic effects, including tachycardia, agitation, sweating, and insomnia; (3) atropinelike effects; (4) orthostatic hypotension, EEG abnormalities, and cardiomyopathies; and (5) tremor and paresthesias.
2. Drug interactions with tricyclics include additive depression of the CNS with other central

depressants, including ethanol, barbiturates, benzodiazepines, and narcotic-analgesics. Tricyclics may also cause a reversal of the antihypertensive action of guanethidine (and possibly methyldopa and clonidine) by blockade of its active accumulation into sympathetic nerve endings.

3. Overdosage of tricyclics is extremely hazardous, and its manifestations include (1) coma, with shock; (2) respiratory depression; (3) hyperpyrexia; (4) agitation, delirium, neuromuscular irritability, and convulsions; and (5) cardiac conduction defects and arrhythmias.
4. Second-generation antidepressants usually have less sedative effect and sometimes less muscarinic blocking action than conventional tricyclics do. Amoxapine is a dopamine receptor blocker and may cause akathisia, parkinsonism, and the amenorrhea-galactorrhea syndrome. Fluoxetine use is reported to lead to agitation and increased suicidal ideation in some patients. This claim is not yet documented. Overdose of amoxapine causes seizures, and with maprotiline both convulsant and cardiotoxic effects occur.
5. Toxic effects of MAO inhibitors include hypertensive reactions, hyperthermia, and CNS stimulation, leading to agitation and convulsions. Hypertensive crisis may occur in patients taking MAO inhibitors who consume food that contains high concentrations of tyramine (eg, fermented food). Overdosage of MAO inhibitors may result in shock, hyperthermia, and seizures.

## DRUG LIST

The following drugs are important members of the group discussed in this chapter. Prototype agents should be learned in detail; the major variants should be known well enough to list the factors that distinguish them from the prototypes and from each other; and the other significant agents should be recognized as belonging to a specific subclass.

| Subclass | Prototype | Major Variants | Other Significant Agents |
|---|---|---|---|
| Tricyclic drugs | Imipramine, amitriptyline | Desipramine, nortriptyline | Doxepin, protriptyline |
| Second-generation drugs | Amoxapine, fluoxetine, maprotiline, trazodone | | |
| MAO inhibitors | Phenelzine | Tranylcypromine | Isocarboxazid |

## QUESTIONS

**DIRECTIONS (items 1–5):** Each numbered item or incomplete statement in this section is followed by answers or by completions of the statement. Select the ONE lettered answer or completion that is BEST in each case.

1. Effects of the tricyclic antidepressant drugs include all of the following EXCEPT
   **(A)** sympathomimetic actions
   **(B)** alpha-adrenoceptor blockade
   **(C)** atropinelike effects
   **(D)** sedation
   **(E)** elevation of the seizure threshold

2. Concerning the proposed mechanisms of action of antidepressant drugs, all of the following statements are accurate EXCEPT:
   (A) The acute effect of amitriptyline is to block the neuronal reuptake of both norepinephrine and serotonin in the CNS
   (B) Neurochemically, endogenous depression has been characterized in terms of decreased functional activity at certain noradrenergic or serotonergic synapses
   (C) Chronic treatment with tricyclics leads to an increase in the number of beta adrenoceptors in the brain
   (D) Phenelzine and tranylcypromine decrease the metabolism of norepinephrine, serotonin, and dopamine

3. Regarding the clinical use of antidepressant drugs all of the following statements are accurate EXCEPT:
   (A) Tricyclics are most likely to be effective in depressions characterized by psychomotor retardation, poor appetite, and weight loss
   (B) In selecting an appropriate drug for treatment of depression, the history of patient response to specific drugs is a valuable guide
   (C) In the treatment of depression imipramine is usually more effective than amitriptyline
   (D) MAO inhibitors are more likely to be effective in depressions with attendant anxiety and phobic features
   (E) Enuresis is an established indication for the use of tricyclics

4. Known drug interactions involving antidepressants include all of the following EXCEPT
   (A) increased antihypertensive effects of clonidine with tricyclics
   (B) hypertensive crisis in patients on MAO inhibitors who ingest foods containing tyramine
   (C) behavioral excitation and hypertension when meperidine is administered to patients on MAO inhibitors
   (D) additive impairment of driving ability when ethanol is ingested by a patient taking a tricyclic antidepressant
   (E) prolongation of tricyclic drug half-life when cimetidine is administered

5. Signs and symptoms of conventional tricyclic drug overdose include all of the following EXCEPT
   (A) neuromuscular irritability and seizures
   (B) respiratory depression, and tendency to sudden apnea
   (C) coma, with shock and sometimes metabolic acidosis
   (D) cardiac conduction defects and arrhythmias
   (E) tremor at rest, dystonic reactions, and akathisia

**DIRECTIONS (items 6–10):** Items 6–10 consist of lettered headings followed by a set of numbered statements. For each numbered statement, select the ONE lettered heading that is most closely associated with it. Each lettered heading may be selected once, more than once, or not at all.

(A) Amoxapine
(B) Amitriptyline
(C) Isocarboxazid
(D) Maprotiline
(E) Fluoxetine

6. A tetracyclic drug with fewer sedative and atropinelike side effects than conventional tricyclic drugs. Seizures may occur at the top of its therapeutic dose range.

7. A newer and more selective blocker of the neuronal reuptake of serotonin. It has been claimed that this drug may promote suicidal thoughts in some depressed patients.

8. This drug is a hydrazide derivative that binds irreversibly to monoamine oxidase types A and B, resulting in prolonged inhibition of amine metabolism.

**9.** This second-generation antidepressant has marked dopamine receptor-blocking action. It may cause dangerous neurotoxicity in overdose.

**10.** Acutely, this drug enhances neurotransmission at both norepinephrine and serotonin receptors in the brain. It has marked sedative and atropinelike effects.

## ANSWERS

**1.** Tricyclics modify sympathetic effects through blockade of norepinephrine reuptake at peripheral neuroeffector junctions and by alpha-adrenoceptor blockade. Sedation and atropinelike side effects are common. In contrast to sedative-hypnotics, tricyclics lower the threshold to seizures. The answer is **(E).**

**2.** Chronic treatment with tricyclic antidepressants results in the down-regulation of beta adrenoceptors, such that receptor number and/or ligand-binding affinity decrease. The answer is **(C).**

**3.** There is no evidence that any individual tricyclic drug is more effective than another in terms of antidepressant efficacy. Although an individual patient may respond more favorably to a specific drug, controlled group comparison studies show that the tricyclic drugs are equivalent in their effectiveness as antidepressants. The answer is **(C).**

**4.** Tricyclic drugs block neuronal uptake of several antihypertensives, including guanethidine, reversing their effects on blood pressure. Although the precise mechanism is not defined, they also block the antihypertensive effects of clonidine. The $H_2$ blocker cimetidine is a potent inhibitor of liver drug-metabolizing enzymes and has been implicated in many drug interactions. The answer is **(A).**

**5.** Tricyclic antidepressant overdose is a medical emergency. Cardiac toxicity is difficult to manage and requires the use of drugs with the least effect on cardiac conductivity (eg, lidocaine, phenytoin). Although neuromuscular irritability and seizures may occur, extrapyramidal dysfunction does not result from overdose with conventional tricyclics. However, akathisia and parkinsonism may occur with amoxapine overdose. The answer is **(E).**

**6.** Maprotiline is chemically similar to desipramine, except that it has a tetracyclic structure. It exerts less sedative and muscarinic receptor-blocking action than conventional tricyclics, but has caused seizures at the top of its recommended dose range. The answer is **(D).**

**7.** Fluoxetine is now used widely in the treatment of depression. It is a selective blocker of serotonin reuptake and has minimal effects on noradrenergic neurotransmission in the brain or periphery. In some patients fluoxetine has been claimed to trigger agitation, mania, and suicidal ideation. The answer is **(E).**

**8.** Isocarboxazid is the only monoamine oxidase inhibitor listed. Unlike tranylcypromine, it binds irreversibly to monoamine oxidase and inhibition may persist after the drug is no longer detectable in the plasma. The answer is **(C).**

**9.** Amoxapine is a metabolite of the antipsychotic drug loxapine and retains dopamine receptor-blocking action. This results in adverse effects commonly associated with antipsychotic drug use, including akathisia, parkinsonian symptoms, and hyperprolactinemia. The answer is **(A).**

**10.** Blockade of neuronal reuptake of both norepinephrine and serotonin, combined with marked sedative and atropinelike effects, are characteristic actions of conventional tricyclic antidepressants such as amitriptyline. The answer is **(B).**

# 30 Opioid Analgesics & Antagonists

## OBJECTIVES

**Define the following terms:**

- Opiate, opioid
- Opiopeptin
- Agonist, antagonist
- Mixed agonist-antagonist
- Tolerance
- Psychologic dependence
- Physical dependence
- Cross-tolerance

**You should be able to:**

- List the receptors affected by opioid analgesics and the endogenous opioid peptides.
- Rank the major opioid analgesic agonists in terms of the relative intensity of their action at receptors.
- Identify the drugs that are opioid receptor antagonists and those that have mixed agonist-antagonist activity.
- Describe the main pharmacodynamic and pharmacokinetic properties of agonist opioid analgesics and list their clinical uses.
- List the main toxic effects of acute and chronic use of opioid analgesics.
- Describe the clinical uses of the opioid receptor antagonists.

## CONCEPTS

**A. Classification:** Opioid analgesics belong to several chemical subgroups, including phenanthrenes (eg, morphine, codeine), phenylheptylamines (eg, methadone), phenylpiperidines (eg, meperidine, fentanyl), morphinans (eg, butorphanol), and benzomorphans (eg, pentazocine). Morphine and other derivatives of the opium poppy are called **opiates.** Compounds that act on the morphine receptor to produce morphinelike effects are called **opioids.** The opioid analgesic and antagonist group can be subdivided in several ways:

1. Strength of analgesia (strong, moderate, and mild agonists).
2. Ratio of agonist to antagonist effects (agonists, mixed agonist-antagonists, and antagonists).
3. Spectrum of effects (analgesics, antitussives, and antidiarrheal drugs).

**B. Pharmacokinetics:** Most drugs in this class are well absorbed, but morphine, hydromorphone, and oxymorphone undergo extensive first-pass metabolism when taken orally. Opioid analgesics cross the placental barrier and exert effects on the fetus that can result in both respiratory depression and physical dependence (with continuous exposure) in neonates. The drugs undergo metabolism by hepatic enzymes, usually to inactive conjugates, prior to their elimination by the kidneys. The duration of their analgesic effects ranges from 2 to 5 hours (longer for methadone), and may increase in patients with hepatic dysfunction.

**C. Mechanism of Action:** The following sections (C through G) apply to most opioids, including the strong agonists.

1. **Receptors.** The effects of opioid analgesics are usually explained in terms of their interactions with specific **opioid receptors** in the CNS and peripheral tissues. Among the several receptor subtypes identified so far, 3 are selectively involved in their actions.
   a. Mu ($\mu$) receptors are responsible for supraspinal analgesia, euphoria, and respiratory and physical dependence effects.
   b. Kappa ($\kappa$) receptors appear to mediate spinal analgesia and the sedative and miotic effects.
   c. Sigma ($\sigma$) receptors may be responsible for hallucinogenic and cardiac stimulant properties.
2. **Peptides.** Opioid receptors are thought to be activated by endogenous chemicals under phys-

iologic conditions. Several naturally occurring peptides **(opiopeptins)** that produce morphinelike effects have been identified; these include 2 pentapeptides (leu-enkephalin and met-enkephalin), a 17-amino acid peptide (dynorphin), and a 31-amino-acid peptide (beta-endorphin). These peptides bind to opioid receptors and can be displaced from binding by opioid antagonists. Although it remains unclear whether these peptides function as classic neurotransmitters, they do appear to modulate synaptic transmission at many sites in the brain.

3. **Second messengers.** The mechanisms involved in the expression of opioid actions subsequent to the activation of their receptors are unclear. Certain opioid receptors are coupled to adenylyl cyclase and may modulate the functions of cyclic AMP. The acute actions of opioids also include inhibition of calcium entry into neurons and an increase in potassium ion conductance. These actions may be relevant to the observed inhibitory effects of both exogenous opioids and opiopeptins on the electrical activity of neurons in many regions of the CNS.

**D. Acute Effects:** The acute effects of opioids include the following:

1. **Analgesia,** through interactions with both spinal cord and brain receptors. These drugs are the most powerful ones available for the relief of pain. Prolonged analgesia, with some reduction in adverse effects, can be achieved with epidural administration of certain opioid analgesics.
2. **Sedation** and **euphoria,** which may occur at low dosage. Some patients experience dysphoria. At higher concentrations the drugs may cause mental clouding and result in a stuporous state called narcosis.
3. **Respiratory depression,** which occurs through inhibition of the respiratory center in the medulla, with decreased response to carbon dioxide challenge. Increased $PCO_2$ may cause cerebral vascular dilatation, with increased blood flow, leading to increased intracranial pressure.
4. **Suppression of the cough reflex,** which is the basis for the clinical use of opioids as antitussives.
5. **Nausea and vomiting,** which result from activation of the chemoreceptor trigger zone. These effects are increased by ambulation.
6. **Constipation,** which occurs through decreased intestinal peristalsis. This effect is the basis for the clinical use of these drugs as antidiarrheal agents.
7. **Smooth muscle effects,** including biliary tract constriction (which may cause biliary colic), increased ureteral and bladder tone, and a reduction in uterine tone that may contribute to a prolongation of labor.
8. **Miosis** (pupillary constriction) is a characteristic effects of opioids.

**E. Chronic Effects:** The effects of chronic use of opioid analgesics include the following:

1. **Tolerance** that develops to the above pharmacologic effects (with the exception of miosis and constipation) may be marked. There is **cross-tolerance** between different opioids.
2. **Dependence** (both psychologic and physical) is part of the basis for the abuse liability of many drugs in this group, particularly the strong agonists. Physical dependence is revealed on abrupt discontinuance as an **abstinence syndrome,** which includes rhinorrhea, lacrimation, chills, gooseflesh, muscle aches, diarrhea, anxiety, and hostility. A more intense state of **precipitated withdrawal** results when an opioid antagonist is administered to a physically dependent individual.

**F. Clinical Use:** The most important clinical uses of these drugs are as follows:

1. Treatment of relatively constant moderate to severe pain. See the Drug List for examples in each category.
2. Cough suppression. Specific drugs include codeine and dextromethorphan.
3. Treatment of diarrhea. Specific drugs include diphenoxylate and loperamide.
4. Management of acute pulmonary edema.
5. Preoperative medications and intraoperative adjunctive agents in anesthesia.
6. Maintenance programs (eg, with methadone) for addicts.

**G. Toxicity:** Most of the adverse effects of the opioid analgesics are predictable from their pharmacologic effects.

1. Overdosage leads to coma with hypotension and marked respiratory depression, with possible fatal consequences if untreated. Suspected overdosage may be confirmed by intravenous in-

jection of the antagonist drug naloxone. Treatment involves the use of antagonists and other therapeutic measures, including respiratory support.

2. The most important **drug interactions** involving opioid analgesics are additive CNS depression with ethanol, sedative-hypnotics, anesthetics, antipsychotic drugs, tricyclic antidepressants, and antihistamines. Concomitant use of certain opioids with MAO inhibitors increases the incidence of hyperpyrexic coma.

**H. Agonist-Antagonist Drugs:** These agents differ from the conventional agonist opioids in several ways.

1. **Analgesic activity.** The analgesic activity of some (eg, buprenorphine, butorphanol, nalbuphine) may be equivalent to that of strong agonists; others have efficacy similar to that of an moderate agonist (eg, pentazocine).
2. **Receptors.** Butorphanol, nalbuphine, and pentazocine are strong kappa agonists. They have weak mu receptor activity (nalbuphine is a mu-receptor antagonist), which leads to unpredictable effects if these drugs are used together with pure agonists. Buprenorphine is a partial agonist at mu receptors. It has a long duration of action since it binds strongly to such receptors, and this property renders its effects resistant to naloxone reversal.
3. **Effects.** These drugs usually cause sedation at analgesic doses, and dizziness, sweating, and nausea may occur. Anxiety, hallucinations, and nightmares are possible adverse effects. Respiratory depression may be less common than with pure agonists. Tolerance develops with chronic use, but is less strong than tolerance to the pure agonists, and there is minimal cross-tolerance. Physical dependence occurs, but the abuse liability of mixed agonist-antagonist drugs is less than that of morphine and meperidine.

**I. Opioid Antagonists: Naloxone** and **naltrexone** are pure opioid receptor antagonists that have few other effects at doses which produce marked antagonism of agonist effects. Their major clinical use is in the management of acute opioid overdosage. At higher doses, naloxone may be useful in the treatment of shock and spinal cord injury. Naloxone has a short duration of action (1–2 hours).

## DRUG LIST

The following drugs are important members of the group discussed in this chapter. Prototype agents should be learned in detail; the major variants should be known well enough to list the factors that distinguish them from the prototypes and each other; and the other significant agents should be recognized as belonging to a specific subclass.

| Subclass | Prototype | Major Variants | Other Significant Agents |
|---|---|---|---|
| Strong agonists | Morphine | Heroin, meperidine, methadone | Fentanyl |
| Moderate agonists | Codeine | | Oxycodone, hydrocodone |
| Weak agonists | Propoxyphene | | |
| Mixed agonist-antagonists | Pentazocine | Nalbuphine | Buprenorphine, butorphanol |
| Antagonists | Naloxone | Naltrexone | |
| Antitussive | Dextromethorphan | | |
| Antidiarrheal | Diphenoxylate | | |

## QUESTIONS

**DIRECTIONS (items 1–6):** Each numbered item or incomplete statement in this section is followed by answers or by completions of the statement. Select the ONE lettered answer or completion that is BEST in each case.

**1.** All of the following statements about opioid analgesics are accurate EXCEPT:
**(A)** They have no significant direct effects on the heart
**(B)** They stimulate the chemoreceptor trigger zone
**(C)** They relax the smooth muscle of the bladder
**(D)** They decrease intestinal peristalsis
**(E)** They cross the placental barrier

**2.** The interaction of opioid analgesics with kappa receptors leads to all of the following EXCEPT
**(A)** sedation
**(B)** cerebral vascular dilatation
**(C)** spinal analgesia
**(D)** pupillary constriction

**3.** Opiopeptins (opioid peptides) are released from larger precursor peptides. Which ONE of the following is released from pro-opiomelanocortin (POMC)?
**(A)** Beta-endorphin
**(B)** Leu-enkephalin
**(C)** Somatostatin
**(D)** Dynorphin
**(E)** Substance P

**4.** With continued use of strong opioid analgesics, tolerance develops to all of the following effects EXCEPT
**(A)** sedation
**(B)** analgesia
**(C)** constipation
**(D)** decreased response to carbon dioxide challenge

**5.** Which of the following is LEAST likely to be a contraindication to the use of morphine?
**(A)** Head injury
**(B)** Borderline respiratory reserve
**(C)** Adrenal insufficiency
**(D)** Pregnancy
**(E)** Pulmonary edema

**6.** Which of the following will most effectively relieve the symptoms of the abstinence syndrome in a heroin addict?
**(A)** Naloxone
**(B)** Codeine
**(C)** Acetaminophen
**(D)** Morphine
**(E)** Dextromethorphan

**DIRECTIONS (items 7–10):** Items 7–10 consist of lettered headings followed by a set of numbered statements. For each numbered statement, select the ONE lettered heading that is most closely associated with it. Each lettered heading may be selected once, more than once, or not at all.

**(A)** Dextromethorphan
**(B)** Nalbuphine
**(C)** Methadone
**(D)** Codeine
**(E)** Naltrexone

7. This drug has analgesic efficacy equivalent to morphine. It is an antagonist at mu receptors.

8. This antagonist drug has been proposed as a maintenance drug for addicts in treatment programs. A single oral dose will block the effects of injected heroin for up to 48 hours.

9. This drug is free of analgesic and addictive properties and only rarely causes constipation. It is an effective antitussive.

10. This drug is a full agonist at opioid receptors. It has analgesic activity equivalent to that of morphine, but its actions are more prolonged. Withdrawal signs on abrupt discontinuance are milder than those with morphine.

## ANSWERS

1. The opioids commonly cause contraction of smooth muscle. They constrict biliary ducts and increase both ureteral and bladder tone. Increased urethral sphincter tone may precipitate urinary retention. Although they increase intestinal smooth muscle tone, they reduce propulsive movements (peristalsis). In contrast, opioids decrease uterine tone—probably via central mechanisms—and may prolong labor. The answer is **(C).**

2. Increases in cerebral blood flow and (possibly) increased intracranial pressure result from the respiratory depressant actions of opioid analgesics. These effects are due to increased arterial $PCO_2$, which results from inhibition of the medullary respiratory center following interaction of opioids with mu receptors. The answer is **(B).**

3. POMC contains both beta-endorphin and met-enkephalin, in addition to adrenocorticotropic hormone and a melanocyte-stimulating peptide. The answer is **(A).**

4. Tolerance does not develop to pupillary constriction and the constipating effects of opioid agonists. The answer is **(C).**

5. Intravenous morphine effectively relieves dyspnea from pulmonary edema associated with left ventricular failure. The mechanism is not clear but may involve a decrease in perception of shortness of breath, relief of anxiety, and reductions in cardiac preload (decreased venous tone) and afterload (decreased peripheral resistance). The answer is **(E).**

6. Prevention of signs and symptoms of withdrawal after chronic use of a strong opiate such as heroin requires replacement with another strong opioid analgesic drug. Codeine is not effective. The antagonist naloxone actually precipitates an abstinence syndrome in a person who is physically dependent on opioids. The answer is **(D).**

7. Mixed agonist-antagonist drugs may have analgesic efficacy equivalent to that of strong agonists. This is the case for nalbuphine despite its antagonist action at mu receptors. Use of drugs in the agonist-antagonist subclass may lead to unpredictable analgesia if combined with full agonists. Although they are less likely to cause respiratory depression than are conventional opioid analgesics, when this does occur it may be difficult to reverse with opioid antagonists. The answer is **(B).**

8. The opioid antagonist naltrexone has a much longer half-life than naloxone, and its effects may last as long as 2 days. A high degree of client compliance would be required if naltrexone were to be of value in treatment programs. The answer is **(E).**

9. Dextromethorphan is the dextrorotatory stereoisomer of levorphanol. It has no appreciable analgesic activity and minimal abuse liability. It causes less constipation than codeine, also an effective antitussive. The answer is **(A).**

**10.** The full agonists fentanyl, hydromorphone, meperidine, methadone, and oxymorphone are all equivalent to morphine in analgesic efficacy. Methadone has the greatest bioavailability of those drugs used orally, and its effects are more prolonged. Tolerance and physical dependence develop more slowly with methadone than with morphine. These properties underlie the use of methadone for detoxification and in maintenance programs. The answer is **(C).**

# Drugs of Abuse 31

## OBJECTIVES

**Define the following terms:**

- Abstinence syndrome
- Controlled substance
- Designer drug
- Functional tolerance
- Metabolic tolerance
- Physical dependence
- Psychologic dependence
- Withdrawal

**You should be able to:**

- List the main factors that contribute to drug abuse.
- Describe the main actions of drugs that are commonly abused in the USA.
- Describe the main signs and symptoms of withdrawal from opioid analgesics and from sedative-hypnotics, including ethanol.
- Identify the most likely cause of fatalities from commonly abused agents.

## CONCEPTS

**A. Drug Abuse:** This term is usually taken to mean the use of an illicit drug, or the excessive or nonmedical use of a licit drug. It also denotes the deliberate use of chemicals that are generally not considered drugs (in the lay public sense of the term) but may be harmful to the user. The motivation for drug abuse appears to be the anticipated feeling of pleasure derived from the CNS effects of the drug. If physical dependence is present, prevention of an abstinence syndrome acts as a reinforcement to continued drug abuse.

**B. Dependence:** Dependence may be psychologic, physical, or both.

1. **Psychologic dependence** consists of the compulsive use of drugs to relieve or prevent the anxiety engendered by their withdrawal.
2. **Physical dependence** consists of an altered state such that withdrawal of the drug causes physiologic disturbances **(an abstinence syndrome)**, which can include both central and peripheral dysfunction.

**C. Tolerance:** This is defined as decreased responsiveness to a drug that develops during continued use.

1. **Metabolic tolerance** may result from an increase in the rate of metabolism of the drug.
2. **Functional tolerance,** which is more common than metabolic tolerance, results from pharmacodynamic alterations that are not well understood but may include down-regulation of drug receptors or compensatory changes in enzymes and other cellular components.

**D. Controlled Substances:** This term denotes drugs that have been categorized by the government on the basis of their abuse liability. Schedules of controlled substances link potential abuse liability to the ways that such drugs can be prescribed legally by practitioners. An example of such a schedule promulgated by the United States Drug Enforcement Agency is shown in Table 31–1. Note that the criteria given by the agency do not always reflect the actual pharmacologic properties of the drugs. Controlled substance schedules are presumed to reflect current attitudes toward substance abuse, and therefore the decision of which drugs are regulated depends, to some extent, on a social judgment.

**E. Designer Drugs:** This term refers to illicitly synthesized compounds that have small structural modifications from standard drugs without any major change in pharmacodynamics. Such chemical congeners, particularly those related to the opioids or the psychostimulant amines, are constantly being produced illegally. The schedules of controlled substances require constant revision to counter these attempts to produce substances that are not currently listed.

## MAJOR CATEGORIES

**A. Sedative-Hypnotics:** This class of drugs is responsible for many cases of drug abuse in the United States, western European countries, and Japan. The group includes **ethanol, barbiturates,** and **benzodiazepines,** all of which are more readily available to the general public than are opioids, cocaine, or hallucinogens. Benzodiazepines are the most commonly prescribed drugs for anxiety and, as Schedule IV drugs, are judged by the US government to have low abuse liability. Ethanol is not listed in schedules of controlled substances with abuse liability since it is rarely prescribed.

1. **Effects.** Sedative-hypnotics are CNS depressants, and their effects are enhanced by concomitant use of opioid analgesics, antipsychotic agents, and antihistamines with sedative properties. Acute overdoses commonly result in death through depression of the medullary respiratory and cardiovascular centers. Sedative-hypnotics reduce inhibitions, suppress anxiety, and produce relaxation. All of these actions are thought to induce development of psychologic dependence.
2. **Withdrawal.** Physical dependence occurs with continued use, and the signs and symptoms of the abstinence syndrome are most pronounced with drugs that have a half-life of less than 24 hours (ethanol, secobarbital, methaqualone). However, they can occur with any sedative-hypnotic, including the longer-acting benzodiazepines. The most important signs of withdrawal derive from excessive CNS stimulation and include anxiety, tremors, nausea and vomiting, delirium, and hallucinations. **Convulsions** are not uncommon and may be life-threatening. Treatment involves substitution with a long-acting sedative-hypnotic (eg, diazepam), with gradual decrement of dosage.

**Table 31–1.** Illustrations from Schedule of Controlled Substances, United States Drug Enforcement Agency.[1]

| Schedule | Criteria | Examples |
|---|---|---|
| I | No medical use; high addiction potential. | Heroin; LSD; mescaline; methaqualone; PCP, DOM; MDA; Marihuana. |
| II | Medical use; high addiction potential. | Strong opiate agonists, short-half-life barbiturates; amphetamine and related drugs; cocaine; cannabinols. |
| III | Medical use; moderate potential for dependence. | Medium strong opiate agonists (codeine); thiopental. |
| IV | Medical use; low abuse potential. | Benzodiazepines; chloral hydrate; meprobamate; weak opiate agonists. |

[1]Adapted, with permission, from Katzung BG (editor): *Basic & Clinical Pharmacology,* 5th ed. Appleton & Lange, 1992.

## B. Opioid Analgesics:

1. **Effects.** The most commonly abused drugs in this group are **heroin, morphine, oxycodone,** and—among health professionals—**meperidine** and **fentanyl.** The effects of intravenous heroin are described by abusers as a "rush" or orgasmic feeling followed by euphoria and then sedation. Intravenous administration of opioid analgesics is associated with rapid development of tolerance and a fast onset of psychologic and physical dependence. Oral administration or smoking of opioids causes milder effects, with a slower onset of tolerance and dependence. Most fatalities from illicit use of opioid analgesics are caused by respiratory depression, in many cases resulting from unintentional overdosage.
2. **Withdrawal.** Deprivation of opioids in physically dependent individuals leads to an abstinence syndrome that includes lacrimation, rhinorrhea, yawning, sweating, weakness, gooseflesh ("cold turkey"), nausea and vomiting, tremor, and hyperpnea. Fatalities are rare during withdrawal from opiates. Treatment involves replacement of the illicit drug with a pharmacologically equivalent agent (eg, methadone), followed by slow "tapering off."

## C. Stimulants:

A chemically heterogeneous class of drugs, the stimulants include caffeine, nicotine, amphetamines, and cocaine.

1. **Caffeine and nicotine**
   a. **Effects.** Caffeine (in beverages) and nicotine (in tobacco products) are legal in most Western cultures even though they have adverse medical effects. In the USA, cigarette smoking is now the major preventable cause of death, and tobacco use is associated with a high incidence of cardiovascular, respiratory, and neoplastic disease. Psychologic dependence on caffeine and nicotine has been recognized for some time. More recently, there has been evidence of physical dependence exhibited by abstinence signs and symptoms.
   b. **Withdrawal.** Withdrawal from caffeine is accompanied by lethargy, irritability, and headache. The anxiety and mental discomfort experienced on discontinuance of nicotine are major impediments to "kicking the habit."
   c. **Toxicity.** Acute toxicity from overdosage of caffeine and nicotine is rare when they are used in their usual forms but includes excessive CNS stimulation and, in the case of nicotine, prominent autonomic signs (Chapters 6 and 7).
2. **Amphetamines**
   a. **Effects.** Amphetamines cause a feeling of euphoria and self-confidence that contributes to the rapid development of psychologic dependence. Drugs in this class include **dextroamphetamine** and **methamphetamine** ("speed"), a crystal form of which ("ice") can be smoked. Chronic high-dose abuse leads to a psychotic state, with delusions and paranoia, that is difficult to differentiate from schizophrenia.
   b. **Tolerance and withdrawal.** Tolerance can be marked, and an abstinence syndrome, characterized by increased appetite, sleepiness, exhaustion, and mental depression, can occur upon withdrawal.
   c. **Congeners of amphetamines.** Several chemical congeners of amphetamines have hallucinogenic properties. These include 2,5-dimethoxy-4-methylamphetamine (**DOM, STP**), methylene dioxyamphetamine (**MDA**), and methylene dioxymethamphetamine (**MDMA, "Ecstasy").** The last compound is purported to facilitate communication in psychotherapy. These derivatives have been reported to be neurotoxic to serotonergic neurons in the brains of animals, with uncertain toxic consequences in humans.
3. **Cocaine.** Cocaine has marked amphetaminelike effects ("super-speed"). Its abuse has reached epidemic proportions in the USA, partly because of the availability of a free-base form ("crack") that can be smoked. The euphoria, self-confidence, and mental alertness produced by cocaine are short-lasting and positively reinforce its continued use.
   a. **Effects.** Overdoses with cocaine commonly result in fatalities from arrhythmias, seizures, or respiratory depression. Cardiac toxicity is due partly to blockade of norepinephrine reuptake by cocaine, and its local anesthetic action contributes to the production of seizures. In addition, the powerful vasoconstrictive action of cocaine may lead to severe hypertensive episodes, resulting in myocardial infarction and strokes.
   b. **Withdrawal.** The abstinence syndrome following withdrawal from cocaine is similar to that following amphetamine discontinuance, with severe depression of mood.

## D. Hallucinogens:

1. **Phencyclidine.** The arylcyclohexylamine drug **phencyclidine** (PCP, "angel dust") is proba-

bly the most dangerous of the currently popular hallucinogenic agents. Psychotic reactions are common with PCP, with impaired judgment leading to reckless behavior. The drug should be classified as a **psychotomimetic.** Overdosage with PCP produces effects that include marked hypertension and seizures, which may be fatal.

2. **Miscellaneous hallucinogenic agents.** Several drugs with hallucinogenic effects have been classified as having abuse liability; these drugs include **lysergic acid diethylamide (LSD), mescaline,** and **psilocybin.** Hallucinogenic effects may also occur with scopolamine. Terms used to describe the CNS effects of such drugs include "psychedelic" and "mind-revealing." The perceptual and psychologic effects of such drugs are usually accompanied by marked somatic effects, particularly nausea, weakness, and paresthesias. Panic reactions ("bad trips") may also occur.

**E. Marihuana:**

1. **Classification.** Marihuana (**"grass"**) is a collective term for the psychoactive constituents present in crude extracts of the plant *Cannabis sativa* (hemp), the active principles of which include the compounds **tetrahydrocannabinol (THC),** cannabidiol (CBD), and cannabinol (CBN). **Hashish** is a partially purified material that is more potent.
2. **Effects.** CNS effects of marihuana include a feeling of being "high," with euphoria, disinhibition, uncontrollable laughter, changes in perception, and achievement of a dreamlike state. Mental concentration may be difficult. Vasodilation occurs, and pulse rate is characteristically increased. Habitual users show a reddened conjunctiva. A mild withdrawal state has been noted only in heavy long-term users of marihuana. The dangers of marihuana use concern its impairment of judgment and reflexes, effects that are potentiated by concomitant use of sedative-hypnotics, including ethanol. The specific hazards of long-term use are unknown. Potential therapeutic effects of marihuana include its ability to decrease intraocular pressure and its antiemetic actions. **Dronabinol** (a controlled-substance pharmaceutical form of THC) is used to combat nausea in cancer chemotherapy.

**F. Inhalants:** Certain gases or volatile liquids are abused because they provide a feeling of euphoria or disinhibition. This class includes the following agents:

1. **Anesthetics** such as nitrous oxide, chloroform, and diethyl ether are hazardous because they affect judgment and induce loss of consciousness. Inhalation of nitrous oxide as the pure gas (no oxygen) has caused asphyxia and death. Ether is highly flammable.
2. **Industrial solvents** and a wide range of volatile compounds are present in commercial products such as gasoline, paint thinners, aerosol propellants, glues, rubber cements, and shoe polish. Because of their ready availability, these substances are most frequently abused by children in their early adolescence. Active ingredients that have been identified include benzene, hexane, methylethylketone, toluene, and trichloroethylene. Many of these are toxic to the liver, kidneys, lungs, bone marrow, and peripheral nerves and cause brain damage in animals.
3. **Organic nitrites** (amyl nitrite and isobutyl nitrite) are referred to as "poppers" and are alleged to be sexual enhancers. Inhalation causes dizziness, tachycardia, hypotension, and flushing. With the exception of methemoglobinemia, few adverse effects of the nitrites have been reported.

## DRUG LIST

The following compounds are important members of the groups discussed in this chapter. The prototypes listed are the most important agents of abuse and should be learned in detail; the major variants and other significant agents should be known well enough for identification and classification.

| Subclass | Prototype | Major Variants | Other Significant Agents |
|---|---|---|---|
| Sedative-hypnotics | Ethanol, pentobarbital, chlordiazepoxide | Secobarbital, diazepam | Methaqualone, meprobamate |
| Opioids | Heroin | Meperidine | Strong agonist-narcotic-analgesics |
| Stimulants | Amphetamine | Methamphetamine, phenmetrazine | DOM, MDA, MDMA |
| | Cocaine, caffeine, nicotine | | |
| Hallucinogens | LSD, phencyclidine | Mescaline | Scopolamine |
| Marihuana | "Grass" | Hashish | Dronabinol |
| Inhalants | Nitrous oxide, toluene | Ether | Chloroform, benzene |
| | Amyl nitrite | Butylnitrite | |

## QUESTIONS

**DIRECTIONS (items 1–6):** Each numbered item or incomplete statement in this section is followed by answers or by completions of the statement. Select the ONE lettered answer or completion that is BEST in each case.

**1.** All of the following statements about the abuse of sedative-hypnotics are accurate EXCEPT:
- **(A)** Withdrawal signs may follow the discontinuance of normal therapeutic doses of benzodiazepines
- **(B)** The abstinence syndrome is more severe following withdrawal from short-acting barbiturates than from phenobarbital
- **(C)** Diazepam is commonly used in the detoxification of alcoholic patients
- **(D)** With chronic use, tolerance to the respiratory depressant effects of barbiturates develops in proportion to tolerance to their sedative effects
- **(E)** Flumazenil is ineffective in overdoses of either ethanol or barbiturates

**2.** All of the following statements about abuse of the opioid analgesics are accurate EXCEPT:
- **(A)** Symptoms of heroin withdrawal may last as long as 6 months
- **(B)** In withdrawal from opioids, clonidine may be useful in reducing symptoms caused by sympathetic overactivity
- **(C)** Lacrimation, rhinorrhea, yawning, and sweating are all early signs of withdrawal from opioid analgesics
- **(D)** Naltrexone may precipitate a severe withdrawal state in abusers of opioid analgesics
- **(E)** Codeine alleviates most of the symptoms of heroin withdrawal

**3.** All of the following statements about the CNS stimulants are accurate EXCEPT:
- **(A)** A paranoid schizophrenic state is characteristic of high-dose amphetamine abuse
- **(B)** Cocaine has potent vasoconstrictor and local anesthetic actions
- **(C)** MDMA is reported to be neurotoxic to brain serotonergic systems
- **(D)** Although psychologic dependence to amphetamines is strong, physical dependence does not occur
- **(E)** Treatment of cocaine overdose includes the use of diazepam and propranolol

**4.** All of the following statements about hallucinogens are accurate EXCEPT:
- **(A)** Mescaline has CNS effects similar to those of LSD
- **(B)** PCP is a basic drug, so its urinary excretion would be accelerated by urinary acidification
- **(C)** Acute psychotic effects are more common with psilocybin than phencyclidine
- **(D)** Dilated pupils, tachycardia, tremor, and alertness are peripheral effects of LSD
- **(E)** Scopolamine can cause ocular dysfunction, dry mouth, and urinary retention

5. Pharmacologic effects of marihuana include all of the following EXCEPT
   (A) increased pulse rate
   (B) pupillary constriction
   (C) hypotension
   (D) conjunctival reddening
   (E) decreased psychomotor performance

6. All of the following statements about inhalants are accurate EXCEPT:
   (A) Fluorocarbons may cause sudden death from cardiac arrhythmias
   (B) Dizziness, hypotension, tachycardia, and flushing last only a few minutes following isobutyl nitrite inhalation
   (C) Methemoglobinemia is a common toxicologic problem following repetitive inhalation of industrial solvents
   (D) Euphoria, numbness, and tingling sensations with visual and auditory disturbances occur in most persons who inhale 35% nitrous oxide
   (E) Abuse of diethyl ether can be a "disinhibiting" experience

## ANSWERS

1. Tolerance develops during chronic illicit or therapeutic use of barbiturates, but its magnitude is not equivalent over the whole range of CNS depressant actions of such drugs. Only a minor degree of tolerance to respiratory depressant actions develops compared with that for sedative effects. Ingestion of ethanol or other respiratory depressants has led to fatalities of chronic users of barbiturates. The answer is **(D)**.

2. Treatment of the withdrawal syndrome following abuse of heroin requires substitution with a pharmacologically equivalent opioid analgesic drug that acts as a full agonist at opiate receptors. Although codeine is an opiate receptor agonist, it is not pharmacologically equivalent to heroin, morphine, meperidine, or methadone. Methadone is commonly used in detoxification of heroin addicts because it is a strong agonist and has high oral bioavailability and a relatively long half-life. The answer is **(E)**.

3. Abuse of amphetamines results in marked tolerance and both psychologic and physical dependence. Withdrawal is manifested by signs and symptoms opposite to those produced by such drugs. On discontinuance, chronic users tend to have a ravenous appetite, they become sleepy and feel exhausted, and their affective state swings to mental depression. The answer is **(D)**.

4. Psilocybin, mescaline, and LSD have similar central and peripheral effects. Although adverse psychologic effects are common, acute psychotic reactions are rare and usually occur in persons with a history of psychotic disorders. In contrast, the abuse of phencyclidine frequently leads to a psychotic state with paranoia and violent behavior. A schizophrenialike state from PCP may last several weeks and necessitate treatment with antipsychotic drugs. Unlike other hallucinogens, PCP overdose may result in seizures. The answer is **(C)**.

5. Two of the most characteristic signs of marihuana use are increased pulse rate and reddening of the conjunctiva. Tolerance to the tachycardia occurs rapidly. Blood pressure may fall, especially in the upright position. Psychologic tests show dose-dependent impairment of memory and of the capacity to carry out tasks requiring multiple mental steps. Depression of psychomotor function is additive with that from ethanol. Pupil size is not changed by marihuana. The answer is **(B)**.

6. Repetitive inhalation of vapors from gasoline, paint thinners, glues, rubber cements, and other common products containing industrial solvents causes many toxic effects. Toxic ingredients including heptane, hexane, methylethylketone, toluene, and trichloroethylene may result in central and peripheral neurotoxicity, liver and kidney damage, and pulmonary disease. Industrial solvents rarely cause methemoglobinemia, but this may occur following excessive use of nitrites. The answer is **(C)**.

# Part VI. Drugs With Important Actions on Blood, Inflammation, & Gout

# Agents Used in Anemias — 32

## OBJECTIVES

**Define the following terms:**

- Colony-stimulating factor
- Erythropoietin
- Hemolytic anemia
- Hypochromic anemia
- Intrinsic factor
- Megaloblastic anemia
- Pernicious anemia
- Transferrin

**You should be able to:**

- Describe the normal mechanism of regulation of iron stored in the body.
- List the major forms of iron used in the therapy of anemias.
- List the anemias for which iron supplementation is indicated and those for which it is contraindicated.
- Describe the acute and chronic toxicity of iron.
- Describe the clinical applications of vitamin $B_{12}$ and folic acid.
- Describe the major hazard involved in the use of folic acid as sole therapy for megaloblastic anemia.

## CONCEPTS

### TYPES OF ANEMIAS

A. **Iron & Vitamin Deficiency Anemias:** Microcytic hypochromic anemia, caused by iron deficiency, is the most common type of anemia. Megaloblastic anemias are caused by a deficiency of vitamin $B_{12}$ or folic acid, cofactors required for the normal maturation of red blood cells. Pernicious anemia, the most common type of vitamin $B_{12}$ deficiency anemia, is caused by a defect in the synthesis of intrinsic factor, a protein required for efficient absorption of dietary vitamin $B_{12}$.

B. **Anemias of Other Causes:** Anemias caused by radiation or cancer chemotherapy involve suppression of bone marrow stem cells. These anemias have been treated—in special cases—by marrow transplantation. Recent development of techniques for recombinant DNA-directed synthesis of marrow growth factors, erythropoietin, and the colony-stimulating factors filgrastim and sargramostim may make possible the treatment of more patients with depressed marrow activity.

### IRON

A. **Role:** Iron is the essential metallic component of heme, the molecule responsible for the bulk of oxygen transport in the blood. Although most of the iron in the body is present in hemoglobin (heme plus globin), an important fraction is bound to transferrin, a transport protein, and to ferritin and hemosiderin, 2 storage proteins. Deficiency of iron occurs most often in women because of menstrual blood loss and in vegetarians or malnourished individuals because of inadequate dietary iron intake.

**B. Regulation of Iron Stores:** Iron content in the body is regulated through modulation of absorption in the intestine (there is no mechanism for the efficient excretion of iron).

1. **Absorption.** The metal is absorbed as the ferrous ion and oxidized in the mucosal cell to the ferric form.
2. **Storage.** Trivalent ferric iron can be stored in the mucosa bound to ferritin or carried elsewhere in the body bound to transferrin. Excess iron is stored in protein-bound form as hemosiderin in the reticuloendothelial system. An accumulation of hemosiderin results from hemolytic anemias (anemias caused by excess destruction of red blood cells) and in hemochromatosis.
3. **Elimination.** Minimal amounts of iron are lost from the body with sweat and saliva and in exfoliated skin and intestinal mucosal cells, but there is no efficient method for excretion of excess iron.

**C. Clinical Use:** Iron deficiency anemia is the only indication for the use of iron. Iron deficiency can be diagnosed from red blood cell changes (microcytic cell size, diminished hemoglobin content of blood) and from measurements of serum and bone marrow iron stores. It is treated by dietary ferrous iron supplementation and, in special cases, by parenteral administration of the metal. Iron should *not* be given in hemolytic anemia, because iron stores are elevated, not depressed, in this type of anemia.

**D. Toxicity:**

1. **Signs and symptoms.** *Acute* iron intoxication is most common in children and occurs as a result of accidental ingestion of iron supplementation tablets. Necrotizing gastroenteritis, shock, metabolic acidosis, coma, and death result. *Chronic* toxicity occurs most often in individuals who must receive frequent transfusions (eg, patients with sickle cell anemia) and in those with hemochromatosis, an inherited abnormality of iron absorption.
2. **Treatment of acute iron intoxication.** Immediate treatment is necessary and usually consists of removal of unabsorbed tablets from the gut, treatment of acid-base imbalance, and administration of iron-complexing agents such as oral phosphate or carbonate salts (to precipitate unabsorbed iron) and parenteral deferoxamine, which chelates circulating iron.
3. **Treatment of chronic iron toxicity.** Treatment of hemochromatosis is usually by phlebotomy, which efficiently removes approximately 250 mg of iron with each unit of blood removed.

## VITAMIN $B_{12}$

**A. Role:** Vitamin $B_{12}$ **(cobalamin),** a cobalt-containing molecule, is a cofactor in the transfer of one-carbon units, a step necessary for the synthesis of DNA. Impairment of DNA synthesis affects all cells, but because red blood cells must be produced continuously, deficiency of either vitamin $B_{12}$ or folic acid is usually manifest first as anemia.

**B. Pharmacokinetics:** Vitamin $B_{12}$ is produced only by bacteria; it cannot be synthesized by multicellular organisms. It is absorbed from the gastrointestinal tract in the presence of intrinsic factor, a product of the parietal cells of the stomach. It is stored in the liver in large amounts; a normal individual has enough to last 5 years. Plasma transport is accomplished by binding to transcobalamin II, a glycoprotein. When parenteral vitamin $B_{12}$ is given, any in excess of the transport protein-binding capacity (about 50–100 μg) is excreted.

**C. Pharmacodynamics:** Vitamin $B_{12}$ is essential in 2 reactions: conversion of methylmalonyl-CoA to succinyl-CoA and conversion of homocysteine to methionine.

**D. Clinical Use & Toxicity:** Vitamin $B_{12}$ is available as **hydroxocobalamin** and **cyanocobalamin,** which have equivalent effects. The major application is in the treatment of naturally occurring pernicious anemia and anemia caused by gastric resection. Because vitamin $B_{12}$ deficiency anemia is almost always caused by inadequate absorption, therapy should be parenteral. Although oral therapy may suffice for maintenance, massive doses must be used. In addition to anemia, an important manifestation of vitamin $B_{12}$ deficiency is the development of neurologic defects, which may become irreversible if not treated promptly. Treatment is by parenteral replacement of vitamin $B_{12}$. Because hydroxocobalamin binds cyanide ion to form cyanocobalamin, hydroxocobalamin has also been used successfully to treat cyanide toxicity caused by nitroprusside. Neither form of vitamin $B_{12}$ has significant toxicity.

### FOLIC ACID

**A. Role:** Folic acid is necessary for the synthesis of purines and for the formation of thymidylic acid.

**B. Pharmacokinetics:** Folic acid is also known as pteroylglutamic acid. It is readily absorbed from the gastrointestinal tract. Only modest amounts are stored in the body, so a decrease in dietary intake is followed by anemia within a few months.

**C. Pharmacodynamics:** Folic acid is necessary for the transfer of one-carbon fragments in the synthesis of purine and pyrimidine bases. Recent studies suggest that deficiency of folic acid during pregnancy may increase the risk of neural tube defects in the fetus.

**D. Clinical Use & Toxicity:** Folic acid deficiency is most often caused by dietary insufficiency or by malabsorption. Anemia due to folic acid deficiency is readily treated by oral folic acid supplementation. Folic acid supplements will correct the anemia but not the neurologic deficits of vitamin $B_{12}$ deficiency. Therefore, vitamin $B_{12}$ deficiency must be ruled out before folic acid is selected as the sole therapeutic agent in megaloblastic anemia. Folic acid has no recognized toxicity.

### ERYTHROPOIETIN & COLONY-STIMULATING FACTORS

These substances are glycoprotein hormones that regulate the differentiation and maturation of stem cells within the bone marrow. Erythropoietin stimulates the production of red cells. **Sargramostim** (granulocyte-macrophage colony-stimulating factor, GM-CSF) stimulates the production of granulocytes and macrophages. **Filgrastim** (granulocyte colony-stimulating factor, G-CSF) stimulates the production of neutrophils. These substances are now available as recombinant DNA-produced, FDA-approved substances and are being evaluated for the treatment of various conditions associated with bone marrow suppression.

## DRUG LIST

The following drugs are important members of the group discussed in this chapter. Prototype agents should be learned in detail; the major variant and the other significant agents should be known well enough to list the factors that distinguish them from the prototypes and from each other.

| Subclass | Prototype | Major Variants | Other Significant Agents |
|---|---|---|---|
| Oral iron supplements | Ferrous sulfate | | Ferrous gluconate, ferrous fumarate |
| Parenteral iron | Iron dextran | | |
| Vitamin $B_{12}$ | Cyanocobalamin | Hydroxocobalamin | |
| Folic acid | Pteroylglutamic acid | | |
| Erythropoietin | Erythropoietin | | |
| Granulocyte colony-stimulating factor | Filgrastim | | |
| Granulocyte-macrophage colony-stimulating factor | Sargramostim | | |

## QUESTIONS

**DIRECTIONS (items 1–3):** Each numbered item or incomplete statement in this section is followed by answers or by completions of the statement. Select the ONE lettered answer or completion that is BEST in each case.

**1.** Important types of anemia and their causes include all of the following EXCEPT:
**(A)** Microcytic hypochromic anemia: Severe hookworm infestation
**(B)** Megaloblastic anemia: Gastrectomy
**(C)** Microcytic hypochromic anemia: Folic acid deficiency
**(D)** Microcytic hypochromic anemia: Pregnancy
**(E)** Aplastic anemia: Cancer chemotherapy

**2.** Optimal treatment of mild iron deficiency anemia associated with pregnancy involves
**(A)** a high-fiber diet
**(B)** parenteral iron dextran injections
**(C)** iron dextran tablets
**(D)** ferrous sulfate tablets
**(E)** folic acid supplements

**3.** Syndromes of toxicity associated with iron include all of the following EXCEPT:
**(A)** Acute oral ingestion of a large overdose causes constipation
**(B)** Chronic iron overload, as in hemochromatosis, causes liver disease
**(C)** Acute overdose may cause metabolic acidosis
**(D)** Hemolytic anemia may cause chronic iron toxicity
**(E)** Overdoses of iron are usually treated, since the body does not have a natural means of excreting this element

**DIRECTIONS (items 4–10):** Each group of items in this section consists of lettered headings followed by a set of numbered phrases. For each numbered phrase, select the ONE lettered heading that is most closely associated with it. Each lettered heading may be used once, more than once, or not at all.

Items 4–7

**(A)** Folic acid
**(B)** Cyanocobalamin
**(C)** Ferrous sulfate
**(D)** Iron dextran
**(E)** Deferoxamine

**4.** Essential for the therapy of neurologic defects in pernicious anemia

**5.** Useful in severe iron deficiency and iron malabsorption syndromes

**6.** Used in the emergency treatment of acute iron intoxication

**7.** Stored in the liver in an amount sufficient for approximately 5 years

Items 8–10

**(A)** Erythropoietin
**(B)** Transferrin
**(C)** Filgrastim
**(D)** Sargramostim
**(E)** Hemosiderin

**8.** Greatly increased in tissues of patients with hemochromatosis

**9.** Granulocyte-macrophage colony-stimulating factor

**10.** Useful in patients with chemotherapy-induced red cell deficiency

## ANSWERS

**1.** Folic acid deficiency causes a megaloblastic anemia similar to that caused by deficiency of intrinsic factor in postgastrectomy or pernicious anemia patients. The answer is **(C)**.

**2.** The anemia usually associated with pregnancy is a simple iron deficiency anemia. Only oral iron supplementation is indicated. The answer is **(D)**.

**3.** Intolerance to normal oral doses of iron is sometimes associated with constipation. However, acute iron overdose causes severe necrotizing gastroenteritis with diarrhea, not constipation. The answer is **(A)**.

**4.** Only vitamin $B_{12}$ reverses the neurologic deficits of pernicious anemia—and only if used early in the course of the disease. The answer is **(B)**.

**5.** Iron dextran can be given parenterally and is useful if iron stores must be replenished rapidly. The answer is **(D)**.

**6.** Deferoxamine is a chelator of iron. It is useful in acute iron intoxication. The answer is **(E)**.

**7.** Vitamin $B_{12}$ is stored in considerable excess in the liver. The answer is **(B)**.

**8.** Hemosiderin is one of the major storage forms of iron. Deposits in the liver, heart, and other tissues cause clinical abnormalities in hemochromatosis. The answer is **(E)**.

**9.** Sargramostim is GM-CSF. The answer is **(D)**.

**10.** Erythropoietin is now used in patients with severe anemia caused by chemotherapy or radiation. The answer is **(A)**.

# 33 Drugs Used in Coagulation Disorders

## OBJECTIVES

**Define the following terms:**

- Clotting cascade
- Coumarin derivatives
- Embolism
- Extrinsic pathway
- Hemophilia
- Intrinsic pathway
- Thrombosis
- Vitamin K-dependent factors

**You should be able to:**

- Compare the oral anticoagulants with heparin in terms of their pharmacokinetics, mechanisms, and toxicities.
- Compare the 4 thrombolytic preparations.
- Compare the antiplatelet drugs.
- List 3 different drugs used to treat disorders of excessive bleeding.

## CONCEPTS

The drugs used in clotting and bleeding disorders fall into 4 groups: thrombolytic agents, antiplatelet drugs, anticoagulants, and drugs used in bleeding disorders. All interact at some point with the clotting process or cascade (as shown in Figure 33–1), a series of enzyme activation steps that originate within the blood itself (intrinsic system) or in tissues (extrinsic system).

### THROMBOLYTIC AGENTS

**A. Classification & Prototypes:** The thrombolytic drugs currently available are **alteplase (tissue plasminogen activator, tPA), anistreplase (APSAC), urokinase,** and **streptokinase.** All are given intravenously. Their properties are listed in Table 33–1.

**B. Mechanism of Action:** Plasmin is the normal endogenous fibrinolytic enzyme. It splits fibrin into fragments, promoting the breakdown and dissolution of the clot. Plasmin must be formed from plasminogen. The thrombolytic enzymes catalyze the conversion of plasminogen to plasmin.

1. **Tissue plasminogen activator.** tPA is a human protein produced in bacteria through recombinant DNA techniques. It directly converts fibrin-bound plasminogen to plasmin.
2. **Anistreplase.** This anisoylated streptokinase activator complex is a pro-drug. As the anisoyl group is hydrolyzed in vivo, the streptokinase-plasmin complex is released and converts endogenous plasminogen to plasmin.
3. **Streptokinase.** Obtained from bacterial cultures, streptokinase forms a complex with plasminogen that catalyzes the rapid conversion of plasminogen to plasmin.
4. **Urokinase.** Extracted from cultured human kidney cells, urokinase directly converts plasminogen to plasmin.

**C. Clinical Use:** The thrombolytic agents are used intravenously in cases of multiple pulmonary emboli and deep venous thrombosis. They have been used by the intra-arterial route in coronary thrombosis but are now used almost exclusively by the intravenous route for this indication as well.

**D. Toxicity:** Bleeding is the most important hazard of the use of these drugs. Even tPA, which should be somewhat more selective for preformed clots, causes a significant increase in cerebral hemorrhage and other serious bleeding. Streptokinase, because it is a foreign protein, may evoke

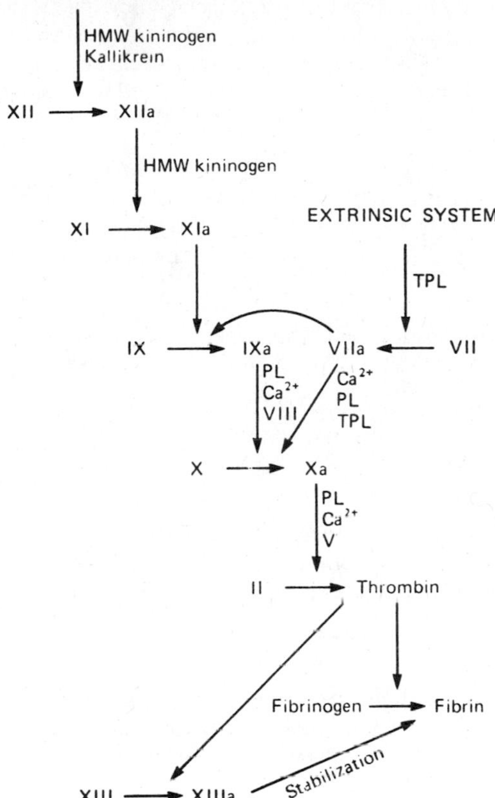


**Figure 33–1.** The clotting mechanism. a, active form of clotting factor; HMW, high-molecular-weight; PL, platelet phospholipid; TPL, tissue thromboplastin. (Reproduced, with permission, from Wessler S, Gitel SN: Warfarin: From bedside to bench. Reprinted by permission of the *New England Journal of Medicine* 1984;311:645.)

the production of antibodies and lose its effectiveness or even induce severe allergic reactions upon subsequent therapy. Patients who have had streptococcal infections may have preformed antibodies to the drug. Urokinase and tPA, because they are human proteins, are not subject to this hazard. However, they are much more expensive than streptokinase and not more effective.

## ANTIPLATELET DRUGS

**A. Classification & Prototypes:** Platelets play a central role in the clotting process and are especially important in clots that form in the arterial circulation. Antiplatelet drugs include **aspirin** and other nonsteroidal anti-inflammatory drugs (NSAIDs), **dipyridamole,** and **sulfinpyrazone.** These drugs increase bleeding time.

**Table 33–1.** Properties of thrombolytic enzymes.

| Agent | Source | Duration of Action | Comments |
|---|---|---|---|
| Alteplase (tPA) | Recombinant human protein | 2–10 min | Active plasminogen activator (converts plasminogen to plasmin); IV infusion required |
| Anistreplase | Pro-drug: streptokinase plus recombinant human plasminogen | 1–2 h | Slowly releases streptokinase-activated plasminogen; single bolus administration provides long duration of action |
| Streptokinase | Bacteria | 20–25 min | Streptokinase combines with plasminogen; the combination activates plasminogen to plasmin; IV infusion required |
| Urokinase | Human kidney cell cultures | <20 min | Active plasminogen activator |

**B. Mechanism of Action:** Aspirin and other NSAIDs inhibit thromboxane synthesis by blocking the enzyme cyclooxygenase. Aspirin is particularly effective because it irreversibly inactivates the enzyme. Because platelets lack the machinery for synthesis of new protein, inhibition by aspirin persists until new platelets are formed. Other NSAIDs cause a less persistent antiplatelet effect. The mechanisms of action of dipyridamole and sulfinpyrazone are not well understood. Some evidence suggests that dipyridamole increases the concentration of cAMP in the platelet by inhibiting phosphodiesterase.

**C. Clinical Use:** Aspirin is used in individuals who have had one or more myocardial infarctions to prevent further infarctions. A large recent study suggested that the drug also reduces the incidence of first infarcts. Dipyridamole is favored for the prevention of thrombosis on artificial heart valves. Sulfinpyrazone is used in rare cases.

**D. Toxicity:** Aspirin and other NSAIDs cause gastrointestinal and CNS effects (see Chapter 35). In addition, antiplatelet drugs significantly enhance the effects of other anticlotting agents.

## ANTICOAGULANTS

**A. Classification & Prototypes:** Anticoagulants reduce the formation of fibrin clots. Two major types of anticoagulants are available: **heparin,** which must be used parenterally, and the orally active **coumarin derivatives.** Whereas heparin is the only member of its group, **warfarin** is one of several coumarin agents. The 2 groups differ in their chemistry, pharmacokinetics, and pharmacodynamics (Table 33–2).

**B. Heparin:**

1. **Chemistry.** Heparin is a naturally occurring sulfated polysaccharide polymer with a molecular weight of about 15,000. It is highly acidic and can be neutralized by basic drugs (eg, protamine). It must be given parenterally (intravenously or subcutaneously). Intramuscular injection is avoided because of hematoma formation.
2. **Mechanism and effects.** Heparin catalyzes the activation of antithrombin III, a factor normally present in an active form in blood. Antithrombin III combines with and inactivates thrombin (activated factor II) and activated factors IX, X, XI, and XII. Low doses of heparin also coat the endothelial wall of vessels, reducing the activation of clotting elements by these cells. Because it acts on blood components, it is active in vitro—almost instantaneously. The action of heparin is monitored by measuring the activated partial thromboplastin time (aPTT).
3. **Clinical use.** Because of its rapid effect, heparin is used when anticoagulation is needed immediately (eg, when starting therapy). It is often used for 1–2 weeks in the period immediately following a myocardial infarction. Because it does not pass the placenta, it is the drug of choice when an anticoagulant must be used during pregnancy.
4. **Toxicity.** Increased bleeding is the most common adverse effect. Additive interactions with other anticoagulants occur. The drug causes moderate transient thrombocytopenia in many patients and severe thrombocytopenia in a small percentage. Prolonged use is associated with osteoporosis.

**C. Coumarin Anticoagulants:**

1. **Chemistry.** The coumarin anticoagulants are small lipid-soluble molecules that are readily absorbed and pass the placenta. Warfarin is the only member of this group of clinical impor-

**Table 33–2.** Properties of heparin and warfarin.

| Property | Heparin | Warfarin |
|---|---|---|
| Structure | Large polymer, acidic | Small lipid-soluble molecule |
| Route of administration | Parenteral | Oral |
| Site of action | Blood | Liver |
| Onset of action | Rapid (seconds) | Slow, limited by half-lives of normal factors |
| Mechanism | Activates antithrombin III | Impairs synthesis of factors II, VII, IX, & X |
| Use | Acute, days | Chronic, weeks or months |

tance in the USA.

2. **Mechanism and effects.** Coumarins interfere with the normal synthesis of clotting factors in the liver, a process that depends on vitamin K. These cofactors include factors II, VII, IX, and X. Because these factors have half-lives of 8–60 hours in plasma, abnormal synthesis is followed by an anticoagulant effect only after sufficient time has passed for the preformed normal factors to decay. Warfarin has no effect on blood clotting in vitro. The action of warfarin can be reversed with vitamin K, but recovery requires the synthesis of new normal clotting factors. More rapid reversal can be achieved by transfusion with fresh or frozen plasma that contains normal clotting factors. The effect of warfarin is monitored by means of the prothrombin time (PT) test.
3. **Clinical use.** Warfarin is used for chronic anticoagulation except in pregnant women (heparin must be used during pregnancy). Warfarin is indicated in established venous thrombosis. It is also often used for 2–6 months following a myocardial infarction.
4. **Toxicity.** Bleeding is the most important adverse effect of warfarin. Like heparin, it interacts with other anticlotting drugs. It also causes bone defects in the developing fetus and therefore is contraindicated in pregnancy. Because it acts in and is metabolized in the liver, warfarin interacts with drugs that influence hepatic drug metabolism.

## DRUGS USED IN BLEEDING DISORDERS

Inadequate blood clotting may result from genetically determined errors in clotting factor synthesis (eg, hemophilia), vitamin K deficiency, a variety of drug-induced conditions, and thrombocytopenia. The most important agents used to treat the first 3 of these conditions are **blood-clotting factors, vitamin K,** and antifibrinolysins, respectively. **Aminocaproic acid** and **tranexamic acid** are orally active agents that inhibit fibrinolysis by inhibiting plasminogen activation. They are sometimes used in hemophilia and other bleeding disorders.

# DRUG LIST

The following drugs are important members of the group discussed in this chapter. Prototype agents should be learned in detail; the major variants should be known well enough to list the factors that distinguish them from the prototypes and from each other; and the other significant agents should be recognized as belonging to a specific subclass.

| Subclass | Prototype | Major Variants | Other Significant Agents |
|---|---|---|---|
| Thrombolytic | Streptokinase | Tissue plasminogen activator (tPA) | Urokinase |
| Antiplatelet | Aspirin | Dipyridamole | Sulfinpyrazone |
| Anticoagulant | Heparin, warfarin | | |
| Vitamin K | Phytonadione ($K_1$) | | |
| Blood factors | Factor VIII | Factor IX | |
| Antifibrinolysin | Aminocaproic acid | | Tranexamic acid |

## QUESTIONS

**DIRECTIONS (items 1–6):** Each numbered item or incomplete statement in this section is followed by answers or completions of the statement. Select the ONE lettered answer of completion that is BEST in each case.

**1.** Activation of plasminogen to plasmin
**(A)** is brought about by heparin
**(B)** is brought about by warfarin
**(C)** is brought about by anistreplase
**(D)** is used preoperatively and during surgery in patients at risk of deep vein thromboses
**(E)** can be reversed by administration of vitamin $K_1$ oxide

**2.** The following changes in plasma concentration of warfarin were observed in a patient when 2 other agents, drugs ***B*** and ***C***, were given on a daily basis at constant dosage starting at the times shown. Which of the following statements most accurately describes what is shown in Graph 33–1?
**(A)** Drug ***B*** displaces warfarin from plasma proteins; drug ***C*** displaces warfarin from tissue binding sites
**(B)** Drug ***B*** stimulates liver metabolism of warfarin; drug ***C*** displaces warfarin from plasma protein
**(C)** Drug ***B*** stimulates renal clearance of warfarin; drug ***C*** inhibits hepatic metabolism of drug ***B***
**(D)** Drug ***B*** stimulates hepatic metabolism of warfarin; drug ***C*** displaces drug ***B*** from tissue binding sites
**(E)** None of the above

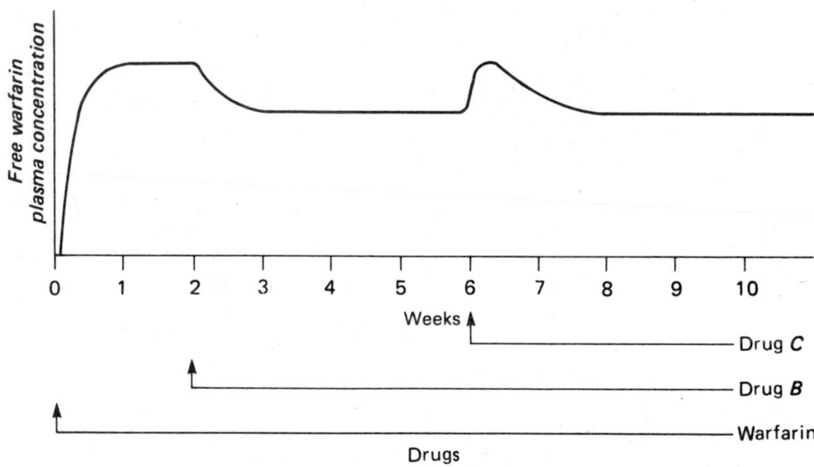


**Graph 33–1.**

**3.** Aspirin should be used cautiously in a patient receiving heparin because aspirin
**(A)** inhibits vitamin K absorption
**(B)** has antithrombin activity
**(C)** inhibits heparin metabolism
**(D)** inhibits platelet aggregation.
**(E)** all of the above

**4.** Which of the following may be of value during the first 2 weeks in the treatment of multiple small pulmonary emboli?
(**A**) Heparin
(**B**) Warfarin
(**C**) Urokinase
(**D**) Streptokinase
(**E**) All of the above

**5.** Concerning anticoagulants, all of the following are correct EXCEPT:
(**A**) Parenteral administration of heparin provides immediate anticoagulation
(**B**) Oral administration of warfarin provides delayed anticoagulation
(**C**) The anticoagulant action of heparin requires the presence of antithrombin III
(**D**) Warfarin is the preferred anticoagulant in pregnant women
(**E**) Heparin overdose can be reversed with the basic protein protamine

**6.** Concerning antithrombotic drugs,
(**A**) the antiplatelet activity of aspirin is probably related to the inhibition of prostacyclin production
(**B**) large doses of aspirin are generally more effective than smaller doses in producing antiplatelet effects
(**C**) both streptokinase and urokinase are orally administered thrombolytic agents
(**D**) a selective fibrinolysin inhibitor should be an effective antiplatelet agent
(**E**) prostacyclin is the primary platelet active agent produced in the endothelium of vessels

**DIRECTIONS (items 7–10):** Items 7–10 consist of lettered headings followed by a set of numbered phrases. For each numbered phrase, select the ONE lettered heading that is most closely associated with it. Each lettered heading may be selected once, more than once, or not at all.

(**A**) Heparin
(**B**) Coumarin agent
(**C**) Protamine
(**D**) Vitamin K
(**E**) Aminocaproic acid

**7.** A positively charged basic amine; a chemical antagonist

**8.** Immediate reversal of effect requires administration of blood or blood extracts

**9.** Large, water soluble salt; active in vitro

**10.** Inhibitor of fibrinolysis; useful in hemophilia

## ANSWERS

**1.** The answer is **(C)**, anistreplase.

**2.** A drug that increases the metabolism (clearance) of the anticoagulant will lower the steady-state plasma concentration (both free and bound forms), whereas one that displaces the anticoagulant will transiently increase the plasma level of the free form until elimination of the drug has again lowered it to the steady-state level. The answer is **(B)**.

**3.** Because aspirin interferes with clotting by a different mechanism (inhibition of platelet aggregation), it has the potential for synergistically interacting with heparin. The answer is **(D)**.

**4.** Urokinase and streptokinase may be useful in the removal of a clot that is already present; heparin (immediately) and warfarin (more slowly) act to prevent the extension of the clot and formation of new ones. The answer is **(E)**.

5. Warfarin is avoided in pregnant women because it crosses the placental barrier and causes teratogenic effects. The answer is **(D)**.

6. Large doses of aspirin inhibit prostacyclin as well as thromboxane synthesis; therefore, low doses are thought to be more effective. Thromboxane is an important contributor to the platelet aggregation process, but it is produced mainly in platelets. Prostacyclin is the major platelet-active product of the endothelium. The answer is **(E)**.

7. Protamine is a small, basic peptide with a strong positive charge. It electrostatically binds heparin (a strongly negatively charged molecule). The answer is **(C)**.

8. Coumarin derivatives, because they cause the synthesis of abnormal clotting factors in the liver, can be reversed immediately only by administration of normal clotting factors. These may be given in the form of fresh whole blood or plasma or as concentrated factors. The answer is **(B)**.

9. Heparin is a large polymer; it is active immediately in vitro as well as in vivo. The answer is **(A)**.

10. Aminocaproic acid is an inhibitor of fibrinolysis. The answer is **(E)**.

# 34 Drugs Used in the Treatment of Hyperlipidemias

## OBJECTIVES

**Define the following terms:**

- Lipoproteins
- Chylomicrons
- FFA, HMG-CoA, ACAT, LCAT, LPL
- HLD, LDL, IDL, VLDL
- Hyperlipoproteinemia
- Hyperlipemia

**You should be able to:**

- Describe the dietary management of hyperlipoproteinemia.
- Describe the mechanism of action and toxic effects of nicotinic acid, lovastatin, clofibrate, and bile acid-binding resins. Describe probucol.

## CONCEPTS

### HYPERLIPOPROTEINEMIA

A. **Pathogenesis:** Premature or accelerated development of atherosclerosis is strongly associated with abnormal levels (above 200 mg/dL) of certain plasma lipoproteins, especially the lipoproteins associated with cholesterol transport. Elevation of the level of low-density lipoproteins (LDL), intermediate-density lipoproteins (IDL), or very low density lipoproteins (VLDL) constitute hyperlipoproteinemias. A depressed level of high-density lipoproteins (HDL) is also associated with increased risk of atherosclerosis, as is hyperlipemia, an elevation of triglycerides. Chylomicronemia, the occurrence of chylomicrons in the serum while fasting (another risk factor), is a recessive trait that can be managed by restriction of total fat intake alone. See Table 34–1.

**B. Mechanism of Action:** Regulation of plasma lipoprotein levels involves a balance between dietary fat intake, hepatic processing, and utilization in peripheral tissues. Primary disturbances in regulation occur in various familial diseases. Secondary disturbances are associated with many endocrine conditions and diseases of the liver or kidneys. Major enzymes involved include:

1. Acyl-CoA:cholesterol acyltransferase (ACAT), which esterifies some cholesterol in the core of chylomicrons
2. Lecithin:cholesterol acyltransferase (LCAT), which esterifies cholesterol and helps transfer it to LDL
3. Lipoprotein lipase (LPL), which hydrolyzes triglycerides to free fatty acids (FFA) and glycerol
4. 3-Hydroxy-3-methylglutaryl–coenzyme A (HMG-CoA), which is essential in the synthesis of cholesterol and other steroids in the liver.

**C. Treatment Strategies:** Treatment always includes dietary management. Drug therapy is added if necessary (Table 34–1).

1. **Diet.** Dietary measures are the first method of management and may be sufficient to reduce lipoprotein levels to a safe range. Cholesterol and saturated fats are the primary dietary factors that contribute to elevated levels of plasma lipoproteins. Alcohol intake raises VLDL levels. Diets are designed to reduce the total intake of these substances.
2. **Drugs.** Drug therapy can reduce fat absorption from the intestine **(resins)**, modify hepatic synthesis **(HMG-CoA reductase inhibitors)** or release of lipoproteins **(niacin)**, increase peripheral clearance of lipoproteins **(clofibrate group)**, and possibly exert other effects **(probucol)**. These drugs are all given orally (Fig 34–1).

**Table 34–1.** The primary hyperlipoproteinemias and their drug treatment.[1]

| | Single Drug[2] | Drug Combination |
|---|---|---|
| Primary chylomicronemia (familial lipoprotein lipase or cofactor deficiency)<br>Chylomicrons, VLDL increased | Dietary management | |
| Familial hypertriglyceridemia<br>Severe<br>Chylomicrons, VLDL increased | Niacin, gemfibrozil, clofibrate | Niacin plus gemfibrozil or clofibrate. |
| Moderate<br>VLDL + chylomicrons increased | Gemfibrozil, clofibrate, niacin | |
| Familial combined hyperlipidemia (multiple type hyperlipoproteinemia)<br>VLDL increased | Niacin, gemfibrozil, clofibrate | |
| LDL increased | Resin, niacin, lovastatin | Niacin plus resin or lovastatin. |
| VLDL, LDL increased | Niacin | Niacin plus resin or lovastatin; clofibrate plus resin. |
| Familial dysbetalipoproteinemia: VLDL remnants, chylomicron remnants increased | Clofibrate, gemfibrozil, niacin | |
| Familial hypercholesterolemia<br>Heterozygous<br>LDL increased | Resin, lovastatin, niacin | Two or 3 of the single drugs. |
| Homozygous<br>LDL increased | Probucol, niacin | Resin plus niacin plus lovastatin; probucol plus agents above. |
| $LP_{(a)}$ hyperlipoproteinemia<br>$LP_{(a)}$ increased | Niacin | Niacin plus lovastatin. |
| Unclassified hypercholesterolemia | Resin, niacin, lovastatin, clofibrate, gemfibrozil | |

[1]Reproduced, with permission, from Katzung BG (editor): *Basic & Clinical Pharmacology,* 5th ed. Appleton & Lange, 1992.
[2]Single-drug therapy should be evaluated before drug combinations are used.

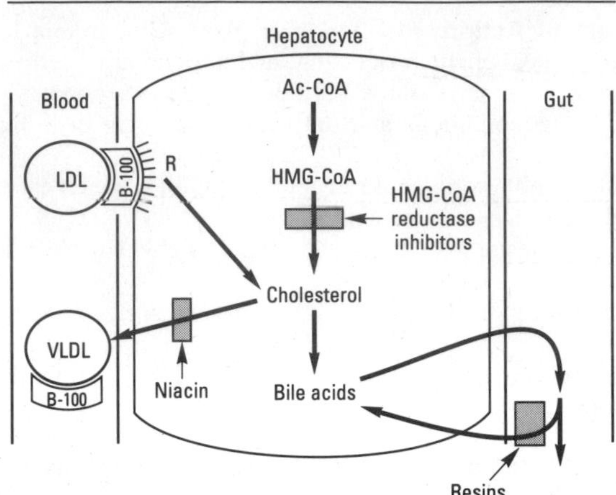


**Figure 34–1.** Sites of action of HMG-CoA reductase inhibitors, niacin, and resins used in treating hyperlipidemias. LDL receptors *(R)* are increased by treatment with resins and HMG-CoA reductase inhibitors. (Reproduced, with permission, from Katzung BG [editor]: *Basic & Clinical Pharmacology,* 5th ed. Appleton & Lange, 1992.)

## RESINS

**A. Prototypes & Chemistry:** Bile acid-binding resins (**cholestyramine** and **colestipol**) are large nonabsorbable polymers that bind bile acids and similar steroids in the intestine. Neomycin, although not a resin, also causes a reduction in bile acid reabsorption.

**B. Mechanism & Effects:** By preventing absorption of dietary cholesterol and reducing reabsorption of bile acids secreted by the liver, these agents enhance the diversion of hepatic cholesterol synthesis to new bile acids, thereby reducing the availability of cholesterol for the production of plasma lipids (Fig 34–1). There is a secondary increase in high-affinity LDL receptors on hepatocytes.

**C. Clinical Applications:** See Table 34–1.

**D. Toxicity:** Adverse effects include bloating, constipation, and impaired absorption of some cationic or neutral drugs. Neomycin is associated with a higher incidence of adverse effects than are the resins.

## HMG-CoA REDUCTASE INHIBITORS

**A. Mechanism & Effects: Lovastatin** (mevinolin) is a pro-drug lactone. In the body, the lactone ring is opened, yielding a structural analog that is a competitive inhibitor of mevalonate synthesis by HMG-CoA, a process essential for cholesterol biosynthesis in the liver (Fig 34–1). There is an increase in high-affinity LDL receptors and increased clearance of VLDL remnants by the liver. Lovastatin may dramatically reduce LDL levels, especially when used in combination with other drugs. **Simvastatin** and **pravastatin** are newer agents that also inhibit HMG-CoA.

**B. Clinical Use:** See Table 34–1.

**C. Toxicity:** Mild elevations of serum transaminase levels are common but are not often associated with hepatic damage. Patients with preexisting liver disease may have more severe reactions. An increase in the level of creatine kinase (released from skeletal muscle) is noted in about 10% of patients, and severe muscle pain and even rhabdomyolysis occurs in a few. Lenticular opacities have also been reported in a few patients.

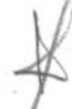

## NIACIN (Nicotinic Acid)

**A. Mechanism & Effects:** Niacin (but not nicotinamide) reduces the secretion of VLDL from the liver (Fig 34–1). Increased clearance of VLDL may also be involved. Consequently, LDL formation is reduced. In addition, the levels of HDL may increase.

**B. Clinical Use:** See Table 34–1.

**C. Toxicity:** Cutaneous flushing is a common adverse effect. Aspirin is said to reduce the intensity of this effect, suggesting that is mediated by prostaglandin release. Tolerance usually develops within a few days. Pruritus and other skin conditions are reported. Moderate elevations of liver enzyme levels may occur.

## CLOFIBRATE & GEMFIBROZIL

**A. Mechanism & Effects:** Clofibrate and gemfibrozil cause a decrease in VLDL levels through a peripheral effect. This effect is probably a stimulation of lipoprotein lipase, resulting in an increase in the clearance of triglyceride-rich lipoproteins. Cholesterol biosynthesis in the liver is secondarily reduced. There may be an increase in HDL levels.

**B. Clinical Use:** See Table 34–1.

**C. Toxicity:** Nausea is the most common adverse effect. Myalgia is reported in patients taking clofibrate, and an antiplatelet effect may result in an interaction with anticoagulants. Skin rashes are common with gemfibrozil.

## PROBUCOL

**A. Mechanism & Effects:** Probucol reduces LDL cholesterol levels by an unknown mechanism. Unfortunately, it often reduces HDL levels as well, which limits its usefulness. However, recent evidence suggests that the drug may inhibit atherogenesis by other mechanisms in addition to its effect on plasma lipids, possibly by an antioxidant effect. The drug distributes into adipose tissue and has a very long half-life.

**B. Clinical Use:** See Table 34–1.

**C. Toxicity:** Probucol causes ECG changes and may precipitate cardiac arrhythmias.

---

# DRUG LIST

The following drugs are important members of the group discussed in this chapter. Prototype agents should be learned in detail; the major variant and the other significant agents should be known well enough to list the factors that distinguish them from the prototypes and from each other.

| Subclass Mechanism | Prototype | Major Variants | Other Significant Agents |
|---|---|---|---|
| Bind bile acids in the intestine | Cholestyramine | | Colestipol |
| Inhibit cholesterol synthesis | Lovastatin | | Simvastatin, pravastatin |
| Reduce VLDL secretion | Niacin | | |
| Increase lipoprotein clearance | Clofibrate | Gemfibrozil | |
| Unknown mechanism | Probucol | | |

## QUESTIONS

**DIRECTIONS (items 1–3):** Each numbered item or incomplete statement in this section is followed by answers or by completions of the statement. Select the ONE lettered answer or completion that is BEST in each case.

**1.** Increased levels of which of the following may be associated with a decreased risk of atherosclerosis?
**(A)** Very low density lipoproteins (VLDL)
**(B)** Low-density lipoproteins (LDL)
**(C)** Intermediate-density lipoproteins (IDL)
**(D)** High-density lipoproteins (HDL)
**(E)** Cholesterol

**2.** Lovastatin has all of the following effects EXCEPT:
**(A)** Increases the synthesis of high affinity LDL receptors
**(B)** Decreases LDL and VLDL plasma levels
**(C)** Increases serum transaminase levels
**(D)** May cause skeletal muscle pain and rhabdomyolysis
**(E)** Stimulates lipoprotein lipase

**3.** Which of the following causes a reduction in absorption of bile acids from the gastrointestinal tract?
**(A)** HMG-CoA reductase inhibitors
**(B)** Colestipol
**(C)** Niacin
**(D)** Probucol
**(E)** All of the above

**DIRECTIONS (items 4–8):** Items 4–8 consist of lettered headings followed by a set of numbered phrases. For each numbered phrase, select the ONE lettered heading that is most closely associated with it. Each lettered heading may be selected once, more than once, or not at all.

**(A)** Clofibrate
**(B)** Nicotinic acid
**(C)** Cholestyramine
**(D)** Probucol
**(E)** Lovastatin

**4.** Associated with cardiac arrhythmias

**5.** Causes cutaneous vasodilatation and reduces VLDL and LDL levels

**6.** Nonabsorbable polymer; acts entirely within the intestine

**7.** Bacterial product that competitively inhibits cholesterol synthesis in the liver

**8.** Activates lipoprotein lipase and increases hydrolysis of triglycerides

## ANSWERS

**1.** An increased level of the lipoproteins is associated with increased risk of atherosclerosis. An increased level of HDL ("good cholesterol"), however, is associated with a decrease in risk. The answer is **(D).**

**2.** Lovastatin can cause all of the effects except stimulation of lipoprotein lipase, a peripheral, not hepatic, enzyme. The answer is **(E).**

**3.** Colestipol (a resin) reduces the absorption of bile acids (see Fig 34–1). The answer is **(B).**

**4.** Probucol has been associated with serious arrhythmias. Nicotinic acid may also occasionally cause arrhythmias, but this is uncommon. The answer is **(D).**

**5.** The answer is **(B),** niacin.

**6.** Cholestyramine slows the absorption of bile acids from the gut. The answer is **(C).**

**7.** The answer is **(E),** lovastatin.

**8.** Clofibrate (and gemfibrozil) activate lipoprotein lipase. The answer is **(A).**

# Nonsteroidal Anti-Inflammatory Drugs, Nonopioid Analgesics, & Drugs Used In Gout

# 35

## OBJECTIVES

**Define the following terms:**

- Antipyretic
- Cyclooxygenase inhibitor
- NSAID
- Prostaglandin
- Uricosuric
- Xanthine oxidase inhibitor

**You should be able to:**

- Describe the effects of aspirin on prostaglandin synthesis.
- List the toxic effects of aspirin.
- Contrast the actions of aspirin and the newer NSAIDs.
- Describe the mechanisms of action of 3 different drug groups used in gout.
- Describe the effects and the major toxicity of acetaminophen.

# CONCEPTS

## ASPIRIN & NEWER NSAIDs

**A. Classification & Prototypes:** Aspirin (acetylsalicylic acid) and the salicylates are traditional drugs used in the treatment of pain, inflammation, and fever. Toxic gastrointestinal effects and, at higher doses, CNS effects limit their use in some patients. The newer NSAIDs (**ibuprofen, indomethacin,** many others) have fewer gastrointestinal effects but may cause renal damage.

**B. Mechanism of Action:** All NSAIDs inhibit cyclooxygenase, the enzyme that converts arachidonic acid into the prostaglandin endoperoxide precursors PGG and PGH (see Chapter 18). As a result, synthesis of prostaglandins and thromboxane is reduced. The major difference between the mechanisms of action of aspirin and the newer NSAIDs is that aspirin acetylates and thereby irreversibly inhibits cyclooxygenase, whereas the inhibition produced by newer agents is reversible.

**C. Effects:** Arachidonic acid derivatives are important mediators of inflammation; cyclooxygenase inhibitors reduce the manifestations of inflammation, although they have no effect on the underlying tissue damage or immunologic reactions. Prostaglandin synthesis in the CNS in response to pyrogenic substances is similarly suppressed by NSAIDs, resulting in reduction of fever (antipyretic action). The analgesic mechanism of these agents is less well understood: Activation of peripheral pain sensors may be diminished as a result of reduced production of prostaglandins in injured tissue; in addition, a central mechanism is operative.

**D. Clinical Use:**

1. **Aspirin.** Aspirin is readily absorbed and is hydrolyzed in blood and tissues to acetate and salicylic acid. Elimination is first-order at low doses, with a half-life of 3–5 hours. At high doses, the half-life increases to 15 hours or more. Excretion is via the kidney. Aspirin is used in fever, moderate pain, and inflammation—especially arthritis. As noted in Chapter 33, aspirin is also indicated for the prevention of platelet aggregation in certain conditions.
2. **Newer NSAIDs.** The most important newer agents are **ibuprofen, indomethacin, naproxen,** and **piroxicam.** They are well absorbed after oral administration and are excreted via the kidneys. Ibuprofen has a half-life of about 2 hours, is relatively safe, and is available as an over-the-counter preparation in the USA. Indomethacin is a potent NSAID with increased toxicity. Naproxen and piroxicam are noteworthy only because of their longer half-lives (12–24 hours), which permits less frequent dosing. Newer NSAIDs are used for pain of dysmenorrhea, inflammation (especially that of rheumatoid arthritis and gout), and patent ductus arteriosus in premature infants.

**E. Toxicity:**

1. **Aspirin.** Possible adverse effects from low doses of aspirin are gastrointestinal disturbances and increased risk of bleeding. Persons with aspirin hypersensitivity (especially that associated with nasal polyps) may experience asthma from the increased synthesis of leukotrienes when prostaglandin synthesis is inhibited. At higher doses, tinnitus and vertigo may occur. At very high doses, the drug causes hyperventilation, respiratory alkalosis, metabolic acidosis, dehydration, collapse, coma, and death. Dialysis is effective in removing salicylates. Children with viral infections are at increased risk of developing Reye's syndrome (hepatic fatty degeneration and encephalopathy) if given aspirin.
2. **Newer NSAIDs.** Like aspirin, these agents may cause significant gastrointestinal disturbance, but the incidence is lower than with aspirin. However, at high dosage, there is a significant risk of renal damage with all the newer NSAIDs. Since they are cleared by the kidneys, renal damage results in higher, more toxic serum concentrations. Phenylbutazone, one of the oldest of this group, should not be used because it causes aplastic anemia and agranulocytosis.

## SLOW-ACTING ANTI-INFLAMMATORY DRUGS

**A. Classification & Prototypes:** This is a heterogeneous group of agents that have anti-inflammatory actions in several connective tissue diseases. The major members of the group are cytotoxic agents, especially **methotrexate;** the **gold compounds,** which are used only as anti-inflammatory agents; the **antimalarials** (eg, **hydroxychloroquine**); and **penicillamine,** which is also used as a chelating agent. **Corticosteroids** may be considered anti-inflammatory drugs with an intermediate rate of action; however, they are too toxic for chronic use (see Chapter 38) and are reserved for temporary control of severe exacerbations of inflammatory joint conditions.

**B. Mechanism of Action:** The mechanisms of action of these drugs are not well understood. Methotrexate is an immunosuppressant drug that probably acts by reducing the number of immune cells available to continue the inflammatory response. Organic gold compounds alter the activity of macrophages, cells that play a central role in inflammation, especially that of arthritis. Gold compounds also inhibit lysosomal enzyme activity, reduce histamine release, and suppress phagocytic activity by polymorphonuclear leukocytes. Antimalarial drugs may interfere with the activity of T lymphocytes, decrease leukocyte chemotaxis, stabilize lysosomal membranes, interfere with DNA and RNA synthesis, and trap free radicals. Penicillamine appears to act by mechanisms similar to those of the antimalarials.

**C. Effects:** These agents have a slow onset of anti-inflammatory action in patients with rheumatoid or other immune complexes in their serum. The action may require several months to become manifest.

**D. Clinical Use:** Slow-acting anti-inflammatory drugs are used in patients with rheumatoid arthritis who do not respond to other agents. Methotrexate, antimalarial drugs, and penicillamine are given orally. Gold compounds are available for parenteral use (gold sodium thiomalate and aurothioglucose) and for oral administration (auranofin).

**E. Toxicity:** All slow-acting agents can cause severe or fatal toxicities. Careful monitoring of any patient on these drugs is mandatory. Methotrexate causes bone marrow suppression, hepatotoxicity, and teratogenic damage to the fetus. The major toxicities of gold compounds include dermatitis and bone marrow suppression. Oral gold compounds cause a high incidence of gastrointestinal disturbances. The antimalarial agents cause dermatitis, bone marrow suppression, and retinal degeneration. Penicillamine causes renal damage and aplastic anemia.

## NONOPIOID NON-ANTI-INFLAMMATORY ANALGESICS

**A. Classification & Prototypes:** **Acetaminophen** is the only member of this group available in the USA. **Phenacetin,** a pro-drug that is metabolized to acetaminophen, is still available in some other countries.

**B. Mechanism of Action:** The mechanism of analgesic action of acetaminophen is unclear. The drug is a weak cyclooxygenase inhibitor in peripheral tissues, accounting for its lack of anti-inflammatory effect. It may be a more effective inhibitor of prostaglandin synthesis in the CNS, resulting in its analgesic and antipyretic action.

**C. Effects:** As noted above, acetaminophen is an analgesic and antipyretic agent but lacks the anti-inflammatory effects of NSAIDs.

**D. Clinical Use:** Acetaminophen is useful as an aspirin substitute, especially in children with viral infections (who are at risk for Reye's syndrome if they take aspirin) and in individuals with any type of aspirin intolerance. Acetaminophen is well absorbed and metabolized in the liver. Its half-life, which is 2–3 hours, is unaffected by renal disease.

**E. Toxicity:** Acetaminophen has negligible toxicity in therapeutic dosages. However, when taken in overdose, it is a very dangerous hepatotoxin (for the reasons described in Chapter 4 under Toxic Metabolism).

## DRUGS USED IN GOUT

**A. Classification & Prototypes:** Gout is associated with increased body stores of uric acid. Acute attacks involve joint inflammation caused by precipitation of uric acid crystals. Treatment strategies include reducing inflammation during acute attacks (with **colchicine** or an **NSAID**); accelerating renal excretion of uric acid with uricosuric drugs (**probenecid** or **sulfinpyrazone**); and reducing the conversion of purines to uric acid by xanthine oxidase (with **allopurinol**).

**B. Mechanism of Action:**

1. **Colchicine** is a selective inhibitor of microtubule assembly. It reduces leukocyte migration and phagocytosis and may also reduce production of leukotriene $B_4$. Potent NSAIDs such as indomethacin are also effective (but not as selective) in inhibiting the inflammation of acute gouty arthritis. They act through the reduction of prostaglandin formation and through the inhibition of crystal phagocytosis by macrophages.
2. **Uricosuric agents** compete with uric acid in the renal tubule for reabsorption by the weak acid carrier mechanism. At low doses, they may also compete with uric acid for secretion by the tubule and can even elevate the serum uric acid concentration. This occurs with aspirin over much of its dose range.
3. **Allopurinol** inhibits xanthine oxidase, which converts hypoxanthine to xanthine and xanthine to uric acid. Urinary concentrations of the more soluble hypoxanthine and xanthine increase, while the concentration of the less soluble uric acid decreases.

**C. Effects:**

1. **Colchicine,** by reacting with tubulin and interfering with microtubule assembly, is a general mitotic poison. Tubulin is necessary for normal cell division and many other processes; therefore, colchicine has systemic toxicity if used in excess.
2. **Uricosuric drugs** act primarily in the kidneys but inhibit the secretion of other weak acids (eg, penicillin) in addition to inhibiting the reabsorption of uric acid.
3. **Allopurinol** is relatively selective but inhibits the purine metabolism of some protozoa and has been used in leishmaniasis as well as gout.

**D. Clinical Use:** All of these drugs are given orally.

1. **Acute gout.** Phenylbutazone, a dangerous NSAID when used chronically, is still sometimes used for short-term management of gouty arthritis. Indomethacin or colchicine is preferred. Colchicine is also of value in the management of "Mediterranean fever," a disease of unknown etiology characterized by fever, peritonitis, pleuritis, arthritis, and, occasionally, amyloidosis.
2. **Chronic gout.** Chronic gout is treated with a uricosuric or allopurinol. These drugs are of no value in acute gouty arthritis and are best withheld for 1–2 weeks after an acute episode.

**E. Toxicity:** Colchicine can severely damage the liver and kidneys. The dosage must be carefully limited and monitored. Therapeutic doses are often associated with gastrointestinal upset, especially diarrhea. Indomethacin may cause renal damage or bone marrow suppression. Phenylbutazone has caused many cases of aplastic anemia. Allopurinol causes gastrointestinal upset and, rarely, peripheral neuritis and vasculitis.

## DRUG LIST

The following drugs are important members of the group discussed in this chapter. Prototype agents should be learned in detail; the major variants should be known well enough to list the factors that distinguish them from the prototypes and from each other, and the other significant agents should be recognized as belonging to a specific subclass.

| Subclass | Prototype | Major Variants | Other Significant Agents |
|---|---|---|---|
| Nonsteroidal anti-inflammatory drugs | Aspirin | Salicylate | |
| | Ibuprofen | Indomethacin | Naproxen, piroxicam |
| | Gold compounds | Hydroxychloroquine | Penicillamine |
| Nonopioid analgesic without anti-inflammatory action | Acetaminophen | | |
| Drugs used in gout | Colchicine | Indomethacin | |
| | Probenecid | | Sulfinpyrazone |
| | Allopurinol | | |

## QUESTIONS

**DIRECTIONS (items 1–5):** Each numbered item or incomplete statement in this section is followed by answers or by completions of the statement. Select the ONE lettered answer or completion that is BEST in each case.

**1.** Important effects of aspirin include all of the following EXCEPT
**(A)** reduction of fever
**(B)** reduction of prostaglandin synthesis in inflamed tissues
**(C)** respiratory stimulation when taken in toxic dosage
**(D)** reduction of bleeding tendency
**(E)** tinnitus and vertigo

**2.** Important effects of ibuprofen include all of the following EXCEPT
**(A)** reversal of joint destruction in rheumatoid arthritis
**(B)** reduction of uterine tone in dysmenorrhea
**(C)** reduction of fever
**(D)** analgesic action in headache
**(E)** reduction in thromboxane synthesis in platelets

**3.** Drugs that are useful in dysmenorrhea include all of the following EXCEPT
**(A)** colchicine
**(B)** ibuprofen
**(C)** aspirin
**(D)** naproxen
**(E)** piroxicam

**4.** Drugs used in the treatment of gout include all of the following EXCEPT
**(A)** indomethacin
**(B)** allopurinol
**(C)** colchicine
**(D)** probenecid
**(E)** aspirin

**5.** Which of the following drug effects is NOT correctly linked with a correct statement about its mechanism of action?
**(A)** Allopurinol action in gout: Inhibition of oxidation of hypoxanthine
**(B)** Aspirin antiplatelet action: Inhibition of cyclooxygenase
**(C)** Hydroxychloroquine antirheumatic action: Interference with T lymphocyte action
**(D)** Probenecid uricosuria: Increased secretion of uric acid by the loop of Henle
**(E)** Indomethacin closure of patent ductus arteriosus: Blockade of PGE production in the newborn ductus

**DIRECTIONS (items 6–10):** Items 6–10 consist of lettered headings followed by a set of numbered phrases. For each numbered phrase, select the ONE lettered heading that is most closely associated with it. Each lettered heading may be selected once, more than once, or not at all.

(A) Aspirin
(B) Acetaminophen
(C) Indomethacin
(D) Hydroxychloroquine
(E) Colchicine

**6.** A potent inhibitor of cyclooxygenase, used to accelerate thc closure of a patent ductus arteriosus

**7.** An antipyretic drug with no anti-inflammatory action

**8.** A drug that has anti-inflammatory effects only in gout and Mediterranean fever

**9.** An antimalarial agent with a slow anti-inflammatory effect in rheumatoid arthritis

**10.** A drug that is metabolized to a hepatotoxic product; the antidote is acetylcysteine

## ANSWERS

**1.** Aspirin may increase the bleeding tendency (by antiplatelet effects). The answer is **(D).**

**2.** It is not clear that any drug actually reverses the joint damage of rheumatoid arthritis, although it has been claimed that gold salts may do so. The answer is **(A).**

**3.** Primary dysmenorrhea is caused by excessive production of $PGF_{2\alpha}$, and NSAIDs that inhibit cyclooxygenase are far more effective in relieving symptoms than other analgesics. Colchicine is not an NSAID. The answer is **(A).**

**4.** Aspirin should not be used in gout because it slows renal secretion of uric acid and raises blood levels of uric acid over part of its dose range. The answer is **(E).**

**5.** Probenecid inhibits the reabsorption of uric acid in the proximal tubule. The answer is **(D).**

**6.** The answer is **(C),** indomethacin.

**7.** The answer is **(B),** acetaminophen.

**8.** Colchicine has a highly selective effect on leukocytes that are partially responsible for the inflammation associated with urate crystal deposition. The answer is **(E).**

**9.** The answer is **(D),** hydroxychloroquine.

**10.** Acetaminophen toxicity is more difficult to treat than aspirin toxicity, but acetylcysteine is effective if given early. The answer is **(B).**

# Part VII. Endocrine Drugs

# Hypothalamic & Pituitary Hormones

# 36

## OBJECTIVES

**Define the following terms:**

- Releasing hormone
- Target gland

**You should be able to:**

- List or describe the major hypothalamic releasing hormones.
- List or describe the major anterior pituitary hormones and their effects.
- List or describe the major posterior pituitary hormones and their effects.

## CONCEPTS

The hypothalamus and pituitary gland synthesize various hormones that regulate other glands and tissues throughout the body. One group of hypothalamic hormones (releasing hormones) regulates the release of anterior pituitary hormones. Two other hypothalamic hormones (oxytocin and vasopressin) are transported to the posterior pituitary and released into the general circulation from that organ to act directly on distant tissues. The hormones currently recognized as most important (and their targets) are included in the Drug List for this chapter. Except for prolactin-inhibiting hormone (dopamine), all of these endocrine agents are peptides.

### HYPOTHALAMIC HORMONES

A. **Growth Hormone-Releasing Hormone (GHRH):** GHRH (also called somatocrinin) has not been precisely characterized. Peptides with GHRH activity have been isolated and synthesized, and 2 of them are available for investigational use. They produce a rapid increase in plasma growth hormone levels and are effective in increasing growth in some short patients. However, most short patients suffer from pituitary insufficiency, not GHRH deficiency. Therefore, the primary use of GHRH preparations appears to be in the diagnosis of growth hormone deficiency.

B. **Somatostatin (Somatotropin Release-Inhibiting Hormone, SRIF):** Somatostatin has been isolated, sequenced, and synthesized. It is found in the pancreas and other parts of the gastrointestinal system as well as in the CNS. In addition to inhibiting the release of growth hormone, it inhibits the release of thyrotropin, glucagon, insulin, and gastrin. Although it can decrease the release of growth hormone in acromegaly, it is of no clinical value because of its short duration of action. **Octreotide** (SMS 201-995), an agent similar to somatostatin, is a synthetic octapeptide with a longer duration of action. It has been found useful in the management of acromegaly, carcinoid, gastrinoma, glucagonoma, and other endocrine tumors.

C. **Thyrotropin-Releasing Hormone (TRH):** TRH is a tripeptide that stimulates release of thyrotropin from the anterior pituitary, possibly through the stimulation of adenylyl cyclase. It also increases prolactin production but has no effect on the release of growth hormone or of ACTH.

**D. Corticotropin-Releasing Hormone (CRH):** This 41-amino-acid peptide stimulates secretion of both ACTH and beta-endorphin (a closely related peptide) from the pituitary. This effect is associated with increased cAMP levels in the gland. The hormone can be used in the diagnosis of abnormalities of ACTH secretion because ACTH secretion by ectopic tumors (eg, of the lungs) does not increase in response to stimulation by CRH, whereas secretion by the pituitary in Cushing's disease does increase.

**E. Gonadotropin-Releasing Hormone (GnRH or LHRH):** GnRH is a decapeptide; **leuprolide** is a synthetic nonapeptide. When given in pulsatile doses (resembling the physiologic cycling), these agents stimulate gonadotropin release. In contrast, steady dosing causes a marked inhibition of gonadotropin release—in effect, a medical castration. GnRH is used in the diagnosis and treatment of hypogonadal states. Leuprolide and several analogues **(nafarelin, buserelin)** are used to suppress gonadotropin secretion (by administration in steady dosage) in patients with prostatic carcinoma or other gonadal steroid-sensitive tumors.

**F. Prolactin-Inhibiting Hormone (PIH): Dopamine** is the physiologic inhibitor of prolactin release. Because of its peripheral effects and the need for parenteral administration, it is not useful in the control of hyperprolactinemia, but **bromocriptine,** an orally active ergot derivative, is effective in reducing prolactin secretion from the normal gland as well as from pituitary tumors. This drug (which is not a hormone) may reduce the secretion of other hormones from such tumors, and, sometimes, regression of the tumor also results.

## ANTERIOR PITUITARY HORMONES

**A. Growth Hormone (Somatotropin):** Growth hormone is a large (191-amino-acid) peptide. In the past it was obtained from the pituitaries of human cadavers. This use was abolished when it was reported that several patients treated with growth hormone from this source developed Creutzfeld-Jakob disease, apparently from slow virus contained in the extracts. Human growth hormone is now produced by recombinant DNA technology and is available in 2 forms: **somatrem** (somatotropin with an extra methionine) and **somatotropin.** These products, which are identical in their biologic properties, are used in the treatment of growth hormone deficiency in children.

**B. Thyroid-Stimulating Hormone (TSH):** This peptide stimulates adenylyl cyclase in thyroid cells and increases iodine uptake and production of thyroid hormones. It has been used as a diagnostic tool to distinguish primary from secondary hypothyroidism. It is still used occasionally to increase $^{131}I$ uptake (and tumoricidal effect) in metastatic thyroid carcinoma.

**C. Adrenocorticotropin (ACTH):** This peptide is formed from a large precursor peptide, proopiomelanocortin. This precursor is also the source of melanocyte-stimulating hormone, beta-endorphin, and met-enkephalin. Although ACTH has been used to increase corticosteroid levels as a therapeutic measure, it is now used almost exclusively for diagnostic purposes in patients with abnormal corticosteroid production. **Cosyntropin,** a synthetic analogue, is usually used for this purpose rather than ACTH itself.

**D. Follicle-Stimulating Hormone (FSH):** FSH is a glycoprotein that stimulates gametogenesis and follicle development in women and spermatogenesis in men. The preparation usually used is **urofollitin,** a product extracted from the urine of postmenopausal women.

**E. Luteinizing Hormone (LH):** LH is the major stimulant of gonadal steroid production. In women, it also regulates follicular development and ovulation. No pure preparation of LH is currently in use. **Human chorionic gonadotropin** (hCG), a product of the placenta with significant LH effect, is available for use (see below).

**F. Menotropins (hMG):** Human menopausal gonadotropins consist of human FSH and LH from postmenopausal urine. The product is often combined with hCG in the treatment of hypogonadal states in both men and women.

**G. Prolactin:** Prolactin, a glycoprotein hormone responsible for lactation, is not used in therapy.

## POSTERIOR PITUITARY HORMONES

**A. Oxytocin:** Oxytocin is a nonapeptide synthesized in cell bodies in the paraventricular nuclei of the hypothalamus and transported to the posterior pituitary, from which it is released into the circulation. It is an effective stimulant of uterine contraction and is sometimes used intravenously to induce or reinforce labor. It also causes contraction of smooth muscle in the myoepithelial cells of the mammary gland and can be used to cause milk "let-down." It is available as a nasal spray for this indication.

**B. Vasopressin (Antidiuretic Hormone, ADH):** Vasopressin is synthesized in the supraoptic nuclei of the hypothalamus and released from the posterior pituitary. As discussed in Chapter 15, it increases the synthesis or insertion of water channels by a cAMP-dependent mechanism, resulting in an increase in water permeability in the collecting tubules of the kidneys. The increased water permeability permits water reabsorption into the hypertonic renal papilla and is responsible for the antidiuretic effect. Vasopressin also causes smooth muscle contraction. The primary use of vasopressin is in the treatment of pituitary diabetes insipidus. Several forms are available, as indicated in the Drug List for this chapter.

# DRUG LIST

The following is a list of the major hormones produced or regulated by the hypothalamus and pituitary gland.

| Hypothalamic Hormone | Pituitary Hormone | Target Organ | Target Organ Hormone |
|---|---|---|---|
| Growth hormone-releasing hormone | Growth hormone (somatotropin) | Liver | Somatomedins |
| Somatostatin | | | |
| Thyrotropin-releasing hormone (TRH) | Thyroid-stimulating hormone (TSH) | Thyroid | Thyroxine, triiodothyronine |
| Corticotropin-releasing hormone (CRH) | Adrenocorticotropin (ACTH) | Adrenal cortex | Adrenal corticosteroids, androgens |
| Gonadotropin-releasing hormone (GnRH or LHRH) | Follicle stimulating hormone (FSH) | Gonads | Estrogen, progesterone, testosterone |
| | Luteinizing hormone (LH) | | |
| Prolactin-inhibiting hormone (PIH, dopamine)[1] | Prolactin (PRL) | Breast | |
| Prolactin-releasing hormone (PRH) | | | |
| Oxytocin | | Smooth muscle, especially uterus | |
| Vasopressin[2] | | Renal tubule, smooth muscle | |

[1]Bromocriptine is an ergot derivative with a dopaminelike effect on the pituitary.
[2]Injectable vasopressin is available as an aqueous solution or suspended in oil. Lysine vasopressin is a similar agent administered as a nasal spray. Desmopressin (DDAVP), another similar agent, is longer-acting and is administered as a nasal powder; it can also be used intravenously and has less action on smooth muscle than vasopressin.

## QUESTIONS

**DIRECTIONS (items 1–5):** Each numbered item or incomplete statement in this section is followed by answers or by completions of the statement. Select the ONE lettered answer or completion that is BEST in each case.

**1.** All of the following are hormones EXCEPT
(A) bromocriptine
(B) somatotropin
(C) thyrotropin
(D) vasopressin
(E) somatomedin

**2.** Drugs useful in the treatment of infertility include all of the following EXCEPT
(A) human chorionic gonadotropin
(B) bromocriptine
(C) gonadotropin-releasing hormone
(D) prolactin
(E) clomiphene

**3.** Hormones that increase cAMP levels in the target organ include
(A) vasopressin
(B) prolactin
(C) thyrotropin-releasing hormone
(D) growth hormone
(E) oxytocin

**4.** Hormones that are synthesized in the hypothalamus include all of the following EXCEPT
(A) corticotropin-releasing hormone
(B) oxytocin
(C) thyrotropin-releasing hormone
(D) luteinizing hormone
(E) vasopressin

**5.** Hormones that are useful in the diagnosis of endocrine insufficiency include
(A) gonadotropin-releasing hormone
(B) thyrotropin-releasing hormone
(C) corticotropin-releasing hormone
(D) cosyntropin, an adrenocorticotropin analogue
(E) all of the above

## ANSWERS

**1.** Bromocriptine is an ergot alkaloid with central dopamine agonist activity. It is not produced in the body. The answer is **(A).**

**2.** Clomiphene is an ovulation-stimulating partial estrogen agonist (see Chapter 39). Prolactin has inhibitory effects on fertility and is never used in infertility. The answer is **(D).**

**3.** Vasopressin acts by increasing cAMP levels. The other hormones act by other mechanisms. The answer is **(A).**

**4.** Luteinizing hormone is synthesized in the anterior pituitary. The answer is **(D).**

**5.** All are correct. The answer is **(E).**

# Thyroid & Antithyroid Drugs

# 37

## OBJECTIVES

**Define the following terms:**

- Graves' disease
- Hypothyroidism
- Iodide organification
- Iodide trapping
- Myxedema
- $T_3$, $T_4$
- Thyrotoxicosis

**You should be able to:**

- List the principal drugs used in the treatment of hypothyroidism.
- List the principal drugs used in the treatment of hyperthyroidism.
- Describe the major toxicities of thyroxine and the antithyroid drugs.

## CONCEPTS

The thyroid secretes two types of hormones: iodine-containing amino acids (thyroxine and triiodothyronine) and a peptide (calcitonin). The first type has very general effects on growth, development, and metabolism. Calcitonin is important in calcium metabolism and is discussed in Chapter 41.

### THYROID HORMONES

**A. Synthesis & Transport of Thyroid Hormones:** The thyroid secretes 2 primary iodine-containing hormones, **triiodothyronine ($T_3$)** and **thyroxine ($T_4$)**. The iodine necessary for the synthesis of these molecules is derived from food or supplements given orally. The uptake of iodine is an active process, and iodide ions are highly concentrated in the thyroid gland. The tyrosine residues of a protein, thyroglobulin, are iodinated in the gland to form monoiodotyrosine (MIT) or diiodotyrosine (DIT). $T_4$ is formed from the combination of 2 molecules of DIT, and $T_3$ contains one molecule of MIT and one of DIT. Whereas $T_3$ is released from the thyroid, much of the circulating $T_3$ is formed by the deiodination of $T_4$ in the tissues. In the blood, both $T_3$ and $T_4$ are bound to **thyroxine-binding globulin,** a transport protein.

Thyroid function is controlled by the pituitary, through the release of thyrotropin, and by the availability of iodide. Higher levels of iodide than normal inhibit iodination of tyrosine. In Graves' disease, lymphocytes release a **thyroid-stimulating immunoglobulin (TSI)** and cause thyrotoxicosis.

**B. Actions of Thyroxine & Triiodothyronine:** $T_3$ is about 10 times more potent than $T_4$, but the 2 drugs have the same effects. Their mechanism of action involves transport into the nucleus and the expression of genes responsible for many metabolic processes. In addition, there may be a separate membrane receptor-mediated effect in some tissues.

1. **Effects.** The organ level actions of the thyroid drugs include normal growth and development of nervous, skeletal, and reproductive systems and control of metabolism of fats, carbohydrates, proteins, and vitamins. The results of excess thyroid activity **(thyrotoxicosis)** and hypothyroidism **(myxedema)** are summarized in Table 37–1. A case of thyrotoxicosis is presented in Case 11 (Appendix I).
2. **Clinical use.** Thyroid hormone therapy can be accomplished with either $T_4$ or $T_3$. Synthetic levothyroxine ($T_4$) is the form of choice for most cases. $T_3$ is faster-acting but has a shorter half-life and higher cost.
3. **Toxicity.** The toxicity is that of thyrotoxicosis (Table 37–1).

**Table 37–1.** Summary of thyroid hormone effects.[1]

| System | Thyrotoxicosis | Hypothyroidism |
|---|---|---|
| Skin and appendages | Warm, moist skin; sweating; heat intolerance; fine, thin hair; Plummer's nails; pretibial dermopathy (Graves' disease). | Pale, cool, puffy skin; dry and brittle hair; brittle nails. |
| Eyes, face | Retraction of upper lid with wide stare; periorbital edema; exophthalmos; diplopia (Graves' disease). | Drooping of eyelids; periorbital edema; loss of temporal aspects of eyebrows; puffy, nonpitting facies; large tongue. |
| Cardiovascular system | Increased peripheral vascular resistance, heart rate, stroke volume, cardiac output, pulse pressure; high-output congestive heart failure; increased inotropic/chronotropic effects; arrhythmias; angina. | Decreased peripheral vascular resistance, heart rate, stroke volume, cardiac output, pulse pressure; low-output congestive heart failure; ECG: bradycardia, prolonged PR interval, flat T wave, low voltage; pericaridal effusion. |
| Respiratory system | Dyspnea; decreased vital capacity. | Pleural effusions; hypoventilation and $CO_2$ retention. |
| Gastrointestinal system | Increased appetite; increased frequency of bowel movements; hypoproteinemia. | Decreased appetite; decreased frequency of bowel movements; ascites. |
| Central nervous system | Nervousness; hyperkinesia; emotional lability | Lethargy; general slowing of mental processes; neuropathies. |
| Musculoskeletal system | Weakness and muscle fatigue; increased deep tendon reflexes; hypercalcemia; osteoporosis. | Stiffness and muscle fatigue; decreased deep tendon reflexes; increased alkaline phosphatase, LDH, SGOT. |
| Renal system | Mild polyuria; increased renal blood flow; increased glomerular filtration rate. | Impaired water excretion; decreased renal blood flow; decreased glomerular filtration rate. |
| Hematopoietic system | Increased erythropoiesis; anemia.[2] | Decreased erythropoiesis; anemia.2 |
| Reproductive system | Menstrual irregularities; decreased fertility; increased gonadal steroid metabolism. | Hypermenorrhea; infertility; decreased libido; impotence; oligospermia; decreased gonadal steroid metabolism. |
| Metabolic system | Increased basal metabolic rate; negative nitrogen balance; hyperglycemia; increased free fatty acids; decreased cholesterol and triglycerides; increased hormone degradation; increased requirements for fat- and water-soluble vitamins; increased drug detoxification. | Decreased basal metabolic rate; slight positive nitrogen balance; delayed degradation of insulin, with increased sensitivity; increased cholesterol and triglycerides; decreased hormone degradation; decreased requirements for fat- and water-soluble vitamins; decreased drug detoxification. |

[1]Reproduced, with permission, from Katzung BG (editor): *Basic & Clinical Pharmacology,* 5th ed. Appleton & Lange, 1992.
[2]The anemia of hyperthyroidism is usually normochromic and caused by increased RBC turnover. The anemia of hypothyroidism may be normochromic, hyperchromic, or hypochromic and may be due to decreased production rate, decreased iron absorption, decreased folic acid absorption, or to autoimmune pernicious anemia.

## ANTITHYROID DRUGS

**A. Thionamides:** **Propylthiouracil** and **methimazole** are small sulfur-containing molecules that inhibit thyroid hormone production by several mechanisms. The most important of their effects is to block iodination of the tyrosine residues of thyroglobulin. In addition, they appear to block coupling of DIT and MIT. They can be used by the oral route and are effective in most patients with uncomplicated hyperthyroidism. Toxic effects include skin rash (common) and severe allergic reactions (rare) such as vasculitis, hypoprothrombinemia, and agranulocytosis. These effects are usually reversible.

**B. Iodide Salts & Iodine:** Iodide salts inhibit organification (iodination of tyrosine) and thyroid hormone release and decrease the size and vascularity of the hyperplastic thyroid gland. These effects are especially desirable if surgical resection of a hyperactive thyroid is planned. The usual forms of this drug are Lugol's solution (iodine and potassium iodide) and a saturated solution of potassium iodide.

**C. Iodinated Radiocontrast Media:** Certain iodinated radiocontrast media effectively suppress the conversion of $T_4$ to $T_3$ in the liver, kidneys, and other peripheral tissues. Inhibition of hormone release from the thyroid may also play a part. **Ipodate** has proved to be very useful in rapidly reducing $T_3$ concentrations in thyrotoxicosis.

**D. Radioactive Iodine:** Radioactive iodine ($^{131}I$) is taken up and concentrated in the thyroid gland so avidly that a dose large enough to severely damage the gland can be given without endangering other tissues. Unlike the thionamides and iodide salts, an effective dose of $^{131}I$ can produce a permanent cure of thyrotoxicosis without surgery.

**E. Other Drugs:** Other agents used in the treatment of thyrotoxicosis include the adrenoceptor-blocking drugs, especially the **beta-blockers.** These agents are particularly useful in controlling the tachycardia and other cardiac abnormalities of severe thyrotoxicosis.

## DRUG LIST

The following drugs are important members of the group discussed in this chapter. Prototype agents should be learned in detail; the other significant agents should be recognized as belonging to a specific subclass.

| Subclass | Prototype | Other Significant Agents |
|---|---|---|
| Thyroid hormones | Thyroxine ($T_4$), triiodothyronine ($T_3$) | |
| Antithyroid drugs | Propylthiouracil, iodide salts, $^{131}I$ (radioactive iodine) | Methimazole, ipodate |
| Miscellaneous | Propranolol | |

## QUESTIONS

**DIRECTIONS (items 1–4):** Each numbered item or incomplete statement in this section is followed by answers or by completions of the statement. Select the ONE lettered answer or completion that is BEST in each case.

**1.** Important drugs used in the treatment of thyrotoxicosis include all of the following EXCEPT
**(A)** propylthiouracil
**(B)** potassium iodide
**(C)** thyroglobulin
**(D)** radioactive iodine
**(E)** methimazole

**2.** Actions of thyroxine include all of the following EXCEPT
**(A)** stimulation of oxygen consumption
**(B)** acceleration of cardiac rate
**(C)** fine tremor of the skeletal muscles
**(D)** decreased glomerular filtration rate
**(E)** increased appetite

**3.** Effects of iodide salts given in large doses include all of the following EXCEPT
**(A)** decreased size of the thyroid gland
**(B)** decreased vascularity of the gland
**(C)** decreased hormone release
**(D)** decreased iodination of tyrosine
**(E)** increased $^{131}I$ uptake

4. Symptoms of hypothyroidism (myxedema) include all of the following EXCEPT
   (A) low heart rate
   (B) dry, puffy skin
   (C) lethargy and sleepiness
   (D) increased appetite
   (E) drooping of the eyelids and large tongue

**DIRECTIONS (items 5–8):** Items 5–8 consist of lettered headings followed by a set of numbered phrases. For each numbered phrase, select the ONE lettered heading that is most closely associated with it. Each lettered heading may be selected once, more than once, or not at all.

(A) Propylthiouracil
(B) $^{131}I$
(C) Triiodothyronine
(D) Ipodate
(E) Propranolol

5. Produced in the peripheral tissues when thyroxine is administered

6. Useful in "thyroid storm" to control cardiac manifestations

7. Radiocontrast medium that is also useful in thyrotoxicosis

8. Produces a permanent reduction in thyroid activity

## ANSWERS

1. Thyroglobulin is a natural product obtained from pigs that contains thyroxin in its protein-bound form. It is now obsolete but was used in hypothyroidism. It would never be used in thyrotoxicosis. The answer is **(C)**.

2. Thyroid hormone increases the glomerular filtration rate. The answer is **(D)**.

3. Iodide has a negative feedback effect on thyroid functioning including iodide uptake. The answer is **(E)**.

4. Appetite decreases in myxedema as the metabolic rate decreases. The answer is **(D)**.

5. $T_4$ is converted into $T_3$ in the periphery. The answer is **(C)**.

6. Beta-blockers are particularly useful in controlling cardiac manifestations of severe thyrotoxicosis ("storm"). The answer is **(E)**.

7. Ipodate is a radiocontrast medium. The answer is **(D)**.

8. Radioactive iodine is the only medical therapy that produces a permanent reduction of thyroid activity. The answer is **(B)**.

# Corticosteroids & Antagonists 38

## OBJECTIVES

**Define the following terms:**

- Addison's disease
- Adrenal androgens, adrenal estrogens
- Circadian rhythm of secretion
- Cushing's syndrome
- Glucocorticoid
- Mineralocorticoid

**You should be able to:**

- Describe the major naturally occurring glucocorticosteroid and its actions.
- List or describe several synthetic glucocorticoids and their differences from the naturally occurring hormones.
- List or describe the actions of the major naturally occurring mineralocorticoid and one synthetic agent in this group.
- List the indications for the use of corticosteroids in adrenal and nonadrenal disorders.
- List or describe the toxic effects of the glucocorticoids when given chronically.

## CONCEPTS

The corticosteroids are the steroid hormones produced by the adrenal cortex. They consist of 2 primary physiologic and pharmacologic groups: (1) **glucocorticoids,** which have important effects on intermediary metabolism, catabolism, and inflammation; and (2) **mineralocorticoids,** which regulate sodium reabsorption in the collecting tubules of the kidney. In addition, some androgenic and estrogenic steroids are synthesized in the adrenal. This chapter reviews the glucocorticoids, mineralocorticoids, and adrenocorticosteroid antagonists.

### GLUCOCORTICOIDS

**A. Cortisol:** The major natural glucocorticoid is **cortisol (hydrocortisone),** a steroid synthesized in the adrenal cortex from 17-hydroxypregnenolone. Its secretion is regulated by ACTH (Fig 38–1) and varies during the day (circadian rhythm), with the peak occurring in the morning and the trough around midnight. In the plasma, it is about 95% bound to corticosteroid-binding globulin. The half-life is approximately 100 minutes, and clearance is primarily by hepatic metabolism. Cortisol is well absorbed from the gastrointestinal tract but has a shorter duration of action than some of its synthetic congeners. Although it diffuses poorly across normal skin, it is readily absorbed across inflamed skin and mucous membranes.

Cortisol and its synthetic analogs enter the cell and bind to cytosolic receptors that transport the steroid into the nucleus, where the complex alters gene expression. The results include the following:

1. **Metabolic effects.** Glucocorticoids stimulate gluconeogenesis. As a result, blood sugar rises, muscle protein is catabolized, and insulin secretion is stimulated. Both lipolysis and lipogenesis are stimulated. If excessive (eg, Cushing's syndrome), there is a net increase of fat deposition in certain areas, eg, face (moon facies) and shoulders and back (buffalo hump).
2. **Catabolic effects.** As noted above, glucocorticoids cause muscle protein catabolism. In addition, lymphoid and connective tissue, fat, and skin undergo wasting under the influence of high concentrations of the corticosteroids. Catabolic effects on bone can lead to osteoporosis. In children, growth is inhibited.
3. **Immunosuppressive effects.** Glucocorticoids inhibit some of the mechanisms involved in cell-mediated immunologic functions, especially those dependent on lymphocytes. They do

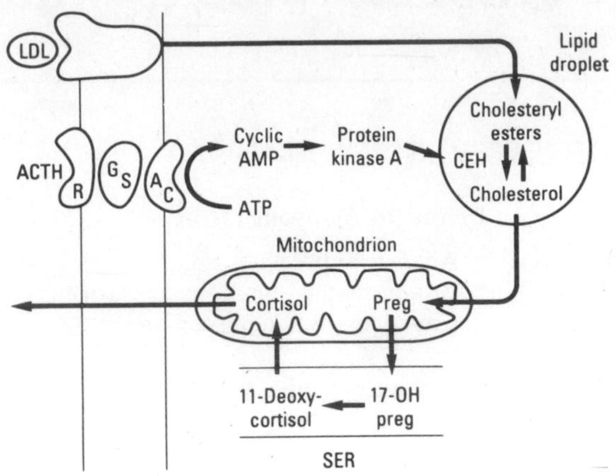


**Figure 38–1.** Mechanism of action of ACTH on cortisol-secreting cells in the inner 2 zones of the adrenal cortex. When ACTH binds to its receptor (R), adenylyl cyclase (AC) is activated via $G_S$. The resulting increase in the AMP level activates protein kinase A, and the kinase phosphorylates cholesterol ester hydrolase (CEH), increasing its activity. Consequently, more free cholesterol is formed and converted to pregnenolone in the mitochondria. Note that in the subsequent steps in steroid biosynthesis, products are shuttled between the mitochondria and the smooth endoplasmic reticulum (SER). Additional corticosterone is also synthesized and secreted. (Reproduced, with permission, from Ganong WF [editor]: *Review of Medical Physiology,* 15th ed. Appleton & Lange, 1991.)

not interfere with the development of normal acquired immunity but delay rejection reactions in patients with organ transplants.

4. **Anti-inflammatory effects.** Glucocorticoids have a dramatic effect on the distribution and function of leukocytes. They increase the number of neutrophils and decrease the number of lymphocytes, eosinophils, basophils, and monocytes. The migration of leukocytes is also inhibited. The mechanism of these effects probably involves synthesis of substances that suppress the production of prostaglandins and leukotrienes in the damaged tissue through inhibition of phospholipase (see Chapter 18).
5. **Renal effects.** Cortisol is required for normal renal excretion of water loads. The molecule also has a small but significant salt-retaining (mineralocorticoid) effect. This is an important cause of hypertension in patients with a corticosteroid-secreting adrenal tumor or a pituitary ACTH-secreting tumor (Cushing's syndrome).
6. **Other effects.** The corticosteroids have effects on the CNS. When given in large doses (especially if given for long periods), they may cause profound behavioral disturbances. Large doses stimulate gastric acid secretion and may decrease resistance to ulcer formation.

**B. Synthetic Glucocorticoids:** Synthetic agents similar to cortisol have been synthesized to achieve 3 goals: to decrease mineralocorticoid effects, to increase the duration of action, and to improve absorption across the skin. The mechanism of action of these agents is identical to that of cortisol. A very large number have been synthesized and are available for use; dexamethasone, prednisolone, and triamcinolone are representative. Their pharmacokinetic properties (when compared with cortisol) include alterations in metabolism, prolongation of half-life and duration of action, and better penetration of lipid barriers.

**C. Clinical Use:**

1. **Adrenal disorders.** Glucocorticoids are essential in chronic severe adrenocortical insufficiency (Addison's disease) to preserve life. They are also often useful in acute adrenal insufficiency associated with life-threatening shock, trauma, etc. Cortisol is also useful in certain types of adrenal hyperplasia, in which synthesis of abnormal forms of corticosteroids is stimulated by ACTH. Administration of cortisol or synthetic agents similar to it may suppress ACTH secretion sufficiently to reduce total steroid synthesis.
2. **Nonadrenal disorders.** Many disorders respond to corticosteroid therapy. Most of these disorders are inflammatory (eg, asthma, collagen diseases, ulcerative colitis), immunologic (eg, hay fever, drug reactions), or neoplastic (eg, leukemia, multiple myeloma). However, the degree of benefit differs considerably in different disorders, and the toxicity of corticosteroids given chronically limits their use. Treatment of one patient with rheumatoid arthritis is described in Case 13 (Appendix III).

**D. Toxicity:** Many of the toxic effects of the glucocorticosteroids are predictable from the effects already described. These include adrenal suppression (from suppression of ACTH secretion), metabolic effects (growth inhibition, diabetes, muscle wasting, osteoporosis), salt retention, and psychosis.

## MINERALOCORTICOIDS

**A. Aldosterone:** The major natural mineralocorticoid is **aldosterone,** which has already been mentioned in connection with hypertension (see Chapter 10) and control of its secretion by angiotensin II (see Chapter 17). Pregnenolone and progesterone are intermediates in its synthesis. The secretion of aldosterone is regulated by ACTH and by the renin-angiotensin mechanisms. It is very important in the regulation of blood volume (see Fig 6–2). Aldosterone has a short half-life and little glucocorticoid activity.

**B. Other Mineralocorticoids:** Other mineralocorticoids include **desoxycorticosterone,** the naturally occurring precursor of aldosterone, and **fludrocortisone.** The latter has significant glucocorticoid activity, and because of its long duration of action it is favored for replacement therapy after adrenalectomy and in other conditions in which mineralocorticoid therapy is needed.

## ADRENOCORTICOSTEROID ANTAGONISTS

**A. Receptor Antagonists:** Spironolactone, an antagonist of aldosterone at its receptor, has been discussed in connection with the diuretics (see Chapter 15). **Mifepristone (RU486)** is an inhibitor at glucocorticoid receptors as well as progesterone receptors (see Chapter 39). It has been used in the treatment of Cushing's syndrome.

**B. Synthesis Inhibitors:** Several drugs are used in the treatment of adrenal cancer when surgical therapy is impractical or unsuccessful because of metastases. The most important of these drugs are **metyrapone, aminoglutethimide,** and **ketoconazole.** The drugs mitotane (a DDT analog) and amphenone B also reduce steroid synthesis in the adrenals but are considered too toxic for human use. Aminoglutethimide is used in the treatment of advanced breast cancer to suppress adrenal secretion of estrogenic steroids. The use of ketoconazole (an antifungal drug) is investigational in the inhibition of steroid synthesis.

# DRUG LIST

The following drugs are important members of the group discussed in this chapter. Prototype agents should be learned in detail; the major variants should be known well enough to list the factors that distinguish them from the prototypes and from each other; and the other significant agents should be recognized as belonging to a specific subclass.

| Subclass | Prototype | Major Variants | Other Significant Agents |
|---|---|---|---|
| Glucocorticoids | Cortisol | Dexamethasone, prednisolone, triamcinolone | Many variants |
| Mineralocorticoids | Aldosterone | Fludrocortisone | |
| Adrenal antagonists | Aminoglutethimide, metyrapone, spironolactone | Mifepristone | Ketoconazole |

## QUESTIONS

**DIRECTIONS (items 1 and 2):** Each numbered item or incomplete statement in this section is followed by answers or by completions of the statement. Select the ONE lettered answer or completion that is BEST in each case.

**1.** Effects of the glucocorticoids include all of the following EXCEPT
**(A)** reduction in circulating lymphocytes
**(B)** increased skin protein synthesis
**(C)** altered fat deposition
**(D)** inhibition of leukotriene synthesis
**(E)** increased blood glucose levels

**2.** Toxic effects of the corticosteroids include all of the following EXCEPT
**(A)** hypoglycemia
**(B)** osteoporosis
**(C)** growth inhibition
**(D)** salt retention
**(E)** psychosis

**DIRECTIONS (items 3–6):** Items 3–6 consist of lettered headings followed by a set of numbered phrases. For each numbered phrase, select the ONE lettered heading that is most closely associated with it. Each lettered heading may be used once, more than once, or not at all.

**(A)** Cortisol
**(B)** Triamcinolone
**(C)** Aldosterone
**(D)** Fludrocortisone
**(E)** Spironolactone

**3.** Naturally occurring mineralocorticoid

**4.** Mineralocorticoid with high salt-retaining potency and long duration of action

**5.** Glucocorticoid with very low mineralocorticoid activity and high topical activity

**6.** Causes salt retention and buffalo hump in patients with Cushing's syndrome

## ANSWERS

**1.** Glucocorticoids stimulate protein breakdown (except in the liver). The answer is **(B)**.

**2.** Corticosteroids may induce hyperglycemia of sufficient magnitude to require insulin therapy. The answer is **(A)**.

**3.** The answer is **(C)**, aldosterone.

**4.** Fludrocortisone has a much longer duration of action than the naturally occurring mineralocorticoids. The answer is **(D)**.

**5.** The answer is **(B)**, triamcinolone.

**6.** Cortisol causes buffalo hump through its effects on fat metabolism and distribution. It also has sufficient salt-retaining activity to cause hypertension. The answer is **(A)**.

# Gonadal Hormones & Inhibitors 39

## OBJECTIVES

**Define the following terms:**

- Anabolic steroid
- Antiestrogen
- Combination, sequential, progestin-only contraceptives
- Oral contraceptive
- Ovulation-inducing agent

**You should be able to:**

- Describe the hormonal changes that occur during the menstrual cycle.
- List the benefits and hazards of oral contraceptives.
- Describe the status of pharmacologic contraception in the male.
- List the benefits and hazards of postmenopausal estrogen therapy.
- Describe the use of sex hormones in the treatment of cancer in women and men.
- List or describe the toxic effects of anabolic steroids used to build muscle mass.

## CONCEPTS

The gonadal hormones include the steroids of the ovary (estrogens and progestins) and testis (chiefly testosterone) and a few other hormones (eg, peptides) of lesser importance. The sex steroids are also synthesized in the adrenal cortex. Because of their importance in oral contraceptive agents, many synthetic estrogens and progestins have been produced. This application constitutes the largest use of these agents. Another important application of agonist and antagonist members of this steroid group is in the treatment of cancer of the breast and prostate.

### OVARIAN HORMONES

The ovary is the primary source of sex hormones in women during the child-bearing years, ie, between puberty and menopause. Under normal regulation by the pituitary, each menstrual cycle consists of the following events: A follicle in the ovary matures, secretes increasing amounts of estrogen, releases an ovum, and is transformed into a progesterone-secreting corpus luteum. If the ovum is not fertilized and implanted, the corpus luteum degenerates; the uterine endometrium (which has proliferated under the stimulation of estrogen and progesterone) is shed as part of the menstrual flow; and the cycle repeats. The mechanism of action of both estrogen and progesterone is by entering cells, binding to a cytosolic receptor that transports them into the nucleus, and there causing modulation of gene expression.

**A. Estrogens:** The major ovarian estrogen in women is **estradiol.** Other estrogens include estrone and estriol, which are produced in other tissues. Almost all of the estrogen in the blood is bound to a sex hormone-binding globulin (SHBG). Estradiol is active by the oral route as replacement therapy but has low bioavailability because of hepatic metabolism. Therefore, semisynthetic derivatives or other estrogens are usually used (see Drug List).

1. **Effects.** Estrogenic action is essential for normal female sexual development. It is responsible for the growth of the genital structures (vagina, uterus, and uterine tubes) during childhood and for the appearance of secondary sexual characteristics and the growth spurt associated with puberty. Estrogens have many metabolic effects: They modify serum protein levels, reduce bone resorption, and enhance nutrient absorption in the gastrointestinal tract. They enhance the coagulability of blood and increase plasma triglyceride levels while reducing alpha-lipoprotein and plasma cholesterol levels. Estrogens are also effective feedback suppressants of pituitary FSH.
2. **Clinical use.** Major therapeutic uses of estrogens are for the treatment of hypogonadism and

the management of postmenopausal genital and bone changes. They are important also as a component of oral contraceptives. Estrogens are sometimes used in the palliative treatment of carcinoma of the prostate. A special use of brief, high-dose therapy is as a "morning-after" contraceptive, ie, to prevent conception as a result of intercourse the night before.

3. **Toxicity.** The primary toxicity of the estrogens relates to their stimulatory effects on vaginal, uterine, and breast tissue. Moderate doses may cause breast tenderness, endometrial hyperplasia, and breakthrough bleeding. When given over long periods, they may contribute to the incidence of endometrial cancer. It is believed that vaginal adenocarcinoma in young women may be caused by the treatment of their mothers early in pregnancy with diethylstilbestrol (DES), a synthetic estrogen. During the 1930s and 1940s, it was erroneously believed that large doses of estrogens reduced the incidence of miscarriage. Estrogen use is also associated with an increased incidence of gallbladder disease.

**B. Progestins: Progesterone** is the major progestin in humans. It is synthesized in the ovaries, testes, and adrenals. It is rapidly metabolized in the liver and therefore has a very low bioavailability and a short half-life. Synthetic agents are used for replacement therapy and in oral contraceptives.

1. **Effects.** Progestins cause development of secretory tissue in the breast and maturation of the uterine endometrium. They have much less effect than the estrogens on plasma protein levels but significantly affect carbohydrate metabolism and stimulate the deposition of fat.
2. **Clinical use.** The major therapeutic use of the progestins is as a component of oral contraceptives. However, they are occasionally used to produce long-lasting ovarian suppression, eg, in endometriosis.
3. **Toxicity.** The toxicity of progestins is rather low. However, they may increase the blood pressure and decrease the level of high-density plasma lipoproteins (HDL).

**C. Oral & Implantable Contraceptives:** Three different types of oral contraceptives for women have been developed: **combination** estrogen-progestin tablets; **sequential** preparations, in which estrogens alone are taken for approximately 2 weeks and followed by progestins; and **progestin-only** preparations. The sequential preparations are not as effective as the other types in preventing pregnancy and are no longer used. An implanted progestin preparation (norgestrel, Norplant) was recently approved. This subcutaneous depot formulation is said to prevent conception for up to 5 years.

1. **Mechanism of action.** The combination agents appear to act through a combination of effects, including inhibition of ovulation (the primary action) and effects on the uterine tubes and endometrium that decrease the likelihood of fertilization and implantation. The progestin-only agents do not inhibit ovulation and probably act through the other mechanisms listed.
2. **Toxicity.** The major toxic effects of the oral contraceptives relate to their actions on blood coagulation. There is a well-documented increase in the risk of thromboembolic phenomena (myocardial infarction, stroke, pulmonary embolism) in older women, in smokers, and in women with a family history of such mishaps. However, the risk incurred by the use of these drugs is usually less than the risk engendered by pregnancy. The other toxicities of the oral contraceptives are much less hazardous and include nausea, breast tenderness, headache, skin pigmentation, acne, and hirsutism. All adverse effects appear to be considerably reduced by the use of preparations containing lower doses of estrogen.

   Numerous studies have been carried out to evaluate the effect of oral contraceptive use on the incidence of cancer. Convincing evidence indicates that these agents reduce the incidence of endometrial and ovarian carcinoma. However, evidence regarding the effects on breast cancer is still confusing. A few studies indicate that women who took the pill for many years after it first became available (ie, in high-dose formulations) may have an increased incidence of breast carcinoma. Most studies show no increase.

**D. Other Hormones Related to the Ovary:**

1. **Danazol.** Danazol is a weak progestational and androgenic synthetic agent that is used in the treatment of endometriosis and fibrocystic disease of the breast. It may act through suppression of ovarian steroid synthesis.
2. **Tamoxifen & clomiphene.** These are synthetic antiestrogenic drugs. Tamoxifen is a nonsteroidal competitive inhibitor of estrogen that is used in the palliative treatment of hormone-sensitive breast cancer. Clomiphene is a partial agonist nonsteroidal estrogen related to DES

and chlorotrianisene. It stimulates ovulation, probably by reducing negative feedback at the pituitary. It is used in anovulatory women who wish to become pregnant.

3. **Mifepristone (RU486).** Mifepristone is an orally active steroid antagonist of progesterone and glucocorticoids. It binds to the cytosolic steroid receptors for these hormones. Its major use thus far (restricted to a few European countries) has been as an abortifacient. When it is given in a single oral dose followed by administration of a PGE or PGF analogue, a very high percentage of complete abortion is achieved with a low incidence of serious toxicity. This drug also appears to have applications in the treatment of several cancers.
4. **Relaxin.** An ovarian **peptide** hormone, relaxin causes relaxation of the pelvic ligaments and softening of the cervix. It may play a physiologic role in parturition but has no documented clinical applications.

## ANDROGENS

**Testosterone** and related androgens are produced in the testes, the adrenals, and, to a small extent, the ovaries. Testosterone is synthesized from progesterone and dehydroepiandrosterone. In the plasma, it is about 65% bound to sex hormone-binding globulin (SHBG), a transport protein. It is converted in many organs to **dihydrotestosterone,** which is the active hormone in those tissues, eg, the prostate. Because of rapid hepatic metabolism, testosterone given by mouth has little effect. It may be given parenterally, or orally active variants may be used (see Drug List).

**A. Mechanism of Action:** Like other steroid hormones, androgens enter cells and react with a cytosolic receptor. The hormone-receptor complex enters the nucleus and modulates the expression of certain genes.

**B. Effects:** Testosterone is necessary for the normal development of the male fetus and infant and is responsible for the major changes in the male at puberty (growth of penis, larynx, and skeleton; development of facial, pubic, and axillary hair; darkening of skin; enlargement of muscle mass). It causes masculinization of the female when used for its anabolic properties. The major effect of androgenic hormones other than the development and maintenance of normal male characteristics is an anabolic action that involves increased muscle size and strength and increased red blood cell production. Excretion of urea nitrogen is reduced ("positive nitrogen balance"). The ratio of androgenic to anabolic potency varies somewhat among the synthetic compounds available, but all retain considerable androgenic effect. Therefore, the use of these hormones by athletes to increase muscle strength is attended by the hazards of unwanted androgenic effects.

**C. Clinical Use:** The clinical uses of the androgens include replacement therapy in hypogonadism and, rarely, suppression of estrogen secretion or function in women. The anabolic effects are used by male and female athletes, especially weight lifters, to increase muscle bulk and strength. The availability of recombinant erythropoietin has rendered obsolete the use of androgens to stimulate red blood cell production in anemias.

**D. Toxicity:** The toxicity of the androgens is largely a result of their masculinizing effects. In addition, they have caused cholestatic jaundice, elevation of SGOT levels, and, in a few cases, hepatocellular carcinoma. Excessive use by athletes and muscle builders is sometimes associated with behavioral changes including unpredictable rage and hostility. Development of dependence and a withdrawal syndrome have been proposed.

## ANTIANDROGENS

**Cyproterone** and its acetate derivative are steroidal competitive inhibitors of testosterone at its receptor. They have been used on an investigational basis to decrease the action of the endogenous hormone. **Flutamide** is a nonsteroidal androgen antagonist sometimes used in prostate cancer. **Ketoconazole**, an antifungal agent, inhibits steroid synthesis. It has been used as an investigational agent to suppress adrenal steroid synthesis in patients with steroid-dependent metastatic tumors. **Finasteride,** a nonsteroid inhibitor of 5α-reductase, the enzyme required for conversion of testosterone to dihydrotestosterone, is used in the treatment of benign prostatic hypertrophy.

### CONTRACEPTION IN THE MALE

**Gossypol** is a cottonseed oil derivative that was serendipitously discovered to reduce spermatogenesis. It reduces fertility in most males by destroying seminiferous cells. However, it is not nearly as reliable a contraceptive as the oral contraceptives used by women. It causes hypokalemia, and the weakness associated with this side effect may limit its use. Androgenic and estrogenic hormones also reduce spermatogenesis, primarily by suppressing pituitary LH and FSH production. However, the low efficacy of these agents and their other hormonal effects have prevented serious consideration of their use as contraceptives.

## DRUG LIST

The following drugs are important members of the group discussed in this chapter. Prototype agents should be learned in detail; the major variants should be known well enough to list the factors that distinguish them from the prototypes and from each other, and the other significant agents should be recognized as belonging to a specific subclass.

| Subclass | Prototype | Major Variants | Other Significant Agents |
|---|---|---|---|
| Estrogens<br>Natural | Estradiol | | Estrone, estriol |
| Orally active | | Ethinyl estradiol, mestranol, chlorotrianisene | Estradiol cypionate |
| Used in cancer | | Diethylstilbestrol | |
| Estrogen antagonists | Tamoxifen | | |
| Partial agonists | Clomiphene | | |
| Progestins<br>Natural | Progesterone | | |
| Orally active | | Norethindrone, Norgestrel, Danazol | |
| Antiprogestin | Mifepristone | | |
| Androgens<br>Natural | Testosterone | | |
| Orally active | Methyltestosterone | Fluoxymesterone | |
| Antiandrogens | Cyproterone | Flutamide, finasteride | |

## QUESTIONS

**DIRECTIONS (items 1–3):** Each of the numbered items or incomplete statements in this section is followed by answers or by completions of the statement. Select the ONE lettered answer or completion that is BEST in each case.

**1.** All of the following agents are useful in oral or implantable contraceptives EXCEPT
**(A)** ethinyl estradiol
**(B)** mestranol
**(C)** clomiphene
**(D)** norethindrone
**(E)** norgestrel

**2.** All of the following are recognized effects of oral contraceptives EXCEPT
**(A)** increased risk of myocardial infarction
**(B)** nausea
**(C)** edema
**(D)** increased risk of endometrial cancer
**(E)** decreased risk of ovarian cancer

**3.** All of the following are recognized effects of natural androgens or androgenic steroids EXCEPT
**(A)** growth of facial hair
**(B)** increased muscle bulk
**(C)** increased milk production in nursing women
**(D)** induction of a growth spurt in pubertal boys
**(E)** cholestatic jaundice and elevation of SGOT levels in the blood

**DIRECTIONS (items 4–8):** Items 4–8 consist of lettered headings followed by a set of numbered phrases. For each numbered phrase, select the ONE lettered heading that is most closely associated with it. Each lettered heading may be selected once, more than once, or not at all.

**(A)** Cyproterone
**(B)** Clomiphene
**(C)** Tamoxifen
**(D)** Mestranol
**(E)** Norgestrel

**4.** A partial agonist estrogen that stimulates ovulation

**5.** A synthetic estrogen that is useful in oral contraceptives of the combined type

**6.** A synthetic progestin used in both combination and progestin-only contraceptives

**7.** A drug that competes with testosterone for its receptor

**8.** A competitive inhibitor of estrogens that is useful in advanced breast cancer

## ANSWERS

**1.** Clomiphene is an antiestrogen and would be of no value in an oral contraceptive. The answer is **(C)**.

**2.** The oral contraceptives are associated with a decreased risk of both endometrial and ovarian cancer. The answer is **(D)**.

**3.** Androgens, like estrogens, suppress the pituitary release of prolactin and suppress lactation. The answer is **(C)**.

**4.** Clomiphene apparently reduces the feedback inhibition by estrogens of the hypothalamus and pituitary, resulting in an increased production of gonadotropins. The answer is **(B)**.

**5.** The answer is **(D)**, mestranol.

**6.** The answer is **(E)**, norgestrel.

**7.** The answer is **(A)**, cyproterone.

**8.** Tamoxifen is a competitive inhibitor of estrogen. It is useful in the treatment of estrogen-dependent breast carcinoma. The answer is **(C)**.

# 40 Pancreatic Hormones & Antidiabetic Agents

## OBJECTIVES

**Define the following terms:**

- A or alpha cell
- B or beta cell
- C-peptide
- Insulin-dependent and non-insulin-dependent diabetes mellitus (IDDM and NIDDM)
- Insulin resistant diabetes
- Oral hypoglycemic agent

**You should be able to:**

- List the sources of insulin in clinical use.
- List the principal types of insulin preparations with different durations of action.
- Describe the effects of insulin on the liver, on muscle, and on adipose tissue.
- Describe the major hazards of insulin therapy.
- Describe the mechanisms of action of the 2 major classes of oral hypoglycemic agents.
- Describe the use of glucagon in diabetes.

## CONCEPTS

The pancreas contains at least 4 different types of endocrine cells, including **A** (alpha, glucagon-producing), **B** (beta, insulin-producing), **D** (delta, somatostatin-producing), and **F** (PP, pancreatic polypeptide-producing). Of these, the B (insulin-producing) cells are predominant. The most common pancreatic disease requiring pharmacologic therapy is diabetes mellitus, a deficiency of insulin production or effect.

### INSULIN

Insulin is synthesized as a prohormone, **proinsulin,** an 86-amino-acid single-chain polypeptide. Cleavage of proinsulin and cross-linking result in the 2-chain 51-peptide insulin hormone and a 31-amino-acid residual **C-peptide.** C-peptide is of clinical interest because it can be measured by immunoassay independently of insulin. Neither proinsulin nor C-peptide appears to have any physiologic actions.

**A. Effects:** Insulin has extremely important effects in almost every tissue of the body. Its actions on the liver, muscle, and adipose tissue are the best documented (Table 40–1). The cell surface insulin receptor is a tyrosine protein kinase that phosphorylates itself and a variety of intracellular proteins. The major target organs for insulin action include the following:

1. **Liver.** Insulin increases the storage of glucose as glycogen in the liver. This involves the increased synthesis of the enzymes pyruvate kinase, phosphofructokinase, and glucokinase and the suppression of several other enzymes. Insulin also decreases protein catabolism.
2. **Muscle.** Insulin stimulates glycogen synthesis and protein synthesis. Glucose (and potassium) transport into the cell is facilitated.
3. **Adipose tissue.** Insulin facilitates triglyceride storage by activating plasma lipoprotein lipase, by increasing glucose transport into cells, and by reducing intracellular lipolysis.

**B. Types of Insulin Available:** Insulin preparations are available from several animal sources (pork, beef), and human insulin is produced by bacterial recombinant DNA technology. The

**Table 40–1.** Endocrine effects of insulin.[1]

| | |
|---|---|
| Effect on liver | |
| Reversal of catabolic features of insulin deficiency | Inhibits glycogenolysis; inhibits conversion of fatty acids and amino acids to keto acids; inhibits conversion of amino acids to glucose |
| Anabolic action | Promotes glucose storage as glycogen (induces glucokinase and glycogen synthase, inhibits phosphorylase); increases triglyceride synthesis and very low density lipoprotein formation |
| Effect on muscle | |
| Increased protein synthesis | Increases amino acid transport; increases ribosomal protein synthesis |
| Increased glycogen synthesis | Increases glucose transport; induces glycogen synthase and inhibits phosphorylase |
| Effect on adipose tissue | |
| Increased triglyceride storage | Lipoprotein lipase is induced and activated by insulin to hydrolyze triglycerides from lipoproteins; glucose transport into cell provides glycerol phosphate to permit esterification of fatty acids supplied by lipoprotein transport; intracellular lipase is inhibited by insulin |

[1]Reproduced, with permission, from Katzung BG (editor): *Basic & Clinical Pharmacology,* 5th ed. Appleton & Lange, 1992.

insulin molecule has a half-life of only a few minutes in the circulation, so many preparations for use in diabetes are formulated to release the hormone slowly into the circulation. The forms available provide 3 durations of effect: short- or rapid-acting **(crystalline zinc [regular], semilente zinc suspension [prompt])**; intermediate-acting **(isophane insulin suspension [NPH insulin], lente zinc suspension)**; and long-acting **(protamine zinc, ultralente)**. The peak and total durations of effect of these preparations are listed in Table 40–2. "Human" insulin is available from 2 sources: bacterial recombinant DNA-induced synthesis and chemical modification of pork insulin.

**C. Hazards of Insulin Use:** Diabetic patients who use insulin are subject to 2 types of complications: hypoglycemia, from excessive insulin effect; and immunologic toxic effects, from the development of antibodies. Hypoglycemia is a very dangerous hazard, because brain damage may result. Prompt administration of glucose (sugar or candy by mouth, glucose by vein) or of glucagon (by intramuscular injection or by nasal spray) is essential.

The most common and important form of insulin-induced immunologic complication is the formation of insulin antibodies, which results in resistance to the action of the drug. Of the forms available, beef insulin is the most antigenic, human the least, and pork intermediate. Lipodystro-

**Table 40–2.** Insulin: Types and activity.[1]

| Pharmacokinetic Type | Species Type | Activity (hours) Peak | Activity (hours) Duration[2] |
|---|---|---|---|
| Rapid-acting | | | |
| Insulin injection USP (regular, crystalline zinc) | Beef, pork, or mixture; or human. | ½–3 | 5–7 |
| Insulin zinc suspension USP (prompt, semilente) | Beef, pork, or mixture; or human. | 1–4 | 12–16 |
| Intermediate-acting | | | |
| Isophane insulin suspension USP (NPH insulin) | Beef, pork, or mixture; or human. | 8–12 | 18–24 |
| Insulin zinc suspension USP (lente) | Beef, pork, or mixture; or human. | 8–12 | 18–24 |
| Long-acting | | | |
| Protamine zinc insulin suspension USP (PZI) | Beef, pork, or mixture. | 8–16 | 24–36 |
| Insulin zinc suspension extended USP (ultralente) | Beef or human. | 8–16 | 24–36 |

[1]Modified and reproduced, with permission, from Katzung BG (editor): *Basic & Clinical Pharmacology,* 5th ed. Appleton & Lange, 1992.
[2]The duration of action is increased with increasing doses.

phy, a change in fatty tissue at the site of injection, was relatively common in the past. Use of purified, less antigenic, forms of insulin has almost eliminated this complication.

## ORAL HYPOGLYCEMIC AGENTS

Two groups of drugs are in use for the oral treatment of diabetes: the **sulfonylureas** and the **biguanides.** Some members of these groups are listed in Table 40–3.

**A. Sulfonylureas:** The primary action of the sulfonylureas is to stimulate the release of endogenous insulin. They are inactive in insulin-dependent diabetes and in adult diabetics who lack functioning islet cells. In addition, it has been proposed that these drugs may reduce glucagon release and increase the number of functional insulin receptors in peripheral tissues. A family of "second-generation" sulfonylureas **(glyburide, glipizide)** is now available. These drugs are considerably more potent and possibly more effective than the older agents **(tolbutamide, chlorpropamide,** etc).

**B. Biguanides:** The biguanides act by an unknown mechanism. They are effective in some patients who lack functional islet cells. Mechanisms that have been proposed include stimulation of glycolysis in peripheral tissues, reduced hepatic gluconeogenesis, reduction of glucose absorption from the gastrointestinal tract, and reduction of plasma glucagon levels. According to some controversial studies, the use of one biguanide **(phenformin)** in the USA was associated with an apparent increase in the incidence of lactic acidosis and no documentation of long-term benefit. It was therefore withdrawn from the market. A newer biguanide, **metformin,** is in clinical trials.

## TREATMENT OF DIABETES MELLITUS

Diabetes is diagnosed on the basis of more than one fasting blood sugar determination in excess of 140 mg/dL. Two major forms of the disease have been identified: **insulin-dependent diabetes mellitus (IDDM,** type I) and **non-insulin-dependent diabetes mellitus (NIDDM,** type II). The clinical history and course of these 2 forms differ considerably, but treatment in both cases requires careful attention to diet and blood sugar levels. Vascular disease is an important complication of IDDM and must be carefully monitored in such patients. IDDM (often called juvenile-onset diabetes) usually has its onset during childhood and results from destruction of the B cells in the pancreatic islets. It is associated with a much higher incidence of ketoacidosis than with the second type. NIDDM usually has its onset in adulthood and is frequently associated with obesity and insulin resistance rather than with insulin deficiency.

**A. Insulin-Dependent Diabetes Mellitus:** Therapy of IDDM involves dietary instruction, parenteral insulin (usually a mixture of shorter- and longer-acting forms to maintain a stable blood sugar level during the day), and careful attention by the patient to factors that change insulin

**Table 40–3.** Oral antidiabetic drugs.

| Drug | Daily Dose | Duration of Action (hours) |
|---|---|---|
| Sulfonylureas | | |
| Tolbutamide | 0.5–2 g in divided doses | 6–12 |
| Tolazamide | 0.1–1 g as single dose or in divided doses | 10–14 |
| Acetohexamide | 0.25–1.5 g as single dose or in divided doses | 12–24 |
| Chlorpropamide | 0.1–0.5 g as single dose | Up to 60 |
| Glyburide | 0.00125–0.02 g | 10–24 |
| Glipizide | 0.005–0.02 g | 3–8 |
| Biguanides | | |
| Phenformin | 0.025–0.15 g as single dose or in divided doses | 4–6 |
| Metformin | 1–3 g in divided doses | 10–12 |

requirements: exercise, infections or other forms of stress, and deviations from the regular diet. A patient with diabetes is discussed in Case 12 (Appendix III).

**B. Non-Insulin-Dependent Diabetes Mellitus:** Therapy of NIDDM starts with attempts to eliminate obesity and lower the blood glucose levels by dietary means. If this regimen is unsuccessful, oral hypoglycemic agents are used. A sulfonylurea agent is given to maximum effect or to the onset of side effects. Insulin is used only if both diet and oral hypoglycemic drugs are unsuccessful in controlling the blood sugar.

## QUESTIONS

**DIRECTIONS (items 1–4):** Each numbered item or incomplete statement in this section is followed by answers or by complications of the statement. Select the ONE lettered answer or completion that is BEST in each case.

**1.** In order to achieve rapid control of severe ketoacidosis in a hospitalized diabetic 13-year-old boy, the appropriate antidiabetic agent to use is
**(A)** crystalline zinc insulin
**(B)** isophane (NPH) insulin
**(C)** protamine zinc or ultralente insulin
**(D)** tolbutamide
**(E)** glyburide

**2.** All of the following act by a similar mechanism EXCEPT
**(A)** tolbutamide
**(B)** tolazamide
**(C)** chlorpropamide
**(D)** glipizide
**(E)** phenformin

**3.** Effects of insulin include all of the following EXCEPT
**(A)** increased glucose transport into cells
**(B)** induction of lipoprotein lipase
**(C)** decreased gluconeogenesis
**(D)** stimulation of glycogenolysis
**(E)** decreased conversion of amino acids into glucose

**4.** Possible complications of insulin therapy include
**(A)** dilutional hyponatremia
**(B)** hypoglycemia
**(C)** pancreatitis
**(D)** increased bleeding tendency
**(E)** all of the above

**DIRECTIONS (items 5–8):** Items 5–8 consist of lettered headings followed by a set of numbered phrases. For each numbered phrase, select the ONE lettered heading that is most closely associated with it. Each lettered heading may be selected once, more than once, or not at all.

**(A)** Human NPH (isophane) insulin (bacterial origin)
**(B)** Porcine regular crystalline zinc insulin
**(C)** Bovine protamine zinc (PZI) insulin
**(D)** Tolazamide
**(E)** Phenformin

C **5.** Longest-acting insulin preparation

**6.** Most antigenic insulin preparation

**7.** Primary action is to release endogenous insulin

**8.** Not dependent on functioning pancreatic islet cells but associated with increased incidence of lactic acidosis

## ANSWERS

**1.** Oral antidiabetic agents are inappropriate in this patient, because he probably has insulin-dependent diabetes mellitus (suggested by his age and the ketoacidosis). The most rapidly acting insulin preparation is needed (Table 40–2). The answer is **(A).**

**2.** Phenformin is a biguanide oral antidiabetic agent; the others are all sulfonylureas (Table 40–3). The answer is **(E).**

**3.** The answer is **(D)** (Table 40–1).

**4.** Hypoglycemia is the most important acute hazard of insulin therapy. The answer is **(B).**

**5.** The answer is **(C)** (Table 40–2).

**6.** Bovine insulin differs from human insulin by 3 amino acids, whereas porcine differs by only one. The answer is **(C).**

**7.** The sulfonylureas are inactive in patients without functioning B cells; ie, they release insulin. In contrast, the biguanides do lower blood sugar in such individuals. The answer is **(D),** tolazamide.

**8.** The answer is **(E),** phenformin, a biguanide.

# 41 Drugs That Affect Bone Mineral Homeostasis

## OBJECTIVES

**You should be able to:**

- List the agents useful in hypercalcemia.
- List the major and minor hormonal regulators of bone mineral homeostasis.
- Describe the major effects of parathyroid hormone on the intestines, kidneys, and bone.
- Describe the major effects of vitamin D and its derivatives on the intestines, kidneys, and bone.
- Describe the therapeutic and toxic effects of fluoride ion.

## CONCEPTS

Calcium and phosphorus are the 2 major elements of bone. They are also important in the metabolism of other cells in the body, and bone therefore functions as a storage reservoir. The 2 hormones of primary importance in the regulation of bone mineral homeostasis are parathyroid hormone (PTH) and vitamin D. Less important endogenous regulators include calcitonin, glucocorticoids, and estrogens. Several drugs that influence bone through other mechanisms are available.

**A. Parathyroid Hormone:** PTH is an 84-amino-acid peptide. It regulates calcium and phosphorus flux across cell membranes in bone and in the renal tubule. At high doses, the hormone increases the blood calcium level and decreases the phosphorus level by increasing net bone resorption. At low doses (physiologic levels), the agent may actually increase net bone formation (Table 41–1). The peptide appears to increase cAMP in cells. A 34-amino-acid agent similar to PTH is under study for the treatment of osteoporosis.

**B. Vitamin D:** Vitamin D, a derivative of 7-dehydrocholesterol, is formed in the skin under the influence of ultraviolet light. It is also found in some foods and is commonly used as a food supplement. Several forms of the hormone occur, differing primarily in the number of hydroxyl groups on the molecule (Table 41–2). Some vitamin D is stored in adipose tissue; the rest is cleared by the liver.

The actions of vitamin D include increased intestinal calcium and phosphorus absorption, decreased renal excretion of these minerals, and a net increase in blood levels of both (Table 41–1). Bone formation may be increased by one of the isomers of the hormone (24,25-dihydroxyvitamin D).

**C. Calcitonin:** Calcitonin is a peptide hormone secreted by the thyroid gland that decreases bone resorption and serum calcium and phosphate levels. Bone formation is not impaired initially, but ultimately is reduced. Therefore, calcitonin is not useful in treating conditions in which bone mass is reduced, eg, osteoporosis. It has been used in conditions in which an acute reduction of serum calcium levels is needed, eg, Paget's disease and hypercalcemia. No disease involving a primary abnormality of calcitonin secretion has been recognized. Although human calcitonin is available, salmon calcitonin is most often selected for clinical use because of its longer half-life and greater potency.

**D. Glucocorticoids:** The adrenal glucocorticoids have several effects (discussed in Chapter 38) that inhibit bone mineral maintenance. As a result, chronic use may be associated with osteoporosis. However, these hormones are useful in the intermediate-term treatment of hypercalcemia.

**E. Estrogens:** The estrogens can prevent or delay bone loss in postmenopausal women. There is some evidence that they may even increase bone density. Their action may involve the inhibition

**Table 41–1.** Actions of PTH and vitamin D on gut, bone, and kidneys.[1]

| | PTH | Vitamin D |
|---|---|---|
| Intestines | Increased calcium and phosphate absorption [by increased $1,25(OH)_2D$ production] | Increased calcium and phosphate absorption [by $1,25(OH)_2D$] |
| Kidneys | Decreased calcium excretion, increased phosphate excretion | Calcium and phosphate excretion may be decreased by 25(OH)D and $1,25(OH)_2D$ |
| Bone | Calcium and phosphate resorption increased by high doses; low doses may increase bone formation | Increased calcium and phosphate resorption by $1,25(OH)_2D$; bone formation may be increased by $24,25(OH)_2D$ |
| Net effect on serum levels | Serum calcium increased, serum phosphate decreased | Serum calcium and phosphate both increased |

[1]Reproduced, with permission, from Katzung BG (editor): *Basic & Clinical Pharmacology,* 5th ed. Appleton & Lange, 1992.

**Table 41–2.** Vitamin D and its clinically available metabolites and analogs.[1]

| Chemical Name | Abbreviation | Generic Name |
|---|---|---|
| Vitamin $D_3$ | D3 | Cholecalciferol |
| Vitamin $D_2$ | D2 | Ergocalciferol |
| 25-Hydroxyvitamin $D_3$ | 25(OH)D3 | Calcifediol |
| 1,25-Dihydroxyvitamin $D_3$ | 1,25(OH)2$D_3$ | Calcitriol |
| Dihydrotachysterol | DHT | Dihydrotachysterol |

[1]Reproduced, with permission, from Katzung BG (editor): *Basic & Clinical Pharmacology,* 5th ed. Appleton & Lange, 1992.

of parathyroid hormone-stimulated bone resorption. They are heavily used in the treatment of postmenopausal osteoporosis.

**F. Other Drugs That Affect Bone or Calcium Homeostasis:** The **diphosphonates** (eg, **etidronate**) are short-chain organic polyphosphate compounds that reduce both the resorption and the formation of bone by an action on the basic hydroxyapatite crystal structure. A recent study suggests that chronic etidronate therapy may halt the progress of postmenopausal osteoporosis and possibly reverse it. **Mithramycin (plicamycin)** is an antibiotic agent used to reduce serum calcium and bone resorption in Paget's disease and hypercalcemia. Appropriate concentrations of **fluoride ion** in drinking water (0.5–1 ppm), or as a dentifrice additive, have a well-documented ability to reduce dental caries. Chronic exposure to the ion may increase new bone synthesis, especially in high concentrations. Results of investigational therapy using fluoride with calcium supplements in osteoporosis have not been encouraging. The **thiazide diuretics** (see Chapter 15) reduce the excretion of calcium by the kidneys and have been used to decrease kidney stone formation.

## QUESTIONS

**DIRECTIONS (items 1 and 2):** Each of the numbered items or incomplete statements in this section is followed by answers or by completions of the statement. Select the ONE lettered answer or completion that is BEST in each case.

**1.** All of the following are useful in the therapy of hypercalcemia EXCEPT
**(A)** calcitonin
**(B)** glucocorticoids
**(C)** thiazides
**(D)** mithramycin
**(E)** parenteral infusion of phosphate

**2.** Characteristics of vitamin D include which of the following?
**(A)** It is a prohormone produced in the liver
**(B)** Active metabolites decrease serum calcium levels
**(C)** Active metabolites increase serum phosphorus levels
**(D)** Active metabolites increase cellular cAMP levels
**(E)** All of the above

**DIRECTIONS (items 3–5):** Items 3–5 consist of lettered headings followed by a set of numbered phrases. For each numbered phrase, select the ONE lettered heading that is most closely associated with it. Each lettered heading may be used once, more than once, or not at all.

**(A)** Parathyroid hormone
**(B)** Vitamin D
**(C)** Calcitonin
**(D)** Estrogen
**(E)** Fluoride

**3.** A hormone secreted by the human thyroid; the more commonly used preparation is obtained from salmon

**4.** An agent that appears to facilitate new, possibly abnormal, bone formation, especially if ingested in high concentrations

**5.** Causes decreased renal calcium excretion and increased plasma phosphorus levels

## ANSWERS

**1.** Thiazides reduce urine calcium levels (see Chapter 15) and are never used in patients with hypercalcemia. Loop diuretics (eg, furosemide), on the other hand, are useful in this condition. The answer is **(C)**.

**2.** Vitamin D is a prohormone whose metabolites increase serum phosphorus levels. They also increase serum calcium levels (Table 41–1). The active metabolites are produced in the skin, not the liver. Parathyroid hormone, not vitamin D, acts via cAMP. The answer is **(C)**.

**3.** The answer is **(C)**, calcitonin.

**4.** The answer is **(E)**, fluoride.

**5.** The answer is **(B)**, vitamin D (Table 41–1).

# Part VIII. Chemotherapeutic Drugs

# Principles of Antimicrobial Drug Action

# 42

## OBJECTIVES

**Define the following terms:**

- Selective toxicity
- Bacteriostatic
- Bactericidal
- Antimetabolite
- Bacterial resistance
- Plasmid-mediated resistance
- R factor
- Cross-resistance

**You should be able to:**

- Describe 4 different mechanisms of action of antimicrobial drugs.
- Classify the major antimicrobial drug groups in terms of their mechanism of action.
- List 4 different mechanisms by which microorganisms become resistant to drugs.
- Identify the major mechanisms responsible for resistance to the antimicrobial drugs commonly used in clinical settings.

## CONCEPTS

### A. Definitions:

1. **Selective toxicity** is a requirement for effective and safe chemotherapy of infections caused by invading organisms. Ideally, an antimicrobial drug should be much more toxic to the microorganism causing infection than to host cells. Selective toxicity may result from the following:
   a. Accumulation of a drug to higher levels in a microorganism than in human cells.
   b. The action of a drug only on cellular structures or biochemical processes that are unique to the microorganism.
   c. Actions of a drug on biochemical processes more critical to the parasite than to host cells.
2. The effects of antimicrobial drugs on bacteria can lead to an inhibition of growth (ie, a **bacteriostatic** effect) that will be reversible upon removal of the drug unless host defense mechanisms have eradicated the organism. Examples of antimicrobial drugs that are usually bacteriostatic include erythromycin and the tetracyclines. Drugs that kill bacteria (ie, **bactericidal** drugs) are less dependent on defense mechanisms for their therapeutic effects. Beta-lactam antibiotics and the aminoglycosides are usually bactericidal.
3. **Resistance** to antimicrobial drugs may develop via both genetic and nongenetic mechanisms. Most resistant organisms emerge through chromosomal or extrachromosomal genetic changes followed by selection processes. **Chromosomal resistance** involves spontaneous mutation at a genetic locus that controls susceptibility to specific drugs. **Extrachromosomal resistance** involves **plasmids (R factors)** that carry genes for resistance to one or more drugs. These plasmids can be transferred between organisms by transduction, transformation, translocation, or, most importantly, bacterial conjugation. **Transposons** may carry genes for resistance from plasmids to chromosomes. **Cross-resistance** can occur between antimicrobial drugs, especially if they are chemically related and have similar mechanisms of action.

## B. Mechanisms of Action:

1. **Inhibition of bacterial cell wall synthesis.** Bacterial cell walls contain complex macromolecules, mucopeptides, and peptidoglycans, formed via biosynthetic pathways that are absent from mammalian cells. The widely used beta-lactam antibiotics (**penicillins** and **cephalosporins**) bind to specific proteins (**penicillin-binding proteins, PBPs**) that are located in the bacterial cytoplasmic membrane. This leads to the inhibition of transpeptidase activities, which are required for cross-linking of the linear peptidoglycan chains, the final step in cell wall synthesis. Inhibition of these enzymes by beta-lactam antibiotics results in decreased cell wall synthesis, and these antibiotics also activate autolytic enzymes that damage the cell wall. In susceptible organisms, these actions are bactericidal.
2. **Inhibition of protein synthesis.** The mechanisms of protein synthesis in microorganisms are not identical to those of mammalian cells. Many of the commonly used antimicrobial drugs selectively inhibit bacterial protein synthesis. **Tetracyclines** block the formation of the 30S initiation complex by binding to a specific site on this ribosomal subunit. **Aminoglycoside antibiotics** also interact with the 30S ribosomal subunit, but with different receptors, and this binding blocks the formation of the 70S initiation complex. The bacterial 50S ribosomal subunit contains specific receptors for **erythromycin,** which can inhibit aminoacyl translocation reactions, and for **chloramphenicol,** which inhibits peptidyltransferase activity. Tetracyclines and chloramphenicol are not totally selective in their actions, since they can inhibit protein synthesis in certain mammalian cells.
3. **Inhibition of nucleic acid synthesis.** A smaller number of drugs act at this level. The **quinolones** and **fluoroquinolones** block nucleic acid synthesis by inhibiting DNA gyrase, the enzyme that converts supercoiled DNA to the relaxed form. **Rifampin** is an inhibitor of DNA-dependent RNA polymerase. Nucleic acid synthesis is dependent on folic acid, which acts as a coenzyme in many biosynthetic reactions. Humans obtain folate in the diet, but many microorganisms must synthesize the coenzyme. **Sulfonamides** inhibit bacterial folate synthesis at the level of dihydropteroate synthetase by acting as antimetabolites of the endogenous substrate *p*-aminobenzoic acid (PABA). Similarly, **trimethoprim** is an antimetabolite of folic acid that selectively inhibits dihydrofolate reductases of bacteria and protozoa.
4. **Disruption of cell membrane permeability.** Although the cell membranes of microorganisms function similarly to those of mammalian cells, their chemical composition is distinctive. This difference permits the selectively toxic action of certain antimicrobial drugs. The **polymyxins** act to disrupt the selective permeability of bacterial cell membranes by insertion into the lipid bilayer to form artificial pores. The **polyene** antimicrobials bind to membrane components, including ergosterol, present only in microbial cells. The **imidazole** antifungal agents act as selective inhibitors of enzymes involved in the synthesis of sterols that are essential components of fungal membranes.

## C. Mechanisms of Resistance:

1. **Production of drug-inactivating enzymes.** This common mechanism causes resistance to many beta-lactam antibiotics. The synthesis of hydrolytic **beta-lactamase** enzymes (**penicillinases),** specific for certain penicillin structures, is characteristic of staphylococci and many gram-negative bacteria. A recent therapeutic strategy to counter such resistance has been administration of a penicillin antibiotic in the "protective custody" of an inhibitor (eg, clavulanic acid, sulbactam) of the penicillinases. Beta-lactamase enzymes that hydrolyze cephalosporins can cause resistance to this class of drugs. Plasmid-mediated resistance to aminoglycosides is caused by the formation of inactivating enzymes **(group transferases)** that catalyze the transfer of acetyl groups and other moieties to the drug molecules.
2. **Changes in receptor structure.** Molecules that act as targets, or receptors, for antimicrobial drugs may undergo changes in molecular structure, rendering them less susceptible to the toxic actions of the drugs. The methylation of a macromolecule that forms part of the erythromycin receptor on the 50S ribosomal subunit is enough to interfere with drug binding and thus lead to resistance. Similarly, apparently minor structural changes in the receptors for aminoglycosides are responsible for marked changes in the drug susceptibility of the organism. The structure of target enzymes may also change, leading to a decrease in the inhibitory effects of antimicrobial drugs. This mechanism has been reported for dihydrofolate reductase in organisms resistant to trimethoprim and for DNA gyrase in resistance to fluoroquinolones. Differences in PBPs may also be responsible for the limited susceptibility of many bacteria to the beta-lactam group of drugs.

3. **Changes in drug permeation and transport.** The antimicrobial action of many drugs depends on their ability to penetrate the cell membranes of an organism and reach effective intracellular concentrations. Aminoglycosides are polar compounds that require oxygen-dependent membrane transport for their intracellular accumulation; thus, anaerobes are resistant to their effects. Tetracycline resistance is a result of decreased intracellular concentrations of such drugs. This may be because of a decrease in microbial membrane permeability, an increase in the activity of mechanisms involved in extrusion of tetracyclines, or a combination of the two.
4. **Development of alternative metabolic pathways.** Of the antibacterial agents, sulfonamides best illustrate the mechanisms of alternative metabolic pathways. Resistant bacterial strains may produce levels of PABA high enough to overcome the inhibition of dihydropteroate synthetase by a sulfonamide. Certain bacteria are able to utilize preformed folic acid from their environment and thus bypass the inhibitory actions of the sulfonamides.

## QUESTIONS

**DIRECTIONS (items 1–4):** Each numbered item or incomplete statement in this section is followed by answers or by completions of the statement. Select the ONE lettered answer or completion that is BEST in each case.

1. Which of the following is NOT an action of the beta-lactam antibiotics on bacteria?
   **(A)** Inhibition of the cross-linking of peptidoglycan chains
   **(B)** Binding to specific proteins in the cytoplasmic membrane
   **(C)** Activation of autolytic enzymes
   **(D)** Inhibition of peptidyl transferase

2. All of the following statements about antimicrobial drugs are accurate EXCEPT:
   **(A)** Transposons can transfer resistance factors from plasmids to bacterial chromosomes
   **(B)** Spontaneous mutation is a frequent cause of clinical resistance during antimicrobial drug therapy in a given patient
   **(C)** Plasmid-mediated resistance is an example of extrachromosomal resistance
   **(D)** R factors are plasmids that carry genes for resistance to one or more drugs

3. The main reason that sulfonamides have a selective action as antimicrobial drugs is:
   **(A)** Sterol synthesis is essential to microbial but not mammalian cells
   **(B)** Bacterial cells do not contain dihydrofolate reductase
   **(C)** The drug sensitivities of dihydrofolate reductases of microbial and mammalian cells are different
   **(D)** Mammalian cells lack dihydropteroate synthetase

4. All of the following antimicrobial agents are inhibitors of protein synthesis EXCEPT
   **(A)** clindamycin
   **(B)** tetracycline
   **(C)** vancomycin
   **(D)** streptomycin
   **(E)** chloramphenicol

**DIRECTIONS (items 5–9):** Items 5–9 consist of lettered headings followed by a set of numbered sentences. For each numbered sentence, select the ONE lettered heading that is most closely associated with it. Each lettered heading may be selected once, more than once, or not at all.

**(A)** Tobramycin
**(B)** Rifampin
**(C)** Erythromycin
**(D)** Ampicillin
**(E)** Tetracycline

5. Plasmid-mediated resistance involves the production of inactivating group transferase enzymes, including those that acetylate this drug

6. Treatment of bacterial infections with this agent as the sole drug often fails because the spontaneous mutation rate is high and can occur with a frequency of $10^{-5}$–$10^{-7}$

7. Resistance to this drug, particularly in staphylococci and gram-negative bacteria, involves the production of beta-lactamases

8. Higher intracellular concentrations of this drug are found in susceptible bacteria than in resistant bacteria

9. Resistance to this drug, an inhibitor of protein synthesis, may occur through small changes in the structure of its receptor on the bacterial 50S ribosomal subunit

## ANSWERS

1. The beta-lactams (penicillins, cephalosporins) bind to specific membrane proteins, inhibit transpeptidases involved in bacterial cell wall synthesis, and activate autolytic enzymes that attack cell walls. They do not interfere with protein synthesis. The answer is **(D)**.

2. Spontaneous mutation usually occurs with a frequency of $10^{-12}$ to $10^{-8}$ and thus is not a frequent cause of emergence of clinical resistance during a course of antimicrobial drug therapy. The answer is **(B)**.

3. Although sterols are essential components of fungal cell membranes, sulfonamides have no effects on sterol synthesis. Statement **(C)** is correct but concerns the selectivity of trimethoprim, not sulfonamides. Mammalian cells do not utilize PABA to synthesize folic acid because they lack dihydropteroate synthetase. The answer is **(D)**.

4. Vancomycin is a glycopeptide antibiotic that inhibits the synthesis of bacterial cell walls by binding to precursor subunits. The other drugs listed all inhibit bacterial protein synthesis, but via different mechanisms. The answer is **(C)**.

5. Resistance to any of the drugs listed may be plasmid-mediated, but production of specific transferase enzyme activities is the mechanism of resistance to aminoglycosides and to chloramphenicol (not listed). The answer is **(A)**.

6. This is an exception to the general rule mentioned in answer to question 2. Chromosomal mutants resistant to rifampin occur with a high frequency, and treatment often fails if the drug is used as the sole agent for bacterial infections. The answer is **(B)**.

7. The inhibitory action of penicillins on bacterial cell wall synthesis requires the intact beta-lactam ring structure. Hydrolysis of the ring via beta-lactamases inactivates ampicillin (and penicillin G). This resistance mechanism is common in staphylococci and in many gram-negative bacteria. The answer is **(D)**.

8. A decrease in the accumulation of tetracyclines is a major characteristic of bacteria that are less susceptible to this class of drugs. This property appears to be responsible for most cases of clinical resistance to the tetracyclines. The answer is **(E)**.

9. The aminoglycosides, erythromycin, and the tetracyclines are all protein synthesis inhibitors. The binding site or receptor for erythromycin is on the 50S ribosomal subunit, and this macromolecule can have a changed structure, via methylation, in resistant bacteria. The answer is **(C)**.

# Penicillins & Cephalosporins 43

## OBJECTIVES

**Define the following terms:**

- Beta-lactam ring structure
- Penicillin-binding proteins
- Peptidoglycan chains
- Beta-lactamase enzyme activity
- Transpeptidases
- Hypersensitivity reactions

**You should be able to:**

- Describe the mechanism of antibacterial action of beta-lactam antibiotics.
- Describe the mechanisms underlying the resistance of bacteria to beta-lactam antibiotics.
- Identify the important drugs in each subclass of penicillins and describe their antibacterial activity and clinical uses.
- Identify the 3 subclasses of cephalosporins and describe their antibacterial activities and clinical uses.
- List the major adverse effects of the penicillins and the cephalosporins.
- Identify the important features of aztreonam and imipenem.

## CONCEPTS

### PENICILLINS

**A. Classification:** All penicillins are derivatives of 6-aminopenicillanic acid and contain a **beta-lactam ring structure** that is essential for antibacterial activity. Penicillin subclasses have additional chemical substituents associated with differences in antimicrobial activity, susceptibility to acid and enzymatic hydrolysis, and biodisposition.

**B. Pharmacokinetics:** Penicillins vary in acid stability and therefore in their oral bioavailability. As polar compounds, they are not metabolized extensively. They are excreted unchanged in the urine via **glomerular filtration** and renal **tubular secretion,** the latter process being inhibited by probenecid. Ampicillin and nafcillin are excreted partly in the bile. The plasma half-lives of most penicillins vary from 0.5 to 1 hour. Procaine and benzathine forms of penicillin G are administered intramuscularly and have long plasma half-lives because the active drug is released very slowly into the bloodstream.

**C. Mechanism of Action:** Beta-lactam antibiotics are bactericidal drugs. They inhibit cell wall synthesis by the following steps (see Fig 43–1): (1) binding of the drug to specific receptors (penicillin-binding proteins, **PBPs**) located in the bacterial cytoplasmic membrane; (2) inhibition of **transpeptidase** enzymes that cross-link linear peptidoglycan chains which form part of the cell wall; and (3) activation of autolytic enzymes that cause lesions in the bacterial cell wall. Enzymatic hydrolysis of the beta-lactam ring of penicillins leads to inactivation of the drug. The formation of **beta-lactamases (penicillinases)** is a major mechanism of bacterial resistance to this class of drugs. Inhibitors of these enzymes (eg, clavulanic acid, sulbactam) are sometimes used in combination with penicillins to prevent their inactivation. Other resistance mechanisms include decreases in membrane permeability to penicillins and changes in membrane PBPs.

**D. Clinical Use:**

1. **Penicillin G** is the prototype of a subclass of penicillins that have a limited spectrum of antibacterial activity and are susceptible to beta-lactamases. Its clinical uses include therapy of infections caused by many streptococci, gonococci, meningococci, gram-positive bacilli, and spirochetes. Most strains of *Staphylococcus aureus* are resistant. Activity against viridans

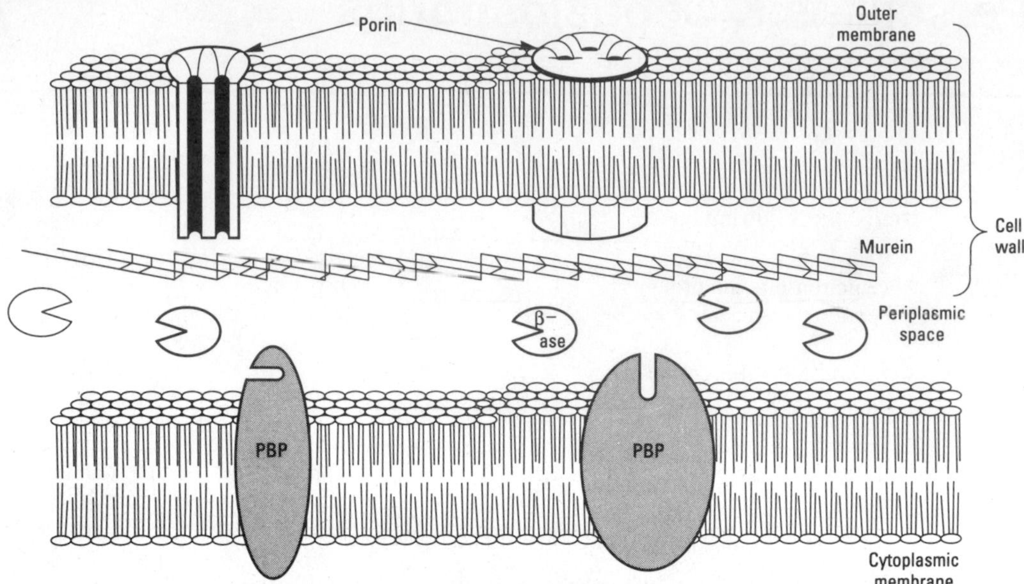


**Figure 43–1.** Beta-lactams and bacterial cell wall synthesis. In this simplified diagram of the bacterial cell envelope, the outer membrane is present only in gram-negative organisms. It is penetrated by proteins (porins) that are permeable to hydrophilic substances such as beta-lactam antibiotics. The peptidoglycan chains (mureins) are cross-linked by transpeptidases located in the cytoplasmic membrane, closely associated with penicillin-binding proteins (PBPs). Beta-lactam antibiotics bind to PBPs and inhibit transpeptidation, the final step in cell wall synthesis. They also activate autolytic enzymes that cause lesions in the cell wall. Beta-lactamases (β-ase), which inactivate beta-lactam antibiotics, may be present in the periplasmic space or on the outer surface of the cytoplasmic membrane. (Reproduced, with permission, from Katzung BG [editor]: *Basic & Clinical Pharmacology,* 5th ed. Appleton & Lange, 1992.)

Streptococcus and *Streptococcus faecalis* is enhanced by aminoglycoside antibiotics. Penicillin V is an oral drug used mainly in common streptococcal infections.

2. **Methicillin** is the prototype of a penicillin subclass that is resistant to the action of penicillinases but has a narrow spectrum of activity. The group includes **nafcillin** and **dicloxacillin.** Their sole use is in the treatment of known or suspected staphylococcal infections. Methicillin-resistant staphylococci may be resistant to multiple antimicrobial drugs.
3. **Ampicillin** and its congener, **amoxicillin,** are penicillins that have a wider spectrum of antibacterial activity than does penicillin G but remain susceptible to penicillinases. Their clinical uses include indications similar to penicillin G and also infections due to *Escherichia coli, Proteus mirabilis,* and *Haemophilus influenzae.* (Some strains of *H influenzae* are resistant.) **Carbenicillin** and congeners have activity against several gram-negative rods, including *Pseudomonas* spp, and are synergistic with aminoglycosides against such organisms. They are susceptible to penicillinases.

## E. Toxicity:

1. **Allergic reactions** include urticaria, severe pruritus, fever, joint swelling, hemolytic anemia, nephritis, and anaphylaxis. About 10–15% of persons with a history of penicillin reaction have an allergic response when given penicillin again. Methicillin causes more nephritis than do other penicillins. Antigenic determinants include degradation products of penicillins, such as penicilloic acid. Complete **cross-allergenicity** between different penicillins should be assumed. Ampicillin frequently causes maculopapular skin rashes that may not be allergic reactions.
2. **Gastrointestinal disturbances,** including nausea and diarrhea, occur with oral penicillins, especially with ampicillin. They may be caused by direct irritation or by overgrowth of gram-positive organisms or yeasts.
3. **Cation toxicity** from $Na^+$ or $K^+$ may occur when high doses of certain penicillin salts are used in patients with cardiovascular or renal disease.

## CEPHALOSPORINS

**A. Classification:** The cephalosporins, which are derivatives of 7-aminocephalosporanic acid, contain the beta-lactam ring structure. Many members of this group are in clinical use. Classified on the basis of their antibacterial activity, they are designated first-, second-, or third-generation drugs according to the time of their introduction into clinical use.

**B. Pharmacokinetics:** Several cephalosporins are available for oral use, but most are administered parenterally. Third-generation drugs are able to enter the brain. Cephalosporins with side-chains may undergo hepatic metabolism, but the major elimination mechanism for drugs in this class is renal excretion via active tubular secretion. Cefoperazone and ceftriaxone are excreted mainly in the bile.

**C. Mechanism of Action:**

1. Cephalosporins inhibit bacterial cell wall synthesis by mechanisms similar to those of penicillins; they are also bactericidal.
2. Structural differences from penicillins render cephalosporins less susceptible to penicillinases produced by staphylococci, but many bacteria are resistant through the production of other beta lactamases that can inactivate cephalosporins.
3. Methicillin-resistant staphylococci are also resistant to most cephalosporins. Other mechanisms of bacterial resistance include changes in permeability and changes in the binding proteins that act as receptors for cephalosporins.

**D. Clinical Use:**

1. **Na cephalothin** and **cefazolin** are examples of **first-generation** drugs that are active against gram-positive cocci, including *S aureus* and common streptococci. Many strains of *E coli* and *K pneumoniae* are also sensitive. Clinical uses include treatment of infections caused by these organisms and surgical prophylaxis in selected cases. They have minimal activity against gram-negative cocci, enterococci, and most other gram-negative rods.
2. **Second-generation** cephalosporins usually have the activities of the first-generation drugs but have expanded gram-negative coverage. Marked differences in activity occur between individual drugs in this subgroup. Examples of clinical uses include infections caused by *Bacteroides fragilis* (**cefoxitin**) and *H influenzae* (**cefuroxime, cefaclor**).
3. Characteristic features of **third-generation** drugs (eg, **cefoperazone, cefotaxime**) include increased activity against resistant gram-negative organisms and the ability to penetrate the blood-brain barrier. Most are active against *Enterobacter* spp, *Providencia* spp, *Serratia marcescens*, and beta-lactamase-producing strains of *H influenzae* and *Neisseria* spp. Individual drugs have activity against *Pseudomonas* spp (**ceftazidime**) and *B fragilis* (**ceftizoxime**). Drugs in this subclass are usually reserved for treatment of serious infections such as those in debilitated, immunocompromised patients.

**E. Toxicity:**

1. Cephalosporin use is associated with a range of **allergic reactions** from skin rashes to anaphylactic shock. Cross-reactivity between penicillins and cephalosporins is not complete (about 5–15%), so penicillin-allergic patients are sometimes treated successfully with a cephalosporin. However, patients with a history of anaphylactic reactions to penicillins should not be treated with a cephalosporin.
2. Cephalosporins may cause pain at intramuscular injection sites and phlebitis after intravenous administration. They may increase the nephrotoxicity of aminoglycosides when the two are administered together.
3. Drugs containing a methylthiotetrazole group (cefamandole, cefoperazone, moxalactam) cause hypoprothrombinemia and may cause disulfiramlike reactions with ethanol. Moxalactam also decreases platelet function and may cause severe bleeding.

## OTHER BETA-LACTAM DRUGS

**A. Aztreonam:** Aztreonam is a monobactam that is resistant to beta-lactamases produced by certain gram-negative rods, including *Klebsiella, Pseudomonas,* and *Serratia* spp. It has no activity against gram-positive bacteria or anaerobes. It is an inhibitor of cell wall synthesis, preferentially binding to PBP subtype 3, and is synergistic with aminoglycosides. The drug is eliminated via renal tubular secretion, and its half-life is prolonged in renal failure. Adverse effects include gastrointestinal upsets with possible superinfection, vertigo and headache, and (rarely) hepatotoxicity. Although skin rashes may occur, there is little cross-allergenicity with penicillins.

**B. Imipenem:** Imipenem is a carbapenem with low susceptibility to beta-lactamases that has wide activity against gram-negative rods and anaerobes. It is inactivated by renal dihydropeptidase I and is administered with an inhibitor of this enzyme, cilastatin. Imipenem is used for infections caused by organisms resistant to other antibiotics. Adverse effects include gastrointestinal distress, skin rashes, and, occasionally, seizures. There is partial cross-allergenicity with the penicillins.

**C. Clavulanic Acid & Sulbactam:** Clavulanic acid and sulbactam have weak antibacterial activities but are effective inhibitors of bacterial beta-lactamases. They prevent inactivation of penicillins when used in combination with them and may enhance their antibacterial actions.

## DRUG LIST

The following drugs are important members of the group discussed in this chapter. Prototype agents should be learned in detail, and the major variants should be known well enough to list the factors that distinguish them from the prototypes and from each other.

| Subclass | Prototype | Major Variants |
|---|---|---|
| Penicillins | | |
| Limited spectrum | Penicillin G | Penicillin V |
| Beta-lactamase-resistant | Methicillin | Nafcillin, oxacillin, dicloxacillin |
| Wider spectrum | Ampicillin, carbenicillin | Amoxicillin, ticarcillin, azlocillin |
| Cephalosporins | | |
| First-generation | Na cephalothin | Cefazolin, cephradine, cephapirin |
| Second-generation | Cefamandole | Cefoclor, cefoxitin, cefuroxime |
| Third-generation | Cefoperazone | Cefotaxime, ceftazidime, moxalactam |

## QUESTIONS

**DIRECTIONS (items 1–5):** Each numbered item or incomplete statement in this section is followed by answers or by completions of the statement. Select the ONE lettered answer or completion that is BEST in each case.

**1.** All of the following statements about the biodisposition of penicillins are accurate EXCEPT:
**(A)** The oral bioavailability of a penicillin drug depends on its acid lability
**(B)** Probenecid increases penicillin excretion by blocking renal tubular reabsorption
**(C)** Penicillins are polar compounds and are not metabolized extensively by liver enzymes
**(D)** Ampicillin undergoes enterohepatic cycling

**2.** The mechanism of antibacterial action of cephalosporins involves
**(A)** inhibition of peptide synthesis
**(B)** interference with the synthesis of ergosterol
**(C)** inhibition of transpeptidase enzymes
**(D)** inhibition of beta-lactamases
**(E)** inhibition of DNA gyrase

**3.** Which of the following drugs is LEAST likely to be effective in the treatment of an infection caused by *S aureus*?
**(A)** Amoxicillin
**(B)** Nafcillin
**(C)** Cefazolin
**(D)** Oxacillin
**(E)** Erythromycin

**4.** All of the following statements about the beta-lactam antibiotics are accurate EXCEPT:
**(A)** Maculopapular rashes are common with ampicillin
**(B)** Aztreonam is not susceptible to most beta-lactamases and has activity against many gram-negative rods
**(C)** The resistance of staphylococci to methicillin is an example of multiple drug resistance
**(D)** Bleeding episodes following moxalactam administration are partly due to interference with platelet function
**(E)** Cefazolin is an appropriate drug for treatment of pneumococcal meningitis

**5.** Which of the following drugs is likely to interfere with vitamin K availability, leading to hypoprothrombinemia and possible bleeding disorders?
**(A)** Na cephalothin
**(B)** Procaine penicillin G
**(C)** Imipenem
**(D)** Cefoperazone
**(E)** Nafcillin

**DIRECTIONS (Items 6–10):** Items 6–10 consist of lettered headings followed by a set of numbered statements. For each numbered statement, select the ONE lettered heading that is most closely associated with it. Each lettered heading may be selected once, more than once, or not at all.

**(A)** Ceftriaxone
**(B)** Penicillin V
**(C)** Dicloxacillin
**(D)** Azlocillin
**(E)** Imipenem

**6.** This drug is often effective in the treatment of infections caused by strains of *Pseudomonas aeruginosa*, although it is susceptible to certain beta-lactamases.

**7.** This drug has a narrow spectrum of activity that does not include gram-negative rods. Although susceptible to penicillinases, it is effective against most streptococci that commonly cause infections. It is stable in gastric acid.

**8.** This drug is used almost exclusively for infections caused by *S aureus*. It has minimal activity against gram-negative rods.

**9.** Cilastatin, an inhibitor of renal dihydropeptidase, must be administered in combination with this drug to prevent the rapid inactivation of the drug.

**10.** The spectrum of activity of this antibiotic includes penicillinase-producing *S aureus* and many gram negative bacteria including meningococci, *E coli*, *Haemophilus influenzae*, and *Klebsiella* spp. Most pseudomonads are resistant. The drug is effective in the empirical treatment of suspected bacterial meningitis in children.

## ANSWERS

1. Probenecid inhibits the tubular *secretion* of beta-lactam antibiotics and thus decreases the elimination rate and prolongs the plasma half-lives of most penicillins and cephalosporins. The answer is **(B)**.

2. As beta-lactam antibiotics, the cephalosporins are bactericidal inhibitors of cell wall synthesis, acting at the peptidoglycan cross-linking stage to inhibit transpeptidation. The answer is **(C)**.

3. It is important to recall that ampicillin and amoxicillin are susceptible to penicillinases. These drugs are unlikely to be effective in infections caused by staphylococci unless they are administered in combination with inhibitors of beta-lactamases. The answer is **(A)**.

4. Cefazolin is probably the most widely used first-generation cephalosporin. None of the drugs in this subclass are able to penetrate the blood-brain barrier, even when the meninges are inflamed, and they are therefore unreliable in the treatment of bacterial meningitis. The answer is **(E)**.

5. This toxicity is associated with use of cephalosporins that contain a methylthiotetrazole group, several of which are third-generation drugs. It can be prevented by administration of vitamin K. The answer is **(D)**.

6. Both imipenem and azlocillin have activity against pseudomonads, but resistance to imipenem develops rapidly when it is used as the sole agent in such infections. Imipenem is not susceptible to beta-lactamases. Although azlocillin is susceptible to hydrolysis by beta-lactamases produced by some organisms (eg, *S aureus*) it is usually active against *Pseudomonas* spp. The answer is **(D)**.

7. Penicillin V is equivalent to penicillin G in terms of its activity against streptococci. Like penicillin G, it has a narrow spectrum of activity and is susceptible to penicillinases. However, it does have activity against many oral pathogens and is widely used in dentistry. Unlike penicillin G, it is stable in gastric acid and is effective when given orally. The answer is **(B)**.

8. Dicloxacillin belongs to a subclass of penicillins that has a narrow spectrum of activity. Methicillin and nafcillin are the prototypes of the group. These drugs are not hydrolyzed by penicillinases produced by gram-positive cocci and are therefore active against most strains of *S aureus*. The answer is **(C)**.

9. Imipenem is resistant to beta-lactamases and has a wide range of antibacterial activity. It is inactivated by renal dihydropeptidases, and cilastatin must be used in combination with the antibiotic to prolong its effects. CNS toxicity has occurred when the dosage of imipenem-cilastatin is not modified in patients with renal failure. The answer is **(E)**.

10. The antibacterial spectrum and clinical use described are those of the third-generation cephalosporin ceftriaxone. The drug is also active against many resistant strains of gonococcus. The answer is **(A)**.

# Chloramphenicol & Tetracyclines 44

## OBJECTIVES

**Define the following terms:**

- Broad-spectrum agent
- Aminoacyl-tRNA
- Gray baby syndrome
- Peptidyltransferase
- Enterohepatic cycling
- Superinfection

**You should be able to:**

- Describe the mechanisms of action of chloramphenicol and tetracyclines.
- Describe the mechanisms responsible for clinical bacterial resistance.
- List the major clinical uses of these drugs.
- Describe the pharmacokinetic features of these agents that are relevant to their clinical use.
- List the main toxic effects of these drugs.

## CONCEPTS

### CHLORAMPHENICOL

**A. Classification & Pharmacokinetics:** This drug has a distinctive chemical structure, and no congeners are used clinically. Effective both orally and parenterally, it is distributed throughout all tissues and crosses both the placental and blood-brain barriers. Chloramphenicol undergoes enterohepatic cycling, and a small fraction of the dose is excreted unchanged in the urine. Most of the drug is inactivated by a liver glucuronosyltransferase.

**B. Mechanism of Action:** Chloramphenicol has a wide spectrum of antimicrobial activity (ie, it is a broad-spectrum drug) and is usually bacteriostatic. It binds to the 50S ribosomal subunit of bacteria and inhibits **peptidyltransferase** (Fig 44–1). This ribosomal enzyme is responsible for peptide bond formation, and in the presence of chloramphenicol protein synthesis is inhibited. Although selectively toxic to bacteria, chloramphenicol can also inhibit mitochondrial protein synthesis in mammalian cells. Resistance to chloramphenicol, which is plasmid-mediated, occurs through the formation of acetyltransferases that inactivate the drug.

**C. Clinical Use:** Because of its toxicity, chloramphenicol is reserved for severe infections caused by *Salmonella* and *Haemophilus* spp and for the treatment of pneumococcal and meningococcal meningitis in penicillin-sensitive persons. Note that some *H influenzae* strains are resistant to

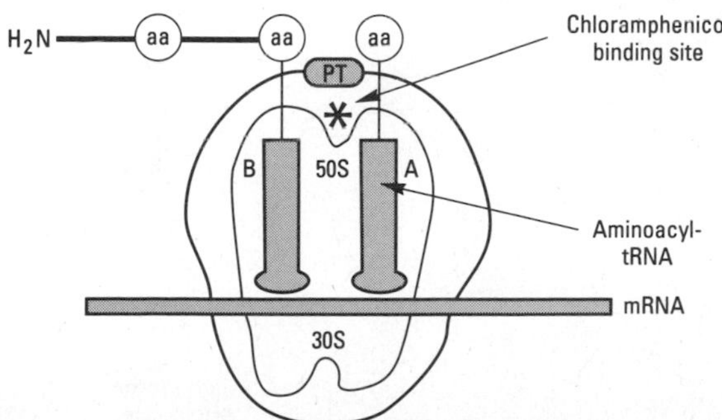


**Figure 44–1.** Chloramphenicol inhibits peptide bond formation. The binding site for chloramphenicol is on the larger ribosomal subunit (50S) of bacteria. It is adjacent to peptidyltransferase (PT), the ribosomal enzyme that catalyzes peptide bond formation. Drug binding interferes with the action of this enzyme, preventing the transfer of amino acids (aa) from aminoacyl-tRNA to the growing peptide chain.

chloramphenicol, and then ceftriaxone or cefuroxime may be preferred. Chloramphenicol is sometimes used for rickettsial diseases and for infections caused by anaerobes such as *Bacteroides fragilis*. It is commonly used as a topical antimicrobial agent because of its broad spectrum.

**D. Toxicity:**

1. **Gastrointestinal disturbances** can occur as a result of direct irritation and from superinfections, especially candidiasis.
2. **Bone marrow dysfunction,** including delayed red cell maturation, can occur; it is dose-dependent and reversible.
3. **Aplastic anemia** is a rare adverse effect (approximately 1 in 25,000–40,000), but it may be fatal.
4. **Gray baby syndrome** involves cyanosis and cardiovascular collapse. This occurs through drug overdosage in neonates who are deficient in glucuronosyltransferase activity.
5. **Inhibition of metabolism** of several drugs, including phenytoin, coumarins, and tolbutamide, can occur.

## TETRACYCLINES

**A. Classification:** Drugs in this class are structural congeners that have a broad range of antimicrobial activity but have only minor differences in their activities against specific organisms. **Tetracycline** is representative of the older drugs; **doxycycline** is a newer agent.

**B. Pharmacokinetics:** Oral absorption is variable, especially for the older drugs, and may be impaired by foods and multivalent cations (calcium, iron, aluminum). The drugs have a wide tissue distribution and enter mammalian cells. They cross the placental barrier, but CNS penetration is limited. All of the tetracyclines undergo enterohepatic cycling, and doxycycline is excreted mainly in feces. The other drugs are eliminated primarily in the urine. The half-lives of doxycycline and minocycline are longer than those of other tetracyclines.

**C. Mechanism of Action:** Tetracyclines are bacteriostatic inhibitors of protein synthesis. They are accumulated intracellularly via energy-dependent transport systems present in bacterial membranes. As shown in Fig 44–2, the binding site for tetracyclines is present on the smaller bacterial ribosomal subunit (30S). The bulky structure of the drug interferes with the binding of **aminoacyl-tRNA** to the A site on the ribosomal complex. This blocking action prevents alignment of the aminoacyl-tRNA anticodons with mRNA, and peptide bond synthesis is inhibited. The selective toxicity of tetracyclines occurs mainly because mammalian cells lack the membrane transport systems that lead to drug accumulation.

Bacterial resistance to tetracyclines is widespread and plasmid-mediated. Tetracycline-resistant organisms show decreased intracellular accumulation of the drugs. The probable mechanisms are decreased activity of the uptake systems and development of mechanisms for active extrusion of tetracyclines out of the organism.

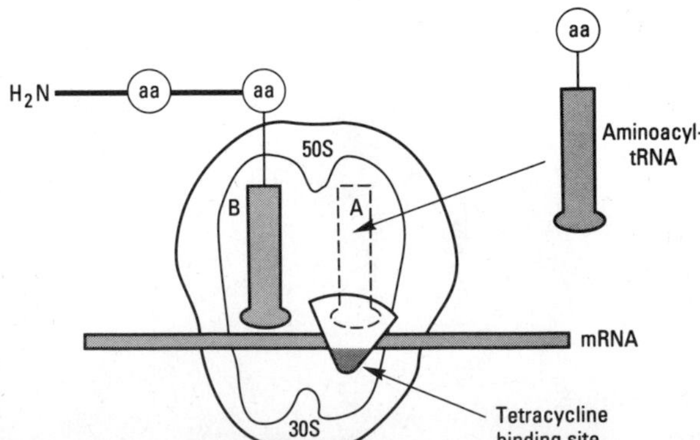


**Figure 44–2.** Tetracyclines inhibit the binding of aminoacyl-tRNA. The interaction of tetracycline with components of the smaller ribosomal subunit (30S) blocks the binding of aminoacyl-tRNA to the A-site on the ribosomal complex, and protein synthesis is inhibited. Compare with Fig 44–1. aa = amino acid.

**D. Clinical Use:**

1. Tetracyclines are the drugs of first choice in the treatment of infections caused by *Mycoplasma pneumoniae,* chlamydiae, and rickettsiae.
2. Tetracyclines are alternative drugs in the treatment of syphilis and gonorrhea (a tetracycline may be required for the accompanying chlamydial infections even if penicillin is used).
3. Tetracyclines are used in the treatment of respiratory infections and in the prophylactic treatment of chronic bronchitis.
4. Specific tetracyclines are used in the treatment of bacterial enteritis (doxycycline) and the meningococcal carrier state (minocycline). Demeclocycline inhibits the renal actions of antidiuretic hormone (ADH) and is used in the management of patients with ADH-secreting tumors. Doxycycline is also used in Lyme disease.
5. Because of their low cost and wide antimicrobial activity, tetracyclines are used in developing countries in the treatment of many diseases, including cholera, brucellosis, leptospirosis, and plague.
6. Tetracyclines continue to be used to suppress acne.

**E. Toxicity:**

1. **Gastrointestinal effects** may range from mild nausea and diarrhea to severe, possibly life-threatening colitis. Disturbances in the gut flora lead to candidiasis (oral and vaginal) and, more rarely, bacterial superinfections by *S aureus* or *Clostridium difficile.*
2. **Pain** at intramuscular injection sites and phlebitis at intravenous injection sites may occur.
3. **Fetal exposure** may lead to tooth enamel dysplasia and irregularities in bone growth.
4. **Photosensitivity reactions** occur, especially with demeclocycline.
5. **Vestibular reactions,** including dizziness and vertigo, have been noted with minocycline.
6. **Hepatotoxic effects** have followed high dosages of tetracyclines in pregnant patients with a history of renal disease.

## DRUG LIST

The following drugs are important members of the groups discussed in this chapter. Prototype agents should be learned in detail; the major variants and the other significant agents should be known well enough to list the factors that distinguish them from the prototypes and from each other.

| Subclass | Prototype | Major Variants | Other Significant Agents |
|---|---|---|---|
| Chloramphenicol | Chloramphenicol | | |
| Tetracyclines | Tetracycline | Demeclocycline | Doxycycline, minocycline |

## QUESTIONS

**DIRECTIONS (items 1–5):** Each numbered item or incomplete statement in this section is followed by answers or by completions of the statement. Select the ONE lettered answer or completion that is BEST in each case.

1. All of the following statements about chloramphenicol are accurate EXCEPT:
   (A) It is completely absorbed following oral administration
   (B) When it is given to neonates, their limited hepatic glucuronosyltransferase activity may result in cyanosis
   (C) It is usually bacteriostatic
   (D) Clinical resistance occurs through changes in the structure of bacterial peptidyltransferase
   (E) The dose should be reduced in patients with hepatic failure

2. Appropriate clinical uses of chloramphenicol include all of the following EXCEPT
   (A) typhoid fever
   (B) topical application for chlamydial infections of the eye
   (C) meningococcal meningitis in a penicillin-allergic person
   (D) initial therapy of meningitis suspected to be caused by *H influenzae*
   (E) sepsis caused by some species of *Bacteroides* spp

3. The mechanism of antibacterial action of tetracyclines involves
   (A) inhibition of the conversion of lanosterol to ergosterol
   (B) inhibition of DNA-dependent RNA polymerase
   (C) blockade of binding of aminoacyl-tRNA to bacterial ribosomes
   (D) selective inhibition of ribosomal peptidyltransferases

4. Appropriate statements about the clinical uses of tetracyclines include all of the following EXCEPT:
   (A) The tetracyclines are drugs of choice in the treatment of rickettsial infections
   (B) Doxycycline is an effective prophylactic drug for Traveler's diarrhea
   (C) The tetracyclines are suitable for the therapy of respiratory infections caused by *Mycoplasma pneumoniae*
   (D) High tissue penetration makes minocycline an appropriate drug for the treatment of osteomyelitis due to methicillin-resistant staphylococci
   (E) At full doses for 7 days, a tetracycline will often be effective in gonorrhea and also control coexisting chlamydial infections

5. All of the following statements about tetracyclines are accurate EXCEPT:
   (A) They cross the placental barrier and are excreted in the milk of nursing mothers
   (B) Suppression of the normal flora by tetracyclines may lead to superinfections from *C albicans* or resistant bacteria
   (C) They are chelating agents that bind to calcium in underdeveloped bone and teeth
   (D) They have minimal activity against most *Pseudomonas* strains
   (E) Clinical resistance is due to formation of enzymes that inactivate tetracyclines

**DIRECTIONS (items 6–10):** Items 6–10 consist of lettered headings followed by a set of numbered statements. For each numbered statement, select the ONE lettered heading that is most closely associated with it. Each lettered heading may be selected only once.

(A) Doxycycline
(B) Minocycline
(C) Chloramphenicol
(D) Tetracycline
(E) Demeclocycline

6. The appearance of markedly vacuolated, nucleated red cells in the marrow, anemia, and reticulocytopenia are characteristic dose-dependent adverse effects of this drug.

7. Decreased renal function has little effect on the rate of elimination of this drug. It has a longer plasma half-life than other drugs in its class.

8. Dizziness, vertigo, nausea, and vomiting are adverse effects of this drug. It is effective in the meningococcal carrier state.

9. Use of this antibiotic has caused abnormal reddening of the skin when exposed to ultraviolet light. It has ADH-inhibiting effects.

10. Studies with oral formulations of this oldest member of its group have shown that milk products, iron tablets, and certain aluminum-containing antacids can interfere with its absorption.

## ANSWERS

1. Clinical resistance to chloramphenicol involves the plasmid-mediated formation of acetyltransferases that inactivate the drug. Although it is usually bacteriostatic, the drug may be bactericidal to some strains of pneumococci and meningococci. The answer is **(D)**.

2. Chloramphenicol penetrates into the aqueous humor and, because of its wide spectrum of activity, is used topically in the treatment of eye infections. However, it is not effective in chlamydial infections. The answer is **(B)**.

3. Tetracyclines inhibit bacterial protein synthesis by interfering with the binding of aminoacyl-tRNA molecules to bacterial ribosomes. Peptidyltransferase is inhibited by chloramphenicol. The answer is **(C)**.

4. Minocycline has greater lipophilicity than other tetracyclines and penetrates tissues effectively. However, staphylococci resistant to methicillin are usually resistant to multiple drugs including the tetracyclines. The answer is **(D)**.

5. The concentration of tetracyclines in sensitive bacteria is much higher than that in resistant organisms. Decreased intracellular accumulation of tetracyclines is the major mechanism involved in the development of resistance to this class of drugs. The development of inactivating transferase enzymes is the mechanism of resistance to chloramphenicol. The answer is **(E)**.

6. Reversible, dose-dependent bone marrow dysfunction occurs with chloramphenicol, as a result of maturation arrest. Elevated serum iron levels result. These actions are unrelated to the rare occurrence of aplastic anemia. The answer is **(C)**.

7. Doxycycline is excreted almost entirely in the feces, mainly via biliary secretion. It is the only tetracycline available that does not require major dosage adjustments in patients with renal impairment. The answer is **(A)**.

8. Vestibular toxicity is associated with the use of minocycline. It is dose-dependent and reversible after drug discontinuance. The answer is **(B)**.

9. Photosensitivity reactions can occur with any tetracycline but appear to be most common with demeclocycline. The answer is **(E)**.

10. Tetracycline acts as a chelating agent for divalent and trivalent cations, and complexed forms of the drug are not well absorbed from the gut. The answer is **(D)**.

# 45 Aminoglycosides & Polymyxins

## OBJECTIVES

**Define the following terms:**

- 30S ribosomal subunit
- Group transferase enzymes
- Ototoxicity
- Ribosomal initiation complex
- Antimicrobial drug synergy
- Membrane lipopolysaccharide

**You should be able to:**

- Describe the probable mechanism of action of aminoglycoside antibiotics and the mechanism by which bacterial resistance to this class of drugs occurs.
- List the major clinical applications of aminoglycosides and describe their main toxic effects.
- Describe the pharmacokinetics of this drug class, with special reference to the importance of renal clearance and its relationship to toxicity.
- Describe the mechanism of action, clinical uses, and major toxic effects of polymyxins.

## CONCEPTS

### AMINOGLYCOSIDES

**A. Classification:** The drugs in this class are all structurally related, containing amino sugars attached by glycosidic linkages. The main differences between individual drugs are in their activities against specific organisms, particularly gram-negative rods.

**B. Pharmacokinetics:** As polar compounds, aminoglycosides are not absorbed orally. They have limited tissue penetration and no significant metabolism. Glomerular filtration is the major mode of excretion, and plasma levels of these drugs are greatly affected by changes in renal function. Individual agents have a particular range ("therapeutic window") of optimal plasma levels below which they have limited antibacterial activity and above which they exert toxic effects. Monitoring of plasma levels of an aminoglycoside is an important requirement for safe and effective dosage adjustment.

**C. Mechanism of Action:** Aminoglycosides are bactericidal inhibitors of protein synthesis. Their penetration through the bacterial cell envelope is partly via oxygen-dependent, active transport, and they have little activity against strict anaerobes. Inside the cell, streptomycin binds to the 30S ribosomal subunit and interferes with the **initiation complex,** preventing its transition to a chain-elongating functional ribosomal complex. The protein-synthesizing machinery becomes "frozen" in the presence of streptomycin. Other aminoglycosides have a similar but not identical mechanism of action.

**Resistance** to aminoglycosides involves the plasmid-mediated formation of inactivating enzymes. As shown in Fig 45–1, these enzymes are **group transferases** that catalyze the acetylation of amine functions and the transfer of phosphoryl or adenylyl groups to the oxygen atoms of hydroxyl groups. Individual aminoglycosides have different susceptibilities to such enzymes. Currently, **amikacin** is susceptible to only a few such enzymes and is active against more strains of organisms than are other aminoglycosides. **Netilmicin** may be even more active.

**D. Clinical Use:**

1. **Aminoglycosides** are primary drugs **(gentamicin, tobramycin, amikacin)** for treatment of serious infections caused by gram-negative bacteria, including *E coli* and *Enterobacter, Klebsiella, Proteus, Pseudomonas,* and *Serratia* spp. Drug choice depends on the susceptibility pattern of the organism isolated from the patient. Aminoglycosides can be used in combi-

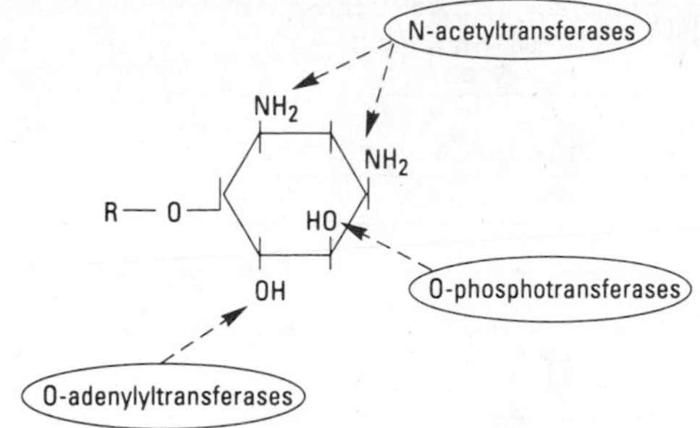


**Figure 45–1.** Sites of action of enzymes involved in aminoglycoside resistance. The structure shown represents an amino sugar typically present in aminoglycoside antibiotic molecules. Both amino and hydroxyl groups may be subject to enzymic attack by at least 3 classes of inactivating bacterial transferases. The metabolites formed have reduced or no antibacterial activities. The relative susceptibility of an individual drug to these enzymes determines its clinical usefulness.

nation with beta-lactam antibiotics, and antibacterial synergy may occur (eg, carbenicillin and gentamicin versus *Pseudomonas* spp).

2. Specific indications for other aminoglycosides include the following:
   a. **Streptomycin:** Tuberculosis, plague, tularemia.
   b. **Neomycin:** Topical antimicrobial use or local use, such as in the gastrointestinal tract.
   c. **Spectinomycin:** Gonorrhea. This drug is an *aminocyclitol.*
   d. **Netilmicin:** A relatively new drug, usually reserved for organisms resistant to other aminoglycosides.

**E. Toxicity:**

1. **Ototoxicity** can include auditory or vestibular damage (or both) and may be irreversible. It is related to high plasma levels of a drug, especially when the dosage has not been modified in cases of renal dysfunction. Ototoxicity may be increased by the use of loop diuretics.
2. **Nephrotoxicity** includes acute tubular necrosis that is usually reversible. It is more common in elderly patients and in those receiving cephalosporin antibiotics.
3. **Neuromuscular blockade** can occur at high doses and leads to respiratory paralysis; it is reversible with calcium and neostigmine.
4. **Allergic** skin reactions (in patients) and contact dermatitis (in personnel handling the drug) may occur, especially with neomycin.

## POLYMYXINS

The polymyxins are fatty acid-containing basic polypeptides that are bactericidal against gram-negative bacteria. They interact with a specific **lipopolysaccharide** component of the outer cell membrane that is also a binding site for calcium. Membrane lipid structure is distorted, with an increase in permeability to polar molecules, resulting in marked changes in cell metabolism. Because of the toxicity of polymyxins, their clinical applications are limited to therapy of resistant gram-negative infections, including those caused by *Enterobacter* and *Pseudomonas* spp. Adverse effects include neurotoxicity (paresthesias, dizziness, ataxia) and acute renal tubular necrosis (hematuria, proteinuria, nitrogen retention).

# DRUG LIST

The following drugs are important members of the group discussed in this chapter. Prototype agents should be learned in detail; the major variants should be known well enough to list the factors that distinguish them from the prototypes and from each other; and the other significant agents should be recognized as belonging to a specific subclass.

| Subclass | Prototype | Major Variants | Other Significant Agents |
|---|---|---|---|
| Aminoglycosides Systemic | Gentamicin | Tobramycin | Amikacin, netilmicin, streptomycin |
| Local | Neomycin | | Kanamycin |
| Aminocyclitols | Spectinomycin | | |
| Polymyxins | Polymyxin B | Colistin (polymyxin E) | |

## QUESTIONS

**DIRECTIONS (items 1–6):** Each numbered item or incomplete statement in this section is followed by answers or by completions of the statement. Select the ONE lettered answer that is BEST in each case.

**1.** All of the following statements about aminoglycosides are accurate EXCEPT:
**(A)** They exert synergistic effects with beta-lactam antibiotics against selected organisms
**(B)** They are bactericidal
**(C)** Their antibacterial action involves binding to the 50S ribosomal subunit and subsequent inhibition of peptidyltransferase
**(D)** Clinical resistance occurs through plasmid-mediated formation of group transferase-inactivating enzymes
**(E)** Staphylococci resistant to methicillin are usually resistant to aminoglycosides

**2.** All of the following statements about the clinical uses of the aminoglycosides are accurate EXCEPT:
**(A)** Streptomycin is the drug of choice for treatment of plague
**(B)** Aminoglycosides are often used in combination with cephalosporins in the empirical treatment of severe bacterial infections
**(C)** Amikacin is more likely to be effective than streptomycin in the treatment of a hospital-acquired infection caused by *Serratia marcescens*
**(D)** The primary indication for spectinomycin is the treatment of iatrogenic gram-negative infections in the immunocompromised patient
**(E)** Gentamicin is used with penicillin G for synergistic effects in the treatment of enterococcal endocarditis

**3.** All of the following statements about the toxic effects of aminoglycosides are accurate EXCEPT:
**(A)** Amphotericin B potentiates the nephrotoxicity of aminoglycosides
**(B)** Muscle paralysis due to aminoglycosides is usually reversed by infusion of calcium gluconate
**(C)** Loop diuretics increase the rate of renal elimination of aminoglycosides and decrease the likelihood of ototoxic effects
**(D)** Headache and vertigo in the upright position are early signs of aminoglycoside neurotoxicity
**(E)** Oral administration of neomycin may lead to intestinal malabsorption and superinfection

**4.** A 70-kg patient with a creatinine clearance of greater than 80 mL/min has a gram-negative infection. You administer amikacin intramuscularly at a dose of 5 mg/kg every 8 hours, and the patient begins to respond. After 2 days, the creatinine clearance declines to 20 mL/min, but you want to continue giving the drug. Assuming that you do not have information on amikacin plasma levels, what would be your approach to modification of the dosage?
**(A)** Decrease the daily dose to a total of 100 mg
**(B)** Decrease the dose to 85 mg every 8 hours
**(C)** Maintain the patient on the present dose and test auditory function
**(D)** Administer 5 mg/kg every 12 hours

**5.** All of the following statements about polymyxins are accurate EXCEPT:
**(A)** They are bactericidal for many gram-negative rods including *Pseudomonas* spp
**(B)** Their activity against gram-positive bacteria is minimal
**(C)** They are effective against intracellular pathogens since they effectively penetrate mammalian cell membranes
**(D)** Paresthesias and incoordination are potential toxic effects of polymyxins
**(E)** Polymyxin-induced injury to renal tubules results in hematuria and proteinuria

**6.** The toxicity of aminoglycosides is enhanced by concomitant administration of all of the following drugs EXCEPT
**(A)** vancomycin
**(B)** cefazolin
**(C)** mannitol
**(D)** penicillin G
**(E)** cisplatin

**DIRECTIONS (items 7–10):** Items 7–10 consist of lettered headings followed by a set of numbered statements. For each numbered statement, select the ONE lettered heading that is most closely associated with it. Each lettered heading may be selected once, more than once, or not at all.

**(A)** Amikacin
**(B)** Clindamycin
**(C)** Neomycin
**(D)** Tobramycin
**(E)** Streptomycin

**7.** The systemic use of this drug has been largely abandoned because of its toxicity. It is used topically and for its local effects in the gastrointestinal tract.

**8.** This drug is used in the treatment of tularemia. When administered in combination with other agents in tuberculosis, it delays the emergence of resistant mycobacteria.

**9.** This drug is active against many gentamicin-resistant bacteria because its metabolism by bacterial enzymes is sterically hindered.

**10.** This drug has a similar spectrum of activity and properties to gentamicin, except that it shows poor activity in combination with penicillin against enterococci.

## ANSWERS

**1.** Bacterial protein synthesis is inhibited by aminoglycosides via their binding to specific components of the 30S ribosomal subunit. This leads to stabilization of the initiation complex and to miscoding when protein synthesis does occur. The answer is **(C).**

**2.** Spectinomycin is an aminocyclitol with limited antibacterial activity. Its only clinical use is the treatment of gonorrhea, as an alternative drug in cases of resistance or patient allergy. The answer is **(D).**

**3.** Aminoglycosides are excreted intact via glomerular filtration, and their rate of elimination is not directly affected by ethacrynic acid or furosemide. However, the loop diuretics are potentially ototoxic and may enhance hearing loss when used with aminoglycosides. Thiazides are preferred when a diuretic is indicated in patients on aminoglycosides. The answer is **(C).**

**4.** This question should remind you of the importance of renal function when aminoglycosides are used. Monitoring the plasma drug levels is important for careful adjustment of dosage to achieve safe and effective therapy. There is a wide interpatient variability in the dose-plasma level relationship. In this case, you would probably decrease the dose in proportion to the decreased creatinine clearance, which has fallen to one-quarter of the starting value. The answer is **(B)**.

5. Polymyxins are cationic basic polypeptides that do not readily penetrate mammalian cell membranes. They have limited activity against intracellular pathogens. The answer is **(C)**.

6. Cephalosporins, cisplatin, mannitol, and vancomycin are reported to increase the incidence of aminoglycoside toxicity. Although penicillins may inactivate aminoglycosides in vitro, and possibly in patients with end-stage renal failure, they do not enhance toxic effects. The answer is **(D)**.

7. When used parenterally, neomycin causes renal damage and ototoxicity. It is used topically and for local actions, including gastrointestinal tract infections, sterilization prior to bowel surgery, and reduction of ammonia intoxication in hepatic coma. The answer is **(C)**.

8. Unlike other aminoglycosides, streptomycin is not usually used for treatment of infections caused by gram-negative rods, since many organisms are resistant. The drug does have selective clinical uses, including the treatment of plague, tularemia, and tuberculosis. The answer is **(E)**.

9. Because of its chemical structure, amikacin is less susceptible than gentamicin to the actions of group transferase enzymes produced by resistant gram-negative organisms. The answer is **(A)**.

10. Tobramycin is almost identical to gentamicin in its properties. However, it is much less active than either gentamicin or streptomycin when used in combination with a penicillin in the treatment of enterococcal endocarditis. The answer is **(D)**.

# 46 Antimycobacterial Drugs

## OBJECTIVES

**You should be able to:**

- Describe the special problems of chemotherapy for mycobacterial infections.
- Describe the pharmacodynamic and pharmacokinetic properties of the first-line drugs used in tuberculosis (isoniazid, ethambutol, pyrazinamide and rifampin).
- Identify the second-line drugs used in tuberculosis and describe their limitations.
- Identify the drugs used in leprosy and describe their toxic effects.

## CONCEPTS

Chemotherapy of infections caused by *Mycobacterium tuberculosis* and *Mycobacterium leprae* is complicated by numerous factors, including the following:

1. Limited information about the mechanisms of action of antimycobacterial agents.
2. The development of resistance.
3. The intracellular location of mycobacteria.
4. The chronic nature of mycobacterial disease, which accentuates drug toxicities.

Chemotherapy almost always involves the use of **drug combinations** to delay the emergence of resistance and to enhance antimycobacterial actions. The major drugs used in tuberculosis are isoniazid, rifampin, ethambutol, and pyrazinamide. The main drug for leprosy is dapsone, but it is commonly given with either rifampin or clofazimine.

## DRUGS FOR TUBERCULOSIS

**A. Isoniazid:** Isoniazid (INH) is the single most important drug and is a structural congener of pyridoxine. Its mechanism of action is not known with certainty but may involve inhibition of mycobacterial cell wall synthesis. Resistance can emerge rapidly, and so INH is usually given with other drugs to delay this, except when used in prophylaxis. The drug is absorbed orally and penetrates cells to act on intracellular mycobacteria. The liver metabolism of INH, via acetylation, is under genetic control, and patients may be "fast" or "slow" inactivators of the drug. Many Asians and Native Americans are "fast" acetylators of INH. Common neurotoxic effects (peripheral neuritis, restlessness, muscle twitching) are alleviated by pyridoxine, which does not block antibacterial effects. Other adverse effects include hepatotoxicity (rare in children), inhibition of drug metabolism, hemolysis in glucose-6-phosphate dehydrogenase deficiency syndromes, and allergies.

**B. Rifampin:** Rifampin, a derivative of rifamycin, is bactericidal to *M tuberculosis* and, if given monthly, delays the emergence of resistance to dapsone in leprosy. It inhibits the DNA-dependent RNA polymerase of many microorganisms, but resistance emerges rapidly if the drug is used alone. Rifampin is orally absorbed, widely distributed to tissues, and eliminated by the liver into the bile. Its adverse effects include hepatotoxicity, thrombocytopenia, skin rashes, decreased antibody responses, and a "flu" syndrome (fever, chills, malaise). Rifampin induces liver drug-metabolizing enzymes and enhances the elimination rate of contraceptive steroids, ketoconazole, methadone, and warfarin.

**C. Ethambutol:** Ethambutol acts on mycobacteria by unknown mechanisms, and resistance occurs rapidly if the drug is used alone. Therefore, it is always used with other drugs. Well-absorbed orally, the drug distributes to most tissues including the CNS. Its elimination half-life is increased in renal failure. The most common adverse effects are dose-dependent visual disturbances, including decreased visual acuity and optic neuritis, which usually regress on drug discontinuance. Other neurotoxic effects include headache, confusion, and peripheral neuritis.

**D. Pyrazinamide:** The mechanism of action of pyrazinamide is not known. It inhibits the growth of *M tuberculosis* at concentrations achievable in body tissues after oral administration. Resistance develops rapidly if the drug is used alone. There is no cross-resistance with other antimycobacterial drugs. Pyrazinamide penetrates most body tissues and enters the CNS, and its plasma half-life is increased in hepatic or renal failure. Adverse effects include gastrointestinal irritation, maculopapular rashes, hepatic dysfunction, hyperuricemia, and photosensitivity reactions.

**E. Alternative Drugs:** The **second-line** antimycobacterial drugs are used in case of resistance to other agents; most are no more effective than the major drugs, and their toxicities are often more serious. **Ethionamide** is a congener of INH, but cross-resistance does not occur. Its major problem is that at doses needed for effective plasma levels, intense gastrointestinal irritation and adverse neurologic effects occur. The aminoglycoside streptomycin delays the emergence of resistance when used in combination therapy. **Aminosalicylic acid (PAS)** is now rarely used because of its toxicity, which includes gastrointestinal irritation, peptic ulceration, hypersensitivity reactions, and effects on kidney, liver, and thyroid function. Other drugs occasionally used include the antibiotics **capreomycin, cycloserine,** and **viomycin.**

## DRUGS FOR LEPROSY

The **sulfones,** particularly diaminodiphenylsulfone **(dapsone),** remain the most active agents against *M leprae*. Their mechanism of action may involve inhibition of folic acid synthesis. Resistance may develop, especially if low doses are given. Dapsone given orally penetrates tissues well, undergoes enterohepatic cycling, and is eliminated in the urine partly as acetylated metabolites. Common adverse effects include gastrointestinal irritation, fever, skin rashes, and methemoglobinemia. Hemolysis may occur in patients with glucose-6-phosphate dehydrogenase deficiency. **Acedapsone** is a repository form that provides inhibitory plasma concentrations for several months. Dapsone is an alternative drug for the treatment of *Pneumocystis carinii* pneumonia in AIDS patients. Alternative drugs for leprosy include rifampin (see above), **clofazimine,** and **amithiozone.** Clofazimine is a phenazine given in cases of dapsone resistance or intolerance. It causes gastrointestinal irritation and marked skin discoloration. Amithiozone is also an alternative to dapsone, but emergence of resistance, together with gastrointestinal and hepatotoxic effects, limits its use.

### DRUGS FOR ATYPICAL MYCOBACTERIAL INFECTIONS

Infections due to atypical mycobacteria (eg, *M marinum, M avium-intracellulare, M ulcerans*), although sometimes asymptomatic, may be treated with the above-described antimycobacterial drugs (eg, ethambutol, rifampin) or with other antibiotics, including erythromycin, or aminoglycosides such as amikacin. *M avium-intracellulare* infections in AIDS patients have been treated with clofazimine.

## DRUG LIST

The following drugs are important members of the group discussed in this chapter. Prototype agents should be learned in detail; the other significant agents should be known well enough to list the factors that distinguish them from the prototypes and from each other.

| Subclass | Prototype | Other Significant Agents |
|---|---|---|
| Drugs for tuberculosis | | |
| Pyridines | Isoniazid | Ethionamide, pyrazinamide |
| Rifamycins | Rifampin | |
| Diamines | Ethambutol | |
| Aminoglycosides | Streptomycin | |
| Others | | Aminosalicylic acid, capreomycin, cycloserine, viomycin |
| Drugs for leprosy | | |
| Sulfones | Dapsone | |
| Phenazines | Clofazimine | |
| Thiosemicarbazones | Amithiozone | |

## QUESTIONS

**DIRECTIONS (items 1–5):** Each numbered item or incomplete statement in this section is followed by answers or by completions of the statement. Select the ONE lettered answer or completion that is BEST in each case.

**1.** The primary reason for the use of drug combinations in the treatment of tuberculosis is to
**(A)** prolong the plasma half-life of each drug
**(B)** lower the incidence of adverse effects
**(C)** enhance activity against metabolically inactive mycobacteria
**(D)** delay the emergence of resistance

**2.** Concerning isoniazid, all of the following statements are accurate EXCEPT:
**(A)** It increases phenytoin plasma levels by inhibiting its liver metabolism
**(B)** With intermittent treatment regimens, Native Americans may require higher doses than other patients
**(C)** It is not used in children because of the high risk of hepatotoxicity
**(D)** Pyridoxine protects against the peripheral neuritis caused by isoniazid

**3.** Concerning the use of rifampin in tuberculosis, all of the following statements are accurate EXCEPT:
**(A)** It may elicit withdrawal symptoms in patients taking methadone
**(B)** Most of its toxic effects result from inhibition of human DNA-dependent RNA polymerase
**(C)** Mutants resistant to rifampin occur at a frequency of $10^{-7}$ or greater
**(D)** It causes a flulike syndrome if administered less often than twice weekly

**4.** Concerning pyrazinamide, all of the following statements are accurate EXCEPT:
**(A)** It is effective orally and penetrates into cerebrospinal fluid
**(B)** It decreases the plasma half-life of warfarin
**(C)** Hepatic dysfunction occurs in 1–5% of patients treated with pyrazinamide
**(D)** Mycobacteria resistant to isoniazid may be sensitive to pyrazinamide

**5.** Concerning drugs used in leprosy, all of the following statements are accurate EXCEPT:
**(A)** The mechanism of action of dapsone probably involves inhibition of folic acid synthesis
**(B)** Single intramuscular injections of acedapsone maintain inhibitory levels of dapsone in tissues for long periods
**(C)** Monthly doses of rifampin delay the emergence of resistance to dapsone
**(D)** Clofazimine should not be given to patients who are intolerant to dapsone or who fail to respond to treatment with dapsone

**DIRECTIONS (items 6–10):** Items 6–10 consist of lettered headings followed by a set of numbered sentences. For each numbered sentence, select the ONE lettered heading that is most closely associated with it. Each lettered heading may be selected once, more than once, or not at all.

**(A)** Ethambutol
**(B)** Ethionamide
**(C)** Dapsone
**(D)** Rifampin
**(E)** Clofazimine

**6.** This drug eliminates a majority of meningococci from carriers, but highly resistant strains may be selected out during treatment

**7.** Periodic testing of visual acuity is advisable during treatment with this drug

**8.** A chemical congener of isoniazid, this drug is poorly tolerated because it causes intense gastric irritation and neurologic symptoms

**9.** Methemoglobinemia is a common side effect of this drug, and hemolysis may occur in patents with glucose-6-phosphate dehydrogenase deficiency

**10.** Active against *M avium-intracellulare* in AIDS patients, this drug may cause red-brown to black skin discoloration

## ANSWERS

**1.** Although it is sometimes possible to achieve synergistic effects against mycobacteria with drug combinations, the primary reason for their use is to delay the emergence of resistance. The answer is **(D)**.

2. The risk of hepatotoxicity from isoniazid increases with age; it rarely occurs in children or young persons under the age of 20 years. The answer is **(C)**.

3. Rifampin inhibits RNA synthesis in bacteria and chlamydiae, but human RNA polymerases are not sensitive to its actions. The answer is **(B)**.

4. Hepatic dysfunction may occur during treatment with pyrazinamide, but the drug is not an inducer of liver drug-metabolizing enzymes. It does not increase the rate of metabolism of other drugs (compare with rifampin). The answer is **(B)**.

5. Clofazimine is not chemically related to dapsone, and there is little cross-resistance. It is used in sulfone-resistant leprosy and in patients who are unable to tolerate dapsone. The answer is **(D)**.

6. Resistance emerges rapidly when rifampin is used as a single agent in the treatment of bacterial infections. When it is used in the meningococcal carrier state, up to 10% of treated carriers may harbor rifampin-resistant organisms. The answer is **(D)**.

7. Decreased visual acuity, optic neuritis, and possible retinal damage are characteristic adverse effects of ethambutol. Ocular toxicity is dose-dependent and is usually reversible when ethambutol use is discontinued. The answer is **(A)**.

8. Ethionamide is chemically related to isoniazid. It has a metallic taste and causes severe nausea, vomiting, and diarrhea unless taken with food to minimize gastric irritation. It is a second-line drug in the treatment of tuberculosis. The answer is **(B)**.

9. Hematologic abnormalities are common with dapsone and can include methemoglobinemia, hemolysis, leukopenia, and thrombocytopenia. The answer is **(C)**.

10. Clofazimine is a phenazine dye that causes skin coloration. Its clinical indications include dapsone-resistant leprosy, erythema nodosum leprosum, and atypical mycobacterial infections. The answer is **(E)**.

# 47 Sulfonamides & Trimethoprim

## OBJECTIVES

**Define the following terms:**

- Dihydropteroate synthetase
- Dihydrofolate reductase
- Sequential blockade
- Antimetabolite
- Antibacterial synergy

**You should be able to:**

- Describe the mechanisms of action of sulfonamides and trimethoprim on bacterial folic acid synthesis.
- Describe the mechanisms of resistance to sulfonamides and trimethoprim.
- List the major clinical uses of sulfonamides and trimethoprim, singly and in combination.
- Indicate the major pharmacokinetic features of sulfonamides and trimethoprim.
- Describe the adverse effects of sulfonamides and trimethoprim.

## CONCEPTS

### A. Classification & Pharmacokinetics:

1. **Sulfonamides.** The sulfonamides are weakly acidic compounds that have a common chemical nucleus resembling *p*-aminobenzoic acid **(PABA).** Members of this group differ mainly in their pharmacokinetic properties. Pharmacokinetic features include modest tissue penetration, hepatic metabolism, and excretion of both intact drug and acetylated metabolites in the urine. Solubility may be decreased in acidic urine, leading to crystalluria. Sulfonamides bind to plasma proteins at sites shared by bilirubin and by other drugs.
2. **Trimethoprim.** This drug is structurally similar to folic acid. It is a weak base, is trapped in acidic environments, and reaches high levels in prostatic and vaginal fluids. A large fraction of the drug is excreted unchanged in the urine.

### B. Mechanism of Action:

1. **Sulfonamides** are bacteriostatic inhibitors of folic acid synthesis (Fig 47–1). Antimetabolites of PABA, they act as competitive inhibitors of **dihydropteroate synthetase.** The selective toxicity of sulfonamides results from the ability of mammalian cells to utilize preformed folic acid present in the diet.
2. **Trimethoprim** is a selective inhibitor of bacterial **dihydrofolate reductase;** it prevents the formation of active forms of folic acid. When sulfonamides are used in combination with trimethoprim, antimicrobial synergy may result from the **sequential blockade** of folate synthesis (Fig 47–1).
3. **Bacterial resistance** to sulfonamides is common and may be plasmid-mediated. It may be caused by decreased intracellular accumulation of the drug, an increased production of PABA by bacteria, or a change in the sensitivity of dihydropteroate synthetase. Clinical resistance to trimethoprim results from the formation of dihydrofolate reductase with reduced affinity for the drug.

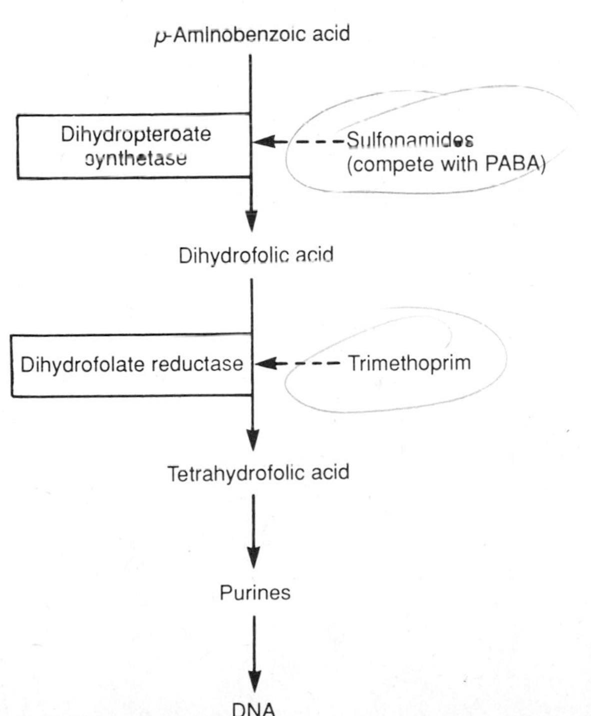


**Figure 47–1.** Inhibitory effects of sulfonamides and trimethoprim on folic acid synthesis. The sequential blockade of the formation of tetrahydrofolic acid by sulfonamides and trimethoprim may lead to antibacterial synergy, with enhanced clinical effectiveness in treatment of bacterial infections. (Reproduced, with permission, from Katzung BG [editor]: *Basic & Clinical Pharmacology,* 5th ed. Appleton & Lange, 1992.)

### C. Clinical Use:

1. The sulfonamides are active against a wide range of gram-positive and gram-negative organisms, chlamydiae, and *Nocardia* spp. As individual drugs, sulfonamides have the following uses:
   a. Simple urinary tract infections, orally **(triple sulfas, sulfisoxazole).**
   b. Ocular infections, topically **(sulfacetamide).**
   c. Burn infections, topically **(mafenide, silver sulfadiazine).**
   d. Ulcerative colitis, orally **(sulfasalazine).**
2. Trimethoprim is used as the sole drug for some urinary tract infections, but its major clinical applications are in combination with **sulfamethoxazole** (as **trimethoprim-sulfamethoxazole, TMP-SMZ**). This combination is the currently accepted treatment for complicated urinary tract infections, *Shigella* enteritis, resistant *Salmonella* infections, *Serratia* sepsis, and *Pneumocystis carinii* pneumonia.

### D. Toxicity:

1. **Adverse effects of sulfonamides** include the following:
   a. **Hypersensitivity reactions,** including skin rashes and fever. Cross-allergenicity between the individual drugs should be assumed. Stevens-Johnson syndrome has occurred.
   b. **Gastrointestinal** disturbances and hepatic dysfunction.
   c. **Hemolysis** in persons with glucose-6-phosphate dehydrogenase deficiency. Anemia is an uncommon effect.
   d. **Nephrotoxicity,** from crystallization in the renal tubules.
   e. **Drug interactions,** from competition with coumarins and methotrexate for plasma protein binding. Displacement of bound bilirubin may cause kernicterus in neonates.
2. **Adverse effects of trimethoprim,** which result from its antifolate effects (megaloblastic anemia, leukopenia, and granulocytopenia), may be ameliorated by folinic acid. AIDS patients given trimethoprim-sulfamethoxazole have a high incidence of adverse effects, including fever, rashes, leukopenia, and diarrhea.

## DRUG LIST

The following drugs are important members of the group discussed in this chapter. Prototype agents should be learned in detail; the major variants and other significant agents should be identifiable on the basis of differences in their pharmacokinetic properties and clinical uses.

| Subclass | Prototype | Major Variants | Other Significant Agents |
|---|---|---|---|
| Sulfonamides<br>Oral agents | Sulfisoxazole | Triple sulfas, sulfamethoxazole | |
| Local agents | | | Sulfacetamide, sulfasalazine, mafenide, sulfadiazine |
| Combination | Trimethoprim-sulfamethoxazole | | |
| Folate reductase inhibitors | Trimethoprim | | Pyrimethamine |

## QUESTIONS

**DIRECTIONS (items 1–5):** Each numbered item or incomplete statement in this section is followed by answers or by completions of the statement. Select the ONE lettered answer or completion that is BEST in each case.

**1.** All of the following statements about sulfonamides are accurate EXCEPT:
**(A)** They inhibit bacterial dihydropteroate synthetase
**(B)** Acute hemolysis may occur in patients with glucose-6-phosphate dehydrogenase deficiency
**(C)** They are antimetabolites of PABA
**(D)** Crystalluria is most likely to occur at high urinary pH

**2.** All of the following statements about the clinical uses of sulfonamides are accurate EXCEPT:
**(A)** Sulfadiazine is effective in acute urinary tract infections due to nonresistant *E coli*
**(B)** Topical sulfacetamide is useful for chlamydial infections of the eye
**(C)** Sulfamethoxazole is effective in Rocky Mountain spotted fever in patients allergic to tetracyclines
**(D)** Sulfisoxazole is not likely to be effective for chronic prostatitis in an elderly patient

**3.** All of the following adverse effects occur with sulfonamide therapy EXCEPT
**(A)** increased anticoagulant effects if given with coumarins
**(B)** Fanconi's aminoaciduria syndrome
**(C)** urticaria
**(D)** kernicterus in the newborn
**(E)** hematuria

**4.** The mechanisms involved in the development of clinical resistance to sulfonamides include all of the following EXCEPT
**(A)** decreased intracellular accumulation of drug
**(B)** changed sensitivity of dihydrofolate reductase
**(C)** increased production of PABA
**(D)** utilization of extracellular sources of folic acid

**5.** All of the following statements about the combination of trimethoprim plus sulfamethoxazole are accurate EXCEPT:
**(A)** It is effective in the treatment of pneumonia due to *Pneumocystis carinii*
**(B)** The drugs produce a sequential blockade of folic acid synthesis
**(C)** Fever and pancytopenia occur frequently in AIDS patients
**(D)** It is appropriate for the treatment of streptococcal pharyngitis
**(E)** It is effective in the management of acute exacerbations of chronic bronchitis

**DIRECTIONS (items 6–9):** Items 6–9 consist of lettered headings followed by a set of numbered statements. For each numbered statement, select the ONE lettered heading that is most closely associated with it. Each lettered heading may be selected once, more than once, or not at all.

**(A)** Trimethoprim
**(B)** Sulfinpyrazone
**(C)** Sulfamethoxazole
**(D)** Sulfasalazine
**(E)** Silver sulfadiazine

**6.** Used orally in ulcerative colitis, this agent has both antibacterial and anti-inflammatory actions.

**7.** When applied topically to burn wounds, this agent is effective in controlling colonization of bacteria including *Pseudomonas* spp.

**8.** This water-soluble drug is used orally as a single agent for simple urinary tract infections. Drug levels in prostatic and vaginal fluids are much lower than those in plasma.

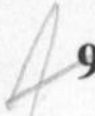

**9.** Supplementary folinic acid may prevent hematotoxicity in folate-deficient persons who use this drug. It is a weak base and achieves tissue levels similar to those in plasma. Resistance may emerge when it is used as the sole drug in urinary tract infections.

## ANSWERS

**1.** The water solubility of sulfonamides is increased by urinary alkalinization, which favors ionization. Crystalluria is more likely to occur if the urine is acidic. The answer is **(D)**.

**2.** Sulfonamides have minimal therapeutic actions in rickettsial infections. Chloramphenicol may be used for Rocky Mountain spotted fever in patients with established allergy or other contraindication to tetracyclines. The answer is **(C)**.

**3.** Renal dysfunction including crystalluria, hematuria, nephrosis, and allergic nephritis occurs with sulfonamides. However, Fanconi's syndrome, characterized by low back pain, aminoaciduria, polydipsia and polyuria, is associated with the use of outdated tetracyclines. The answer is **(B)**.

**4.** Several mechanisms of bacterial resistance to sulfonamides have been documented, and resistance may be plasmid-mediated. The sulfa drugs are not specific inhibitors of dihydrofolate reductase, and there is no evidence that changes in sensitivity of this enzyme are responsible for resistance to sulfonamides. The answer is **(B)**.

**5.** The combination of trimethoprim and sulfamethoxazole is often effective in respiratory infections due to susceptible *S pneumoniae* and *H influenzae*. However, in streptococcal pharyngitis the organisms are not eradicated. The answer is **(D)**.

**6.** The name should help! Sulfasalazine is converted by intestinal microflora to yield sulfapyridine, which is antibacterial, and 5-aminosalicylate, which has anti-inflammatory activity. The answer is **(D)**.

**7.** Silver sulfadiazine and mafenide (not listed) are used prophylactically as topical agents in burn wounds to prevent bacterial colonization. The answer is **(E)**.

**8.** Highly soluble, rapidly excreted sulfonamides are used for the oral treatment of uncomplicated urinary tract infections. These agents include sulfadiazine, sulfisoxazole, and sulfamethoxazole. The sulfonamides are weak acids, which generally do not achieve high drug levels in prostatic and vaginal secretions. Sulfinpyrazone is an antiplatelet drug. The answer is **(C)**.

**9.** Trimethoprim is the only basic compound listed. As a weak base with high lipid solubility at blood pH, trimethoprim penetrates membrane barriers more effectively than sulfonamides. Because prostatic fluid and vaginal fluid are usually more acidic than blood, levels of the drug in these organs are similar to—and often higher than—those in plasma. (The opposite is true of sulfonamides, which are weak acids.) Leukopenia and thrombocytopenia may occur in folate deficiency when the drug is used alone or in combination with sulfamethoxazole. The answer is **(A)**.

# Antifungal Agents 48

## OBJECTIVES

**You should be able to:**

- Describe the probable mechanisms of action of griseofulvin and the antifungal agents used for systemic infections.
- Describe the clinical uses and pharmacokinetics of amphotericin B, flucytosine, fluconazole, griseofulvin, and ketoconazole.
- Indicate the major toxic effects of systemic antifungal drugs and griseofulvin.
- Identify the main topical antifungal agents.

## CONCEPTS

### A. Drugs for Systemic Fungal Infections:

1. **Amphotericin B,** a polyene antibiotic related to nystatin, is the most important antifungal drug. It binds to ergosterol, a sterol specific to fungal cell membranes, to change the permeability and transport properties of the membranes. Resistance can occur via a decreased level of, or structural change in, membrane ergosterol. The drug is active against *Blastomyces, Coccidioides, Cryptococcus,* and *Histoplasma* spp and *Candida albicans* and is usually given by slow intravenous infusion. Penetration into the CNS is minimal, and the drug has a long plasma half-life. Toxic effects are extensive and include fever and chills, electrolyte imbalance, hypotension, neurologic symptoms, nephrotoxicity, and cardiac toxicity. Dose reduction (with lowered toxicity) may be possible in some fungal infections if rifampin or a tetracycline is used concomitantly. A liposomal preparation of amphotericin B may have reduced toxic effects.
2. **Flucytosine (5-fluorocytosine)** is activated in fungal cells by cytosine deaminase-mediated conversion to 5-fluorouracil (5-FU), which, when incorporated into RNA, causes functional changes. Selective toxicity occurs because mammalian cells have low levels of permease (for uptake of the drug) and deaminase. Resistance can occur rapidly and involves decreases in permease or deaminase levels. When given with amphotericin B, resistance is decreased and synergistic effects may occur. The antifungal spectrum is limited to *Cryptococcus* spp and *C albicans.* Oral bioavailability is good, and the drug enters the CNS. Its principal toxic effect is reversible bone marrow depression.
3. **Ketoconazole** is an azole antifungal agent that decreases ergosterol formation by inhibiting 14α-demethylation of lanosterol. The drug is active against systemic infections caused by certain *Blastomyces, Coccidioides,* and *Histoplasma* strains as well as *C albicans.* In disseminated blastomycoses it is the drug of choice. It is orally active and undergoes liver metabolism and biliary excretion. Oral absorption of ketoconazole may be impaired by antacids, cimetidine, or rifampin. Adverse effects include gastrointestinal irritation, fever, chills, hepatic dysfunction, and hormonal effects due to inhibition of steroid synthesis.
4. **Fluconazole** is a new azole that is more reliably absorbed via the oral route than ketoconazole. The drug is distributed widely in the body, readily enters the CNS, and undergoes renal elimination. It is used for local and systemic candidiasis, and it can suppress cryptococcal meningitis in immunodeficient patients. Adverse effects include gastrointestinal irritation, rashes, and impairment of liver function. Fluconazole may increase the plasma levels of phenytoin, oral hypoglycemics, and warfarin.
5. The azoles **miconazole** and **clotrimazole** have also been used (intravenously) for systemic mycoses. They are more commonly used topically for fungal infections of the skin and mucous membranes. Although they are effective in some infections, when used systemically they appear to be more toxic than ketoconazole and fluconazole.

**B. Systemic Drugs for Superficial Fungal Infections:** **Griseofulvin,** the major systemic drug for superficial fungal infections, inhibits the growth of dermatophytes and *C albicans* by mechanisms that may involve interference with microtubule function, resulting in decreased mitosis. Sensitive fungi take up the drug by an energy-dependent mechanism, and resistance can occur via a decrease in this transport. Oral absorption is aided by high-fat foods, and the drug is distributed to the stratum corneum, where it binds to keratin. Adverse effects include headaches, mental confusion, gastrointestinal irritation, and changes in liver function. A drug interaction may result from enhanced coumarin metabolism. Griseofulvin may be teratogenic or carcinogenic. Oral **ketoconazole** is also effective against dermatophytes.

**C. Topical Drugs for Superficial Infections:** A number of antifungal drugs are used topically for superficial infections caused by *C albicans* and dermatophytes. **Nystatin** is a polyene antibiotic that disrupts fungal membranes by binding to ergosterol. It is commonly used topically to suppress local *Candida* infections and has been used orally to eradicate gastrointestinal fungi in patients with impaired defense mechanisms. Other topical antifungal agents include the azole compounds **miconazole** and **clotrimazole** and the nonazoles **haloprogin, tolnaftate,** and **undecylenic acid.**

## DRUG LIST

The following drugs are important members of the group discussed in this chapter. Information about amphotericin B, flucytosine, fluconazole, griseofulvin, and ketoconazole should be learned in detail. You should be able to identify the topical drugs.

| Subclass | Prototype | Other Significant Agents |
|---|---|---|
| Drugs for systemic mycoses | Amphotericin B | Flucytosine, fluconazole, ketoconazole |
| Drugs for superficial infections | | |
| Oral | Griseofulvin | Ketoconazole |
| Topical | Nystatin | Miconazole, clotrimazole, tolnaftate |

## QUESTIONS

**DIRECTIONS (items 1–4):** Each numbered item or incomplete statement in this section is followed by answers or by completions of the statement. Select the ONE lettered answer or completion that is BEST in each case.

**1.** Each of the following statements about ketoconazole is accurate EXCEPT:
**(A)** It is the drug of choice in disseminated blastomycosis
**(B)** It is effective in the treatment of fungal meningitis
**(C)** It inhibits ergosterol synthesis
**(D)** It inhibits the synthesis of endogenous steroids
**(E)** It is effective against dermatophytes

**2.** Each of the following statements about the adverse effects of individual antifungal agents is accurate EXCEPT:
**(A)** Cardiotoxicity occurs with rapid intravenous administration of amphotericin B
**(B)** Headache, lethargy, and mental confusion are common side effects of griseofulvin
**(C)** Flucytosine causes gynecomastia
**(D)** Ketoconazole is not recommended during pregnancy because it has teratogenic potential
**(E)** Fluconazole may enhance the actions of oral hypoglycemics

**3.** Each of the following statements about griseofulvin is accurate EXCEPT:
- **(A)** It acts on microtubules to decrease mitosis
- **(B)** It is not active against *C albicans*
- **(C)** It may reduce the efficacy of some oral contraceptives
- **(D)** It is effective topically against many dermatophytes
- **(E)** In animal studies it is teratogenic and carcinogenic

**4.** All of the following statements about antifungal drugs are accurate EXCEPT:
- **(A)** Flucytosine is deaminated and converted to a metabolite that inhibits fungal thymidylate synthetase
- **(B)** Fever and azotemia are common adverse effects of intravenous amphotericin B
- **(C)** The metabolism of ketoconazole is inhibited by rifampin
- **(D)** Ketoconazole is the preferred treatment for chronic mucocutaneous candidiasis

**DIRECTIONS (items 5–8):** Items 5–8 consist of lettered headings followed by a set of numbered statements. For each numbered statement, select the ONE lettered heading that is most closely associated with it. Each lettered heading may be selected once, more than once, or not at all.

- **(A)** Flucytosine
- **(B)** Nystatin
- **(C)** Amphotericin B
- **(D)** Ketoconazole
- **(E)** Clotrimazole

**5.** This polyene antifungal agent is too toxic for systemic use. It is applied topically, or given orally for its local actions in the gastrointestinal tract.

**6.** With chronic use this drug causes hypochromic, normocytic anemia and renal dysfunction leading to the wasting of $K^+$ and $Mg^{2+}$. When used to treat fungal meningitis it must be administered via intrathecal infusion.

**7.** After oral administration of this drug the cerebrospinal fluid levels achieved are almost as high as the plasma levels. Resistance may emerge during the treatment of systemic mycoses if the drug is used as the sole antifungal agent.

**8.** The oral absorption of this drug is impaired by antacids and by histamine $H_2$ receptor-blocking agents. Elevation of plasma aminotransferase activity is common, and progressive hepatotoxicity may develop following high doses.

## ANSWERS

**1.** Levels of ketoconazole achievable in the cerebrospinal fluid in fungal meningitis are less than 1% of that in the plasma. Therefore, the drug has limited effectiveness in such infections. The answer is **(B)**.

**2.** Adverse effects of prolonged treatment with flucytosine include reversible bone marrow depression, alopecia, and gastrointestinal distress. Although hormonal changes may occur, gynecomastia has not been reported with flucytosine; it is a known adverse effect of treatment with ketoconazole. The answer is **(C)**.

**3.** Topical application of griseofulvin has minimal antifungal effects. In the treatment of dermatophytic infections the drug must be given orally. Absorption is increased by using ultramicrosize particles or by taking griseofulvin with a fat-containing meal. Note that griseofulvin may increase the activity of liver drug-metabolizing enzymes, leading to drug interactions. The answer is **(D)**.

**4.** When rifampin is used in the treatment of tuberculosis, fungal infections may not respond to conventional doses of ketoconazole. Rifampin induces liver drug-metabolizing enzyme and decreases the plasma half-life of a number of drugs, including ketoconazole. The answer is **(C)**.

**5.** Two polyene antifungal drugs are listed. Despite the introduction of the azole antifungals, amphotericin B remains the drug of choice for most deep mycotic infections. Nystatin is as active as amphotericin B, but is too toxic for parenteral use. The answer is **(B)**.

**6.** The characteristics described should permit identification of amphotericin B. A markedly depressed hematocrit probably results from decreased production of erythropoietin. Renal dysfunction occurs in up to 80% of patients on chronic therapy, it includes tubular acidosis and electrolyte imbalance. Note that amphotericin B does not cross the blood-brain barrier and therefore must be administered intrathecally in fungal meningitis. The answer is **(C)**.

**7.** Flucytosine is an antifungal agent that reaches high levels in the cerebrospinal fluid after oral administration. The rapid emergence of resistant strains of fungi restricts its use as a single agent. Flucytosine is used mainly in combination with amphotericin B. The answer is **(A)**.

**8.** An acidic environment is required for the dissolution of ketoconazole, and its oral absorption is impaired by antacids and drugs that decrease gastric acidity. Mild, asymptomatic liver dysfunction is common, and severe hepatitis has occurred in some patients. The answer is **(D)**.

# 49 Antiviral Chemotherapy & Prophylaxis

## OBJECTIVES

**You should be able to:**

- Identify the main steps in viral replication.
- Describe the mechanisms of antiviral actions of purine and pyrimidine antimetabolites (idoxuridine, vidarabine, acyclovir, and azidothymidine), amantadine, and the interferons.
- Describe the clinical uses of the antimetabolites, amantadine, and the interferons and list the toxic effects of drugs that are used systemically.
- Identify the less commonly used antiviral agents (methisazone, rifampin) and the newer drugs dideoxyinosine, disoxaril, foscarnet, ganciclovir, and ribavirin.

## CONCEPTS

### A. Mechanism of Action:

1. **Adsorption and penetration of the virus.** The first steps in viral replication involve adsorption to the mammalian cell membrane, penetration intracellularly, and viral particle uncoating. Drugs that act at this stage include the **immune (gamma) globulins,** which contain specific antibodies to viral antigens and can block cell penetration. The process of fusion of the viral particle with the endosomal membrane requires low pH. **Amantadine** inhibits this step, partly because it is basic and raises the endosomal pH. At low concentrations, amantadine

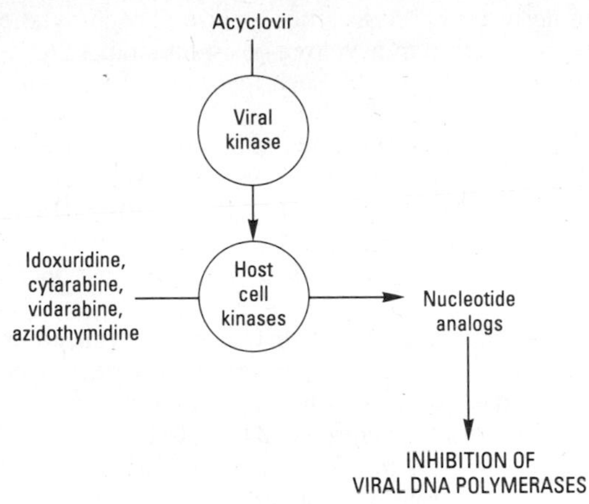


**Figure 49–1.** Antiviral actions of purine and pyrimidine analogues.

also binds to a specific protein in the surface coat of the influenza virus to prevent fusion. The investigational drug **disoxaril** binds to and stabilizes the surface coat of some viruses, preventing uncoating, so that the viral genome is not released into the infected cell.

2. **Early protein synthesis.** Biguanides inhibit viral RNA polymerases and thus interfere with the synthesis of nonstructural proteins and enzymes. Resistance to these compounds occurs rapidly, and no clinically useful drugs act at this stage in viral replication.
3. **Nucleic acid synthesis.** Many useful antiviral drugs are structurally similar to purine or pyrimidine bases and act as **antimetabolites.** As shown in Fig 49–1, these drugs undergo phosphorylation by host cell kinases to form nucleotide analogues, which may inhibit viral **DNA polymerases** or act as substrates for viral enzymes (or both), resulting in their incorporation into viral nucleic acids. Selective toxicity may result, because viral DNA polymerases are more sensitive to inhibition by these antimetabolites than are mammalian polymerases. The selective antiherpetic action of acyclovir is partly a result of its initial phosphorylation by a viral thymidine kinase that is absent in uninfected cells. The **interferons** exert multiple actions that affect viral RNA and DNA synthesis. They induce the formation of enzymes, including a protein kinase that phosphorylates a factor which blocks peptide chain initiation, a phosphodiesterase that degrades terminal nucleotides of tRNA, and enzymes that activate RNase.
4. **Late protein synthesis and viral assembly.** Few clinically useful drugs act at the later stages of viral replication. **Methisazone** interferes with synthesis of a late structural protein in variola virus (the agent of smallpox), resulting in blockade of particle assembly. **Rifampin** blocks a step in the formation of viral envelopes, preventing the assembly of enveloped mature particles.

### B. Clinical Use & Toxicity:

1. **Topical antiviral drugs.** Several antiviral agents with marked systemic toxicity (bone marrow, hepatic, renal) are used mainly as topical drugs for herpes simplex virus eye infections, including corneal keratitis. These drugs include the antimetabolites **idoxuridine, cytarabine,** and **trifluorothymidine.**
2. **Vidarabine.** The purine nucleoside analogue vidarabine is useful in herpes simplex virus diseases, including encephalitis, keratitis, and neonatal herpes, but has no effect on genital lesions. It also prevents the dissemination of varicella-zoster virus in immunocompromised patients. It is available for topical use but is used intravenously in serious infections. Systemic toxic effects include gastrointestinal irritation, paresthesias, tremors, convulsions, and hepatic dysfunction.
3. **Acyclovir (acycloguanosine).** Acyclovir is active against herpes simplex virus type 1, Epstein-Barr virus, and varicella-zoster virus. Clinical uses include treatment of mucocutaneous and genital herpes lesions and prophylaxis in immunocompromised patients (eg, those undergoing heart or kidney transplants). It is active by the topical, oral, and intravenous routes. Systemic toxic effects include delirium, tremor, seizures, hypotension, and nephrotoxicity.

**Foscarnet,** a simple phosphonoformate derivative that does not require phosphorylation for antiviral activity, inhibits herpes DNA polymerase in acyclovir-resistant strains that are thymidine kinase-deficient. Given intravenously, it suppresses such resistant herpetic infections in patients with AIDS.

4. **Ganciclovir.** The guanine derivative ganciclovir is an antimetabolite that is phosphorylated by cellular kinases to form a nucleotide which inhibits DNA polymerases of cytomegalovirus (CMV). It is used intravenously in immunocompromised patients (eg, those with AIDS and those undergoing cancer chemotherapy or organ transplantation). Resistant strains of CMV can emerge during prolonged treatment. Systemic toxic effects include leukopenia, thrombocytopenia, renal dysfunction, and seizures.
5. **Azidothymidine (AZT, zidovudine).** AZT is an antimetabolite that is phosphorylated and inhibits DNA polymerase (reverse transcriptase) of the retrovirus human immunodeficiency virus (HIV). The viral enzyme is about 100 times more susceptible to inhibition than are mammalian DNA polymerases. AZT is active orally and is eliminated by both hepatic metabolism and renal excretion. The drug temporarily reduces mortality and morbidity in patients with AIDS and AIDS-related complex and slows the rate of progression to AIDS in asymptomatic HIV-positive individuals. Toxic effects include bone marrow suppression (which may require transfusions), granulocytopenia, thrombocytopenia, headaches, agitation, and insomnia. Drugs that are metabolized via glucuronyltransferase, including acetaminophen, NSAIDs, and sulfonamides, increase the toxicity of AZT. Newer drugs with activity against AZT-resistant strains of HIV include **dideoxyinosine (DDI)** and **dideoxycytidine (DDC).** Both drugs cause peripheral neuropathies, and DDI may cause pancreatitis.
6. **Ribavirin.** Ribavirin inhibits the replication of both RNA and DNA viruses by interfering with guanidine monophosphate formation and subsequently nucleic acid synthesis. It is used for respiratory syncytial virus infections and may shorten the duration of symptoms of influenza A and B virus infections. Ribavirin interferes with the action of AZT in HIV infection.
7. **Amantadine.** Amantadine is active against influenza A and rubella viruses. It is prophylactic (not curative) in influenza but may modify symptoms if given early. Drug-resistant influenza A virus mutants can emerge and infect contacts. It is orally active and is eliminated unchanged in the urine at a rate proportionate to creatinine clearance, and dose modification is required in renal insufficiency. Toxic effects include dizziness, ataxia, and slurred speech. **Rimantadine** is equally effective and requires no dose adjustment in renal failure.
8. **Interferons.** Interferons are glycoproteins originating from human leukocyte (IFN-$\alpha$), fibroblast (IFN-$\beta$), or immune (IFN-$\gamma$) cells and now produced by recombinant DNA technology. Clinical uses include prevention of herpes zoster virus dissemination in cancer patients, suppression of viremia with hepatitis B virus, and cancer chemotherapy. Toxic effects include gastrointestinal irritation, fatigue, anemia, myalgia, mental confusion, and cardiovascular dysfunction.

## DRUG LIST

The following drugs are important members of the group discussed in this chapter. Prototype drugs should be learned in detail; the other significant agents that act as systemic antiviral agents should be known well enough to list the factors that distinguish them from the prototypes and from each other.

| Subclass | Prototype | Other Significant Agents |
|---|---|---|
| Purine and pyrimidine analogues: | | |
| Topical | Idoxuridine | Trifluorothymidine, cytarabine |
| Systemic | Acyclovir | Vidarabine, azidothymidine, dideoxyinosine, ganciclovir, ribavirin |
| Tricyclic symmetric amines | Amantadine | Rimantadine |
| Proteins | Immune globulin, interferon | |

## QUESTIONS

**DIRECTIONS (items 1–4):** Each numbered item or incomplete statement in this section is followed by answers or by completions of the statement. Select the ONE lettered answer or completion that is BEST in each case.

**1.** Each of the following statements about the mechanisms of action of antiviral drugs is accurate EXCEPT:
**(A)** The initial step in activation of vidarabine is its phosphorylation by viral thymidine kinase
**(B)** The reverse transcriptase of HIV is 50–100 times more sensitive to inhibition by azidothymidine than are host cell DNA polymerases
**(C)** Increased activity of host cell phosphodiesterases that degrade tRNA is one of the antiviral actions of interferons
**(D)** Rimantadine inhibits the fusion of viral particles with the endosomal membrane

**2.** This drug has activity against herpes simplex virus type 1 and is used only topically. Systemic administration results in bone marrow depression, hepatic dysfunction, and nephrotoxicity.
**(A)** Ganciclovir
**(B)** Acyclovir
**(C)** Amantadine
**(D)** Vidarabine
**(E)** Idoxuridine

**3.** Each of the following statements about antiviral agents is accurate EXCEPT:
**(A)** Interferons may prevent dissemination of herpes zoster virus in cancer patients and reduce CMV shedding after renal transplantation
**(B)** The oral absorption of acyclovir is slow and incomplete, but is not affected by foods
**(C)** Since amantadine is eliminated mainly via hepatic metabolism, dose modification is not required in renal insufficiency
**(D)** Foscarnet is active against resistant herpesvirus strains that are thymidine kinase-deficient

**4.** Each of the following statements about the effects of antiviral drugs is accurate EXCEPT:
**(A)** Treatment with acyclovir does not prevent transmission of herpes during sexual intercourse
**(B)** Dideoxyinosine has activity against certain HIV strains resistant to azidothymidine
**(C)** AIDS patients treated with azidothymidine should take acetaminophen to relieve neurologic symptoms
**(D)** Topical use of vidarabine requires caution during pregnancy because systemic absorption occurs and the drug is potentially mutagenic and teratogenic

**DIRECTIONS (items 5–8):** Items 5–8 consist of lettered headings followed by a set of numbered statements. For each numbered statement, select the ONE lettered heading that is most closely associated with it. Each lettered heading may be selected once, more than once, or not at all.

**(A)** Interferon
**(B)** Acyclovir
**(C)** Ribavirin
**(D)** Cytarabine
**(E)** Azidothymidine

**5.** Although used primarily as a topical agent in herpes simplex virus ocular infections, this drug may also be administered systemically for its antineoplastic effects.

**6.** The antiviral actions of this drug include inhibition of both RNA and DNA synthesis. It is used for the treatment of severe respiratory syncytial virus infections in neonates.

**7.** At the initiation of therapy with this drug, most patients experience a flulike syndrome. Its clinical uses include the treatment of Kaposi's sarcoma, hairy-cell leukemias, and genital warts.

**8.** Over 90% of this drug is excreted intact in the urine. Since its urinary solubility is low, patients should be well hydrated to prevent nephrotoxicity.

## ANSWERS

**1.** Initial phosphorylation by viral thymidine kinase is a distinctive feature of the bioactivation of acyclovir. Vidarabine and other antiviral agents that act as antimetabolites are activated exclusively by host cell kinases. The answer is **(A).**

**2.** Because of its systemic toxicity, idoxuridine is used as a topical agent for the treatment of herpesvirus ocular infections. When applied to the cornea, it does not penetrate the deep stroma and is not absorbed into the bloodstream to a significant extent. The answer is **(E).**

**3.** Amantadine is eliminated in the urine via renal tubular secretion. In patients with normal renal function, the drug has a half-life of 24 hours, but in renal insufficiency the half-life may be prolonged to 10 days. The answer is **(C).**

**4.** In the management of AIDS patients on AZT, one should avoid drugs that are substrates for hepatic glucuronosyltransferase since they interfere with AZT metabolism and elevate plasma levels of the drug. Acetaminophen increases the toxicity of AZT by this mechanism. The answer is **(C).**

**5.** Herpes simplex virus infections of the eye that are resistant to idoxuridine may respond to cytarabine. The drug is sometimes used intravenously in acute leukemias, but causes dose-dependent neuritis, peripheral neuropathy, and depression of bone marrow. The answer is **(D).**

**6.** The antiviral actions of ribavirin include inhibition of RNA polymerases, inhibition of DNA and RNA synthesis, and interference with viral coating. It is used by aerosol inhalation for respiratory syncytial virus infections in premature infants and children with cardiopulmonary disease. The answer is **(C).**

**7.** Headache, fever, chills, and muscle aches are common side effects of treatment with interferons. Patients are advised to take acetaminophen, since aspirin aggravates gastrointestinal irritation and may promote bleeding. Interferons may also cause neurotoxicity, cardiovascular dysfunction, and bone marrow depression. The answer is **(A).**

**8.** Acyclovir is eliminated in the urine via filtration and by active tubular secretion, which is inhibited by probenecid. Nephrotoxic effects including hematuria and crystalluria are enhanced in patients who are dehydrated, or who have preexisting renal dysfunction. The answer is **(B).**

# Miscellaneous Antimicrobial Agents & Urinary Antiseptics

# 50

## OBJECTIVES

**Define the following terms:**

- macrolide
- DNA gyrase

**You should be able to:**

- Describe the mechanisms of antibacterial action of clindamycin, erythromycin, fluoroquinolones, and vancomycin.
- Describe the clinical uses of clindamycin, erythromycin, vancomycin, and fluoroquinolones; the significant features of their biodisposition; and their main toxic effects.
- Identify the antibacterial uses of metronidazole and bacitracin.
- Identify the drugs commonly used as urinary antiseptics and describe their toxic effects.

## CONCEPTS

**A. Erythromycin:** Erythromycin is a macrolide antibiotic, ie, a large (16–18 member) lactone ring with antimicrobial activity. It inhibits protein synthesis by binding to a **23S rRNA** component of the 50S ribosomal subunit to prevent ribosomal translocation. Resistance can result from plasmid-mediated formation of enzymes that methylate this receptor, preventing drug binding. Among coliforms a transmissible plasmid occurs that specifies an esterase which hydrolyzes the lactone ring of erythromycin, thereby inactivating the drug. The drug can be bacteriostatic or bactericidal. Its clinical uses include infections caused by gram-positive cocci (including beta-lactamase-producing staphylococci) and by *Neisseria, Mycoplasma, Chlamydia,* and *Legionella.* Oral absorption is variable, and wide tissue distribution occurs. Excretion is primarily via the bile. Toxic effects are minor but include gastrointestinal irritation, skin rashes, eosinophilia, and possible hypersensitivity-based acute cholestatic hepatitis with erythromycin estolate. The drug inhibits hepatic cytochrome P-450 and can increase plasma levels of the anticoagulants, carbamazepine, digoxin, and theophylline. It is widely used as an alternative to penicillin G in persons allergic to penicillins. Newer macrolides include **azithromycin** and **clarithromycin,** which have expanded activity against gram-negative organisms.

**B. Lincosamines: Lincomycin** and **clindamycin** have few clinical uses. They inhibit bacterial protein synthesis via a mechanism similar to that of erythromycin and are usually bacteriostatic. The activity and clinical uses of clindamycin are limited to gram-positive cocci and anaerobes such as *Bacteroides* spp. Good tissue penetration occurs after absorption. The lincosamines are eliminated partly via metabolism and partly by biliary and renal excretion. The toxicity of clindamycin includes marked gastrointestinal irritation, skin rashes, neutropenia, hepatic dysfunction, and possible superinfections such as *C difficile* pseudomembranous colitis.

**C. Fluoroquinolones: Norfloxacin, ciprofloxacin,** and newer members of this group are fluorinated agents similar but far superior to nalidixic acid. These drugs inhibit DNA gyrase and prevent the conversion of supercoiled DNA to the relaxed DNA forms. Clinical uses include treatment of urogenital, respiratory, and soft tissue infections caused by gram-negative organisms such as *Enterobacter, Neisseria, Pseudomonas,* and *Salmonella* spp. They may also be useful for prophylaxis in neutropenic patients and for treatment of infectious diarrhea caused by toxigenic coliforms. Resistance mechanisms include changes in the drug sensitivity of the target enzyme and decreased drug accumulation. After oral absorption, the drugs are well distributed to body tissues. Elimination is partly via metabolism and mainly through the kidneys via active tubular secretion (blocked by probenecid). Toxic effects include gastrointestinal irritation, skin rashes, headache, and dizziness. Superinfections with streptococci and *Candida* spp may occur. The drugs may enhance theophylline toxicity and can interfere with collagen metabolism.

**D. Vancomycin:** This drug is used for serious infections caused by drug-resistant gram-positive organisms, including beta-lactamase-producing staphylococci and *C difficile*. It is a bactericidal inhibitor of the synthesis of cell wall mucopeptides, and resistance is minimal. The drug is not absorbed from the gastrointestinal tract, but may be given orally for bacterial enterocolitis. When given parenterally, vancomycin penetrates most tissues and is eliminated unchanged in the urine. Dose modification is necessary in patients with renal impairment. Toxic effects following parenteral use include chills, fever, phlebitis, ototoxicity, and nephrotoxicity. Rapid intravenous infusion may cause diffuse flushing (red man syndrome).

**E. Metronidazole:** An antiprotozoal agent, metronidazole is also active against *Gardnerella vaginalis* and anaerobes such as *Bacteroides* and *Clostridium* spp. Its bactericidal actions result from the formation of toxic metabolites in the bacterial cell. The drug is effective orally and penetrates most tissues, including abscesses and the CNS. Its toxic effects include gastrointestinal irritation, headache, vestibular dysfunction, and disulfiramlike reactions with ethanol. It is teratogenic in some animals.

**F. Urinary Antiseptics:** These agents act in the urine to suppress bacteriuria. They lack systemic antibacterial effects but may be toxic. They are often administered with acidifying agents, since bacterial growth in urine is inhibited at a low pH.

1. **Nitrofurantoin** is active against many urinary tract pathogens (not *Proteus* or *Pseudomonas* spp), and resistance emerges slowly. The drug is active orally and is excreted in the urine via filtration and secretion; it may reach toxic levels in the blood of patients with renal dysfunction. Adverse effects include gastrointestinal irritation, skin rashes, neuropathies, and hemolysis in patients with glucose-6-phosphate dehydrogenase deficiency.
2. **Nalidixic acid** is a quinolone that acts against many gram-negative organisms (not *Proteus* or *Pseudomonas* spp) by mechanisms that may involve acidification or inhibition of DNA gyrase. Resistance emerges rapidly. The drug is active orally and is excreted in the urine partly unchanged and partly as the inactive glucuronide. Toxic effects include gastrointestinal irritation, glycosuria, skin rashes, photosensitization, visual disturbances, and CNS stimulation.
3. **Methenamine** mandelate and hippurate combine acidification with the release of the antibacterial compound formaldehyde at pH levels below 5.5. They are not usually active against *Proteus* spp because of urinary alkalinization by these organisms. Insoluble complexes form between formaldehyde and sulfonamides, and the drugs should not be used together.
4. **Cycloserine** inhibits the incorporation of D-alanine into cell wall mucopeptides. It is active against coliforms, mycobacteria, and *Proteus* spp. Its clinical use is limited by serious toxicity, including headache, tremors, vertigo, convulsions, and psychotic reactions.

   ***Note:*** Many systemically active antimicrobial agents are effective in the treatment of urinary tract infections; these agents include penicillins, cephalosporins, sulfonamides, trimethoprim-sulfamethoxazole, and aminoglycosides.

## DRUG LIST

The following drugs are important members of the group discussed in this chapter. Prototype agents should be learned in detail; the major variants should be known well enough to list the factors that distinguish them from the prototypes and from each other.

| Subclass | Prototype | Major Variants |
|---|---|---|
| Macrolides | Erythromycin | Azithromycin |
| Lincosamines | Lincomycin | Clindamycin |
| Glycopeptides | Vancomycin | |
| Nitrofurans | Nitrofurantoin | |
| Fluoroquinolones | Ciprofloxacin | Norfloxacin |
| Quinolones | Nalidixic acid | Cinoxacin |
| Methenamine salts | Methenamine mandelate | Methenamine hippurate |
| Cycloserine | Cycloserine | |

## QUESTIONS

**DIRECTIONS (items 1–5):** Each numbered item or incomplete statement in this section is followed by answers or by completions of the statement. Select the ONE lettered answer or completion that is BEST in each case.

**1.** Each of the following statements about erythromycin is accurate EXCEPT:
**(A)** Children rarely develop cholestatic hepatitis with erythromycin estolate
**(B)** It is excreted mainly in the bile
**(C)** Resistance can occur through methylation of a receptor on 23S rRNA
**(D)** It is used for pneumococcal infections in penicillin-allergic patients
**(E)** It is active against methicillin-resistant staphylococci

**2.** Each of the following statements about the fluoroquinolones is accurate EXCEPT:
**(A)** They are often effective in the treatment of urogenital infections caused by multiresistant organisms
**(B)** Resistance may involve changes in the drug sensitivity of DNA gyrase
**(C)** They must be administered parenterally as a result of their low oral bioavailability
**(D)** They may enhance theophylline toxicity
**(E)** Modification of the dosage is required in renal insufficiency

**3.** All of the following statements about the lincosamines are accurate EXCEPT:
**(A)** Lincomycin and clindamycin are bacteriostatic inhibitors of protein synthesis
**(B)** They are active versus *S aureus* and common streptococci
**(C)** Lincomycin is effective in the treatment of infections caused by *B fragilis*
**(D)** They are excreted mainly in the bile
**(E)** Clindamycin use may lead to pseudomembranous colitis

**4.** Each of the following statements about vancomycin is accurate EXCEPT:
**(A)** It inhibits the synthesis of bacterial cell wall precursor molecules
**(B)** It does not achieve effective plasma levels after oral administration
**(C)** Rapid infusion may cause the "red man" syndrome
**(D)** Resistance emerges rapidly if it is given as a single agent
**(E)** It may be used for severe infections caused by resistant *S aureus*

**5.** Each of the following statements about metronidazole is accurate EXCEPT:
**(A)** Its activity includes a wide range of aerobic bacteria
**(B)** It is effective orally and penetrates into the CNS
**(C)** It may cause peripheral neuropathies
**(D)** Caution is advised during pregnancy because metronidazole has teratogenic potential
**(E)** It interacts with ethanol

**DIRECTIONS (items 6–10):** Items 6–10 consist of lettered headings followed by a set of numbered statements. For each numbered statement, select the ONE lettered heading that is most closely associated with it. Each lettered heading may be selected once, more than once, or not at all.

**(A)** Methenamine
**(B)** Erythromycin
**(C)** Nalidixic acid
**(D)** Vancomycin
**(E)** Nitrofurantoin

**6.** This drug has activity against gram-negative bacteria in urinary tract infections, but resistance may develop during the course of treatment. There is cross-resistance with cinoxacin. The drug should be used with caution in patients with seizure disorders.

**7.** A urinary antiseptic, this drug is not effective in the treatment of urinary tract infections due to *Proteus* spp. It releases formaldehyde, which may form an insoluble complex with sulfonamides.

**8.** Important clinical uses of this drug include the treatment of infections caused by *M pneumoniae,* chlamydiae, and gram-positive cocci.

**9.** This drug may be used to treat endocarditis caused by viridans streptococci in patients allergic to penicillins. In combination with an aminoglycoside, it is also effective in enterococcal endocarditis, but ototoxicity may occur.

**10.** Neuropathies are more likely to occur with this drug when it is used in patients with renal dysfunction. It may cause acute hemolysis in patients with glucose-6-phosphate dehydrogenase deficiency.

## ANSWERS

**1.** Methicillin-resistant staphylococci are also resistant to many commonly used antimicrobial drugs including erythromycin. For infections caused by such organisms vancomycin is the drug of choice. The answer is **(E).**

**2.** The fluoroquinolones are well absorbed following oral administration, achieving tissue levels effective in the treatment of infections caused by many aerobic gram-negative organisms. The answer is **(C).**

**3.** The antibacterial activity of lincomycin is essentially restricted to gram-positive cocci including penicillinase-producing staphylococci. It has minimal activity against anaerobes. However, clindamycin is active versus *B fragilis* and continues to be used for infections caused by strains of this organism. The answer is **(C).**

**4.** The occurrence of mutants that are resistant to vancomycin is very rare. The incidence of *S aureus* resistance has not risen appreciably since the drug was introduced over 30 years ago. The answer is **(D).**

**5.** In addition to its use as an antiprotozoal agent metronidazole is active against anaerobic cocci and bacilli. It has minimal activity against aerobes, because anoxic or hypoxic conditions are necessary for the formation of cytotoxic metabolites. The answer is **(A).**

**6.** Nalidixic acid, a quinolone, is structurally related to cinoxacin. Both drugs are used in the treatment of urinary tract infections, and cross-resistance may occur. Quinolone derivatives may lower the seizure threshold in susceptible individuals. The answer is **(C).**

7. Methenamine is a urinary antiseptic with antibacterial actions that are mainly due to release of formaldehyde at acidic pH. Sulfonamides may form complexes with formaldehyde, resulting in mutual antagonism. The answer is **(A).**

8. Too easy? Erythromycin is equivalent to tetracyclines in the treatment of most infections caused by *M pneumoniae* and chlamydiae. It is active against penicillinase-producing staphylococci and is an alternative drug for streptococcal infections in patients allergic to beta-lactam antibiotics. The answer is **(B).**

9. In addition to its important clinical use in staphylococcal infections, vancomycin is effective in bacterial endocarditis. It causes auditory impairment, which may be irreversible, and this occurs more frequently when vancomycin is administered with other ototoxic drugs. The answer is **(D).**

10. Acute hemolytic reactions in glucose-6-phosphate dehydrogenase deficiency occur with drugs that are oxidizing agents, including antimalarials, nalidixic acid, sulfonamides, and the furans. Severe polyneuropathies with both motor and sensory nerve degeneration may occur with nitrofurantoin. They are more likely to occur in patients with renal dysfunction. The answer is **(E).**

# Disinfectants & Antiseptics 51

## OBJECTIVES

**Define the following terms:**

- Antiseptic
- Disinfectant
- Sterilization
- Chlorine demand

**You should be able to:**

- Identify the compounds used as antiseptics and disinfectants.
- Describe the advantages and disadvantages of the most commonly used antiseptics and disinfectants.

## CONCEPTS

Although the terms are often used interchangeably, **disinfectant** usually denotes a compound used to kill microorganisms in an inanimate environment, whereas **antiseptic** refers to a compound that safely inhibits bacterial growth both in vitro and in vivo. Disinfectants and antiseptics do not have selective toxicity, and their clinical use is confined to topical application (with the exception of urinary antiseptics; see Chapter 50). Most antiseptics delay wound healing. **Sterilization** usually refers to procedures that kill microorganisms and spores on instruments and dressings; they include dry heat, autoclaving, and exposure to ethylene oxide.

A. **Alcohols, Aldehydes, & Acids: Ethanol** (70%) and **isopropanol** (70–90%) are effective skin antiseptics, since they precipitate microbial proteins. **Formaldehyde,** which also precipitates proteins, is too irritating for topical use but is a disinfectant for instruments. **Acetic acid** (0.25–1%) is used in surgical dressings and has activity against gram-negative bacteria when used as a urinary irrigant and in the external ear. **Salicylic acid** and **undecylenic acid** are useful antidermatophytes.

**B. Halogens: Iodine tincture** is an effective antiseptic for intact skin and is commonly used in preparing the skin before taking blood samples, although it can cause dermatitis. Iodine complexed with povidone (**povidone-iodine**) is widely used, particularly as a preoperative skin antiseptic, but solutions can become contaminated with gram-negative bacteria. **Hypochlorous acid,** formed when chlorine dissolves in water, is antimicrobial. This is the basis for the use of chlorine and halazone in water purification. Organic matter binds chlorine, thus preventing antimicrobial actions. In a given water sample, this process is referred to as the **"chlorine demand,"** since the chlorine-binding capacity of the organic material must be exceeded before bacterial killing is accomplished. Many preparations of chlorine for water purification do not eradicate all bacteria or *Entamoeba* cysts.

**C. Heavy Metals: Mercuric ions** precipitate proteins and inactivate sulfhydryl groups of enzymes. They are toxic if ingested but may be used as skin antiseptics. Organic mercurials such as **nitromersol** and **thimerosal** are more effective and less toxic than inorganic salts. **Merbromin** is a very weak antiseptic. **Silver** is a protein precipitant and inhibitor of microbial metabolism, but it can be irritating to tissues. Its uses, as the nitrate salt, include the prevention of neonatal gonococcal ophthalmia and the treatment of burns. **Silver sulfadiazine** (a sulfonamide) is also used to decrease bacterial colonization in burns.

**D. Chlorinated Phenols:** Phenol, the first substance to be used as an antiseptic, is irritating to tissues and is now used only as a disinfectant of inanimate objects. Chlorinated phenolic compounds are less irritating. **Hexachlorophene** is widely used in surgical scrub routines and in deodorant soaps. It forms antibacterial deposits on the skin if used routinely. It has also been used to protect against staphylococcal infections in neonates, but repeated use on the skin in infants can lead to absorption of hexachlorophene, which can cause CNS white matter degeneration. Antiseptic soaps may also contain other chlorinated phenols such as **triclocarban** and **chlorhexidine.** Although the latter compound is not very effective against *Pseudomonas* or *Serratia* strains, it is commonly used in hospital scrub routines or to disinfect skin sites preoperatively. All antiseptic soaps may cause allergies or photosensitization. **Lindane** (gamma benzene hexachloride) is used to treat infestations with mites or lice, and it is also an agricultural insecticide. It may be absorbed through the skin and cause toxic effects, including blood dyscrasias and convulsions, if excessive amounts are applied.

**E. Cationic Surfactants: Benzalkonium chloride** and **cetylpyridinium chloride** are used as antiseptics of skin and surgical instruments. Their antimicrobial action is antagonized by soaps. A serious disadvantage of their use is that certain gram-negative bacteria (eg, *Pseudomonas*) may not be eradicated. **Nitrofurazone** is an antimicrobial agent often used on skin lesions. Although it does not impair wound healing, it can cause allergic reactions. **Hydrogen peroxide** and **potassium permanganate** are oxidizing agents with limited uses.

## DRUG LIST

The following agents are important members of the group discussed in this chapter. Prototype agents should be learned in detail, and major variants should be identifiable.

| Subclass | Prototype | Major Variants |
|---|---|---|
| Alcohols, aldehydes, and acids | Ethanol, formaldehyde, acetic acid | Isopropanol, glutaraldehyde, salicylic acid |
| Halogens | Iodine, chlorine | Povidone-iodine, halazone |
| Heavy metals | Silver nitrate, mercury bichloride | Silver sulfadiazine, nitromersol, thimerosal |
| Chlorinated phenols | Hexachlorophene | Triclocarban, chlorhexidine |
| Cationic surfactants | Benzalkonium chloride | Cetylpyridinium chloride |

## QUESTIONS

**DIRECTIONS (items 1 and 2):** Each numbered item or incomplete statement in this section is followed by answers or by completions of the statement. Select the ONE lettered answer or completion that is BEST in each case.

**1.** All of the following statements about antiseptics and disinfectants are accurate EXCEPT:
**(A)** Povidone-iodine is an effective antibacterial agent, killing vegetative forms and clostridial spores
**(B)** Chlorhexidine disrupts bacterial cell membranes, especially those of gram-positive organisms
**(C)** Mercury interacts with sulfhydryl groups to inactivate microbial enzymes
**(D)** Benzalkonium chloride effectively eradicates *Pseudomonas* and other gram-negative bacteria when applied to the skin
**(E)** Dilute (0.25%) acetic acid is particularly active against aerobic gram-negative bacteria

**2.** All of the following statements about antiseptics and disinfectants are accurate EXCEPT:
**(A)** Most soaps are anionic surfactants that form strongly alkaline solutions in water
**(B)** "Chlorine demand" refers to the chlorine-binding capacity of a water sample
**(C)** Merbromin is an effective topical antiseptic that acts to promote wound healing
**(D)** Ninety percent isopropanol is an effective skin antiseptic
**(E)** Although too irritating for use on tissues, formaldehyde is widely employed as a disinfectant for instruments

**DIRECTIONS (items 3–7):** Items 3–7 consist of lettered headings followed by a set of numbered statements. For each numbered statement, select the ONE lettered heading that is most commonly associated with it. Each lettered heading may be selected once, more than once, or not at all.

**(A)** Hexachlorophene
**(B)** Silver nitrate
**(C)** Halazone
**(D)** Benzalkonium chloride
**(E)** Chlorhexidine

**3.** This compound is used in tablet form to purify drinking water but is not effective if a large quantity of organic material is present. It does not eradicate cysts of *Entamoeba histolytica.*

**4.** This agent can reduce infection of burn wounds and decrease the mortality rate in burn cases. It is irritating to tissues and can be reduced by bacterial enzymes to form a compound that causes methemoglobinemia.

**5.** Daily use of this agent results in a deposit on the skin that is bacteriostatic. The compound may be absorbed and has caused neurotoxic effects in neonates when used as an antistaphylococcal agent.

**6.** Incorporated into soaps, this agent is used as an antiseptic hand-washing preparation in surgical scrub procedures.

**7.** The antimicrobial actions of this antiseptic are antagonized by soaps.

## ANSWERS

**1.** Cationic surfactants cannot be used safely as skin antiseptics. Applied to the skin, they form a film under which microorganisms can survive. Infections due to *Pseudomonas* spp and other gram-negative organisms occur. The answer is **(D).**

2. No antiseptic in current use is able to promote wound healing. In fact, most agents do the opposite. In general, cleansing of abrasions and superficial wounds with soap and water is just as effective as, and less damaging than, the application of topical antiseptics. The staining of tissues that follows merbromin application looks "effective," but the compound has negligible antiseptic properties. The answer is **(C)**.

3. The addition of 4–8 mg of halazone/L will sterilize most water samples in about 30 minutes but will not kill cysts of *Entamoeba histolytica*. The answer is **(C)**.

4. Silver nitrate destroys many microorganisms upon contact and is used to prevent neonatal gonococcal ophthalmia and to reduce infections of burn wounds. Reduction of nitrate to nitrite by microorganisms may cause methemoglobinemia. The answer is **(B)**.

5. Repeated bathing of newborns with hexachlorophene to prevent staphylococcal colonization may permit systemic absorption, leading to neurotoxic effects, including spongiform degeneration of white matter. The answer is **(A)**.

6. Chlorhexidine is a bisdiguanide that disrupts bacterial cytoplasmic membranes, especially of gram-positive organisms. It is less effective against *Pseudomonas* and *Serratia* spp. Hospital uses include hand-washing procedures (incorporated in soap), wound cleansing, and preparation of skin sites for operative procedures. The answer is **(E)**.

7. Cationic surfactant agents, including benzalkonium and cetylpyridinium salts, are antagonized by anionic agents and are thus incompatible with soaps. The answer is **(D)**.

# 52 Clinical Use of Antimicrobials

## OBJECTIVES

**Define the following terms:**

- Antimicrobial chemoprophylaxis
- Antimicrobial synergism and antagonism
- Bacteriostatic, bactericidal
- Empiric (presumptive) therapy
- Minimum inhibitory concentration (MIC)
- Susceptibility testing

**You should be able to:**

- List the steps that should be taken prior to the initiation of empiric antimicrobial therapy.
- Describe the importance of susceptibility testing and analyses of serum drug levels, or bactericidal titers, in antimicrobial chemotherapy.
- Identify the antimicrobial drugs that require major modifications of dosage with changes in renal or hepatic function (or both) or with the use of dialysis.
- Describe the valid reasons for use of antimicrobial drugs in combination and the probable mechanisms involved in drug synergy.
- Describe the principles underlying valid antimicrobial chemoprophylaxis and give examples of surgical and nonsurgical prophylaxis.

## CONCEPTS

**A. Guidelines to Antimicrobial Therapy: Empiric antimicrobial therapy** is antimicrobial therapy begun before a specific pathogen has been identified. It is based on the presumption of an infection that requires immediate drug treatment. Prior to initiation of such therapy, accepted practice involves making a clinical diagnosis of microbial infection, obtaining specimens for laboratory analyses, making a microbiologic diagnosis, deciding whether treatment should precede the results of laboratory tests, and, finally, selecting the optimum drug or drugs. *The Medical Letter on Drugs and Therapeutics* publishes annually an updated list of antimicrobial drugs of choice for specific pathogens. This can provide a useful guide to empiric therapy based on presumptive microbiologic diagnosis.

**B. Principles of Antimicrobial Therapy:** Antimicrobial therapy in established infections is guided by the following principles:

1. **Susceptibility testing.** The results of susceptibility testing establish the drug sensitivity of the organism. These most commonly predict the **minimum inhibitory concentrations (MICs)** of a drug for comparison with anticipated blood or tissue levels.
2. **Blood drug concentration.** The measurement of drug concentration in the blood may be necessary for a number of reasons, including use of agents of low therapeutic index (eg, aminoglycosides) and investigation of poor clinical response to a drug treatment regimen.
3. **Serum bactericidal titers.** In certain microbial infections in which host defenses may contribute minimally to cure, the estimation of serum bactericidal titers can confirm the appropriateness of the choice of drug and dosage. Serial dilutions of serum are incubated with standardized quantities of the pathogen isolated from the patient, and killing at a dilution of 1:8 is generally considered satisfactory.
4. **Route of administration.** Parenteral therapy is preferred in most cases of serious microbial infections. Chloramphenicol, the fluoroquinolones, and trimethoprim-sulfamethoxazole may be effective orally.
5. **Monitoring of therapeutic response.** Therapeutic responses to drug therapy should be monitored clinically and microbiologically to detect the development of resistance or superinfections. With few exceptions, the duration of drug therapy is determined empirically.

**C. Clinical Failure of Antimicrobial Therapy:** Inadequate clinical or microbiologic response to antimicrobial therapy can result from multiple causes, including laboratory testing errors and problems with the drug (eg, incorrect choice, poor tissue penetration, inadequate dose), the patient (poor host defenses, undrained **abscesses**), and the pathogen (resistance, superinfection).

**D. Factors Influencing Antimicrobial Drug Use:**

1. **Status of drug elimination mechanisms.** Changes in hepatic and renal function, and the use of dialysis techniques, can influence the pharmacokinetics of antimicrobials and may necessitate dosage modifications. In patients with anuria, the elimination half-life of many drugs is increased; this is true of all penicillins, all cephalosporins (except cefoperazone), all aminoglycosides, all tetracyclines (except doxycycline), the fluoroquinolones, and trimethoprim-sulfamethoxazole. Erythromycin, clindamycin, chloramphenicol, rifampin, and the antifungal drugs (amphotericin B, griseofulvin, and ketoconazole) are notable exceptions, requiring no change in dosage in patients with renal failure. Dialysis, especially hemodialysis, may also have marked effects on the plasma levels of many antimicrobials, including ampicillin, most antipseudomonal penicillins, cephalosporins, and fluoroquinolones.
2. **Pregnancy and the newborn.** Antimicrobial therapy requires special consideration during pregnancy and the neonatal period. Tetracyclines cause tooth enamel dysplasia and inhibition of bone growth. The sulfonamides, trimethoprim, and metronidazole may exert fetal toxicity. Sulfonamides, by displacing bilirubin from serum albumin, may cause kernicterus in neonates. Chloramphenicol may cause the "gray baby" syndrome.
3. **Drug interactions.** Interactions sometimes occur between antimicrobials and other drugs. These include enhanced nephrotoxicity or ototoxicity when aminoglycosides are given with loop diuretics, vancomycin, or cisplatin. Several interactions with sulfonamides are based on competition for plasma protein binding, including hypoglycemia with sulfonylureas and increased hypoprothrombinemia with warfarin. Disulfiramlike reactions to ethanol with metronidazole and several newer cephalosporins can also occur. Many drug interactions have been

reported for rifampin, which decreases the effects of digoxin, ketoconazole, oral contraceptives, propranolol, quinidine, and warfarin by increasing their clearance by the liver.

**E. Antimicrobial Drug Combinations:** Therapy with multiple antimicrobials may be indicated in the following clinical situations:

1. In emergency situations (empiric therapy to provide greater coverage, eg, sepsis, meningitis).
2. To delay the emergence of resistance (isoniazid plus rifampin in tuberculosis).
3. To obtain synergistic effects (beta-lactam plus aminoglycoside in *Pseudomonas aeruginosa* infections; amphotericin B plus flucytosine in cryptococcal meningitis).
4. In mixed infections (eg, bacterial and fungal).

In terms of bactericidal actions, the outcomes of combined use of 2 antimicrobials may be **indifference** (additive effects); **synergism** (actions greater than simple addition of the 2 individual drug effects); or **antagonism** (actions less than those achievable by either of the 2 drugs used individually). Such actions are more readily demonstrated in vitro than at the clinical level. Mechanisms that may account for synergism include the following:

1. Sequential blockade of reactions in a metabolic pathway; eg, trimethoprim and sulfamethoxazole inhibit different steps in the formation of tetrahydrofolic acid.
2. Blockade of drug-inactivating enzymes; eg, clavulanic acid and sulbactam inhibit penicillinases that can inactivate penicillin G, ampicillin, and the antipseudomonal penicillins.
3. Enhanced uptake of drug, eg, that resulting from increased permeability to aminoglycosides after exposure of certain bacteria to cell wall-inhibiting antimicrobials such as the beta-lactams.

**F. Antimicrobial Chemoprophylaxis:** The general principles of antimicrobial chemoprophylaxis can be summarized as follows:

1. Direct the prophylaxis toward a *specific* pathogen.
2. Use a drug to which the pathogen does not become rapidly *resistant.*
3. Limit the *duration* of drug use.
4. Use conventional (therapeutic) *doses.*
5. Use only in situations of documented *efficacy.*

Situations in which nonsurgical antimicrobial prophylaxis is of benefit (or commonly used) include contacts in cases of meningococcal infections, gonorrhea, syphilis, and plague; prophylaxis against streptococcal infections in patients with rheumatic heart disease; animal or human bite wounds; and recurrent otitis media. Prophylaxis against postsurgical infections should embody the above principles, with drug selection based on the likely infecting organism and treatment initiated just prior to surgery and continued for no more than 48 hours. Ideally, the agent should be nontoxic and not essential for treatment of severe microbial infections. Situations in which surgical antimicrobial prophylaxis is of benefit (or commonly used) include gastrointestinal procedures, vaginal hysterectomy, cesarean section, joint replacement, open fracture surgery, and dental procedures in patients with valvular heart disease.

## QUESTIONS

**DIRECTIONS (items 1–9):** Each numbered item or incomplete statement in this section is followed by answers or by completions of the statement. Select the ONE lettered answer or completion that is BEST in each case.

**1.** Antimicrobial treatment of a severely neutropenic patient with fever and evidence of bacterial infection should not be initiated before
(A) the pathogen has been identified by the microbiology laboratory
(B) the results of a Gram stain are available
(C) specimens have been taken for laboratory tests and examinations
(D) antipyretic drugs have been given to lower the body temperature
(E) the results of antibacterial drug susceptibility tests are available

**2.** In the systemic use of aminoglycosides in the treatment of bacterial infections, monitoring of serum levels of such drugs is important because
**(A)** if administered orally they are unstable in gastric acid
**(B)** their antibacterial actions are antagonized by cephalosporins
**(C)** they have a narrow "therapeutic window"
**(D)** they do not readily penetrate into the cerebrospinal fluid
**(E)** they may cause aplastic anemia

**3.** Clearance of antimicrobial drugs from the body usually depends on renal function. However, the elimination half-lives of ONE pair of drugs listed below are not significantly altered in anuria (creatinine clearance of less than 5 mL/min).
**(A)** Trimethoprim, sulfamethoxazole
**(B)** Clindamycin, nafcillin
**(C)** Amikacin, gentamicin
**(D)** Cefazolin, cefoxitin
**(E)** Tetracycline, minocycline

**4.** All of the following drugs should be avoided (or used with extreme caution) in pregnancy because of possible teratogenic or toxic effects on the fetus, EXCEPT
**(A)** metronidazole
**(B)** demeclocycline
**(C)** cefazolin
**(D)** sulfisoxazole
**(E)** chloramphenicol

**5.** A relatively common drug interaction that occurs with the use of antimicrobial drugs, particularly those that have a wide antibacterial spectrum of activity, is
**(A)** antabuselike reactions when ethanol is ingested
**(B)** decreased efficacy of oral contraceptives
**(C)** enhancement of the anticoagulant effects of warfarin
**(D)** increased adverse effects if acetaminophen is administered as an antipyretic
**(E)** hypertension with ingestion of red wine and cheese

**6.** Examples of antimicrobial drug synergism, established at the clinical level, include all of the following EXCEPT
**(A)** enterococcal endocarditis (penicillin and vancomycin)
**(B)** cryptococcal meningitis (amphotericin B and flucytosine)
**(C)** pseudomonal urethritis (carbenicillin and gentamicin)
**(D)** bacterial meningitis (penicillin and tetracycline)
**(E)** recurrent urinary tract infections (trimethoprim and sulfamethoxazole)

**7.** Nonsurgical antimicrobial prophylaxis is of established benefit in all of the following situations EXCEPT
**(A)** contacts of index case in gonorrhea
**(B)** recurrent otitis media
**(C)** contacts of the index case in mycoplasmal pneumonia
**(D)** recurrent urinary tract infection
**(E)** tuberculin convertors

**8.** Established mechanisms of antimicrobial synergy include all of the following EXCEPT:
**(A)** Drug A induces enzymes that convert drug B to a more polar form
**(B)** Drugs A and B block successive steps in a bacterial metabolic pathway
**(C)** Drug A promotes the intrabacterial accumulation of drug B
**(D)** Drug A inhibits an enzyme that inactivates drug B

**9.** General principles of surgical antimicrobial prophylaxis include all of the following EXCEPT:
**(A)** It is indicated when the infection rate exceeds 5% under optimal conditions
**(B)** Drugs should be administered at least 24 hours prior to surgery
**(C)** It is justified in surgical procedures involving implantation of a foreign body
**(D)** Treatment should not be continued for more than 12–48 hours after surgery

## ANSWERS

1. To delay therapy until laboratory results are available is inappropriate in serious bacterial infections, but specimens for possible laboratory identification must be obtained before drugs are administered. The answer is **(C)**.

2. Monitoring plasma levels is important during systemic treatment with aminoglycosides because the drugs have a low therapeutic index. The "therapeutic window" for aminoglycosides is narrow, such that toxicity occurs when plasma levels are only 2–3 times higher than those needed for antibacterial action. Decreases in renal function may elevate the plasma concentrations of aminoglycosides to toxic levels within a few hours. The answer is **(C)**.

3. Almost all antimicrobial drugs require dose modification in renal failure. Notable exceptions are erythromycin, cefoperazone, clindamycin, doxycycline, isoniazid, ketoconazole, and nafcillin. These antimicrobial agents are eliminated via hepatic metabolism, or biliary excretion, depending on the individual drug. The answer is **(B)**.

4. Several groups of antimicrobial drugs are relatively safe in pregnancy, including penicillins, cephalosporins, erythromycin, and lincomycin. The answer is **(C)**.

5. Disturbance of the gut microbial flora often leads to decreased availability of vitamin K, with enhancement of the anticoagulant effects of coumarins. The answer is **(C)**. Can you name the drugs in the other drug interactions listed?

6. Combinations of antimicrobial drugs are not always synergistic. When synergy occurs at the clinical level, it is worth noting. In the treatment of bacterial meningitis 2 drugs may not be better than one. For example, the combination of penicillin and a tetracycline cures fewer patients with pneumococcal meningitis than does the same dose of penicillin used alone. Similarly, the combination of chloramphenicol and ampicillin may result in more treatment failures in baceterial meningitis than occur with ampicillin alone. The answer is **(D)**.

7. The efficacy of antimicrobial drug prophylaxis is good to excellent in all of the situations listed except that involving mycoplasmal pneumonia. Tetracycline has been administered to subjects exposed to the index case, but the effectiveness of such treatment has not been documented. The answer is **(C)**.

8. Increased activity of enzymes that make drugs more polar is likely to inactivate an antimicrobial drug and will not lead to synergy. Specific examples of mechanisms that do lead to synergy include **(B)** the combination of trimethoprim and sulfamethoxazole, **(C)** the combination of a penicillin and an aminoglycoside, and **(D)** the combination of clavulanic acid and amoxicillin. The answer is **(A)**.

9. Antimicrobial surgical prophylaxis should be initiated only 1 or 2 hours before surgery and continued for no longer than 48 hours. The answer is **(B)**.

# Basic Principles of Antiparasitic Chemotherapy

# 53

## OBJECTIVES

**Define the following terms:**

- Selective toxicity
- Sequential blockade
- Hydrogenosome
- Purine and pyrimidine salvage
- Salvage enzymes
- Suicide substrate
- Glycosome
- Microtubule

**You should be able to:**

- Describe the mechanisms of action of drugs whose targets are enzymes unique to parasites.
- Describe the mechanisms of action of drugs whose targets are enzymes indispensable to parasites.
- Describe the mechanisms of action of drugs whose targets are biochemical functions common to host and parasite cells.

## CONCEPTS

Rational approaches to antiparasite chemotherapy involve exploitation of **selective toxicity;** this involves taking advantage of biochemical and physiologic differences between parasite and host cells. The mechanisms of action of antiparasitic agents include enzyme targets that are unique to, or indispensable to, parasites; some agents also affect cellular functions common to both host and parasite cells.

### A. Mechanisms Involving Enzymes Unique to Parasites:

1. **Dihydropteroate synthetase.** Sporozoans (*Plasmodium, Toxoplasma,* and *Eimeria* spp) lack the ability to utilize exogenous folate and therefore possess enzymes for its synthesis; these enzymes can be inhibited by drugs. **Sulfonamides,** which are antimetabolites of PABA, inhibit dihydropteroate synthetase. Metachloridine, used in malaria, and 2-ethoxy-p-aminobenzoate, used in chicken parasitic disease, are other drugs that inhibit dihydropteroate synthesis. **Sequential blockade** can be achieved with a sulfonamide and an inhibitor of dihydrofolate reductase (eg, **pyrimethamine**), and such drug combinations are effective in malaria and toxoplasmosis.
2. **Pyruvate:ferredoxin oxidoreductase.** Certain anaerobic protozoans (*Trichomonas, Entamoeba* spp) lack mitochondria and possess a pyruvate:ferredoxin oxidoreductase of low redox potential that generates acetyl-CoA via electron transport. In trichomonal flagellates this enzyme is coupled to a hydrogenase in a membrane-limited organelle called a **hydrogenosome.** Under anaerobic conditions, electron transport results in the formation of hydrogen. The system also transfers electrons from pyruvate to the nitro groups of drugs that are 5-nitroimidazoles (eg, **metronidazole**), forming cytotoxic products that bind to proteins and DNA to inhibit parasite growth.
3. **Nucleoside phosphotransferases.** Protozoan parasites depend critically on purine salvage pathways because they are unable to synthesize purine nucleotides de novo. In *Leishmania* spp purine nucleoside phosphotransferase, a **salvage enzyme** that transfers phosphate groups to the 5′ position of purine nucleosides, also phosphorylates purine nucleoside analogues **(allopurinol riboside, formycin B, thiopurinol riboside).** The triphosphate derivatives of these drugs may be incorporated into nucleic acids or may inhibit enzymes in purine metabolism. Toxicity is low because mammalian cells lack this salvage enzyme. Trichomonads must salvage pyrimidine (as well as purines), since they lack dihydrofolate reductase and thymidylate synthase. They have only a single pathway to convert exogenous thymidine to thymidine

5′-phosphate by the action of a thymidine phosphotransferase. This enzyme can be selectively inhibited by antimetabolites (eg, **guanosine**).

4. **Trypanothione reductase.** In kinetoplastidans glutathione exists largely in the form of trypanothione, a unique conjugate with spermidine. Trypanothione, via the action of a specific reductase, plays a central role in maintaining the reduced state of intracellular thiols and is essential for survival of such parasites. **Nifurtimox** and certain trivalent arsenicals used as antitrypanosomal agents inhibit trypanothione reductase.

### B. Mechanisms Involving Enzymes Indispensable to Parasites:

1. **Purine phosphoribosyltransferases.** Hypoxanthine-guanine phosphoribosyltransferase (HGPRTase) is a key enzyme in purine synthesis in many parasites, including *Leishmania, Schistosoma,* and *Trypanosoma* spp. **Allopurinol** is a good substrate for this enzyme in certain parasites (but not for the mammalian enzyme), and the drug is metabolized to the ribotide, which, after phosphorylation, is incorporated into RNA forms that do not allow normal growth. Purine salvage in *Giardia* spp depends critically on the enzyme adenine and guanine phosphoribosyltransferase. Unlike mammalian forms of these enzymes, the parasitic enzymes do not utilize hypoxanthine, xanthine, or adenine as substrates and are thus amenable to inhibition by a designed inhibitor.
2. **Ornithine decarboxylase.** This enzyme, which controls the formation of the polyamine putrescine, appears to be more critical for growth of certain parasites than of mammalian cells. **Alpha-difluoromethylornithine (DFMO)** is a **suicide inhibitor** of ornithine decarboxylase and has antiparasitic activity against *Trypanosoma, Plasmodium,* and *Giardia* spp. DFMO transforms *Trypanosoma brucei* into a nondividing form that is eliminated by the host immune response.
3. **Glycolytic enzymes.** The bloodstream form of the African trypanosome *T brucei* is entirely dependent on glycolysis for generation of ATP. The enzymes involved are arranged in close proximity in membrane-bound organelles called glycosomes. Glycerol-3-phosphate oxidase is a key enzyme that can be inhibited by **salicylhydroxamic acid (SHAM),** bringing the parasite into an anaerobic state. The addition of glycerol inhibits the reversed glycerol kinase reaction, which stops glycolysis and results in death of the parasite. Biogenesis of glycosomes may also be a target for antiparasitic drugs. Suramin binds to glycolytic enzymes via its sulfonyl groups and may prevent their incorporation into the glycosome.

### C. Mechanisms Involving Biochemical Functions Common to Host and Parasite:

1. **Thiamine transporter.** Carbohydrate metabolism is the primary energy source in coccidia. Inhibition of the cellular transport of thiamine by the structurally similar agent **amprolium** leads to a deficiency of this cofactor in coccidia.
2. **Mitochondrial electron transporter.** Anticoccidial drugs that are **4-hydroxyquinolines** (eg, **buquinolate**) interact with unidentified components of the respiratory chain specific to *Eimeria* spp and inhibit electron transport in mitochondria. Mammalian mitochondrial respiration and that of other parasites is not inhibited by these drugs.
3. **Microtubules.** The microtubules of the cytoskeleton and mitotic spindle consist of tubulin polymers. These tubulins are heterogeneous between species. Structural features of alpha tubulins in helminths may account for the selective toxicity of benzimidazole drugs (eg, **mebendazole**). These agents bind to microtubules in helminths to block transport processes.
4. **Neurotransmission.** The antiparasitic effects of nicotinic agonist drugs (eg, **levamisole, pyrantel pamoate**) in nematodes is caused by stimulation of neuromuscular transmission, leading to muscle contraction. **Piperazine** acts as a GABA receptor agonist in nematodes, causing flaccid paralysis, and facilitation of the actions of GABA appears to underlie the actions of milbemycins and **avermectins.** These natural products do not cross the blood-brain barrier in mammalian hosts and are relatively nontoxic. **Praziquantel,** an antischistosomal and antitapeworm agent, stimulates $Ca^{2+}$ entry into the muscles of these parasites, inducing contraction.

# QUESTIONS

**DIRECTIONS (items 1–8):** Each numbered item or incomplete statement in this section is followed by answers or by completions of the statement. Select the ONE lettered answer or completion that is BEST in each case.

**1.** Certain anaerobic protozoan parasites lack mitochondria and generate energy-rich compounds, such as acetyl-CoA, by enzymes present in organelles called hydrogenosomes. An important enzyme involved is
**(A)** cytochrome P-450
**(B)** glycerol-3-phosphate oxidase
**(C)** pyruvate:ferredoxin oxidoreductase
**(D)** hypoxanthine-guanine phosphoribosyltransferase
**(E)** thymidylate synthase

**2.** This compound is a good substrate for hypoxanthine-guanine phosphoribosyltransferase in trypanosomes (but not mammals) and is eventually converted into metabolites that are incorporated into RNA.
**(A)** Alpha-difluoromethylornithine
**(B)** Salicylhydroxamic acid
**(C)** Allopurinol
**(D)** Mebendazole
**(E)** Glycerol

**3.** One chemotherapeutic strategy used to eradicate the bloodstream form of African trypanosomes is based on the absolute dependence of the organism on
**(A)** mitochondrial respiration
**(B)** cytochrome-dependent electron transfer
**(C)** lactate dehydrogenase
**(D)** glycolysis
**(E)** dihydropteroate synthesis

**4.** This drug enhances GABA actions on the neuromuscular junctions of nematodes and arthropods.
**(A)** Pyrantel pamoate
**(B)** Avermectin
**(C)** Picrotoxin
**(D)** Glutamic acid
**(E)** Thiamine

**5.** This antitrypanosomal drug is an antimetabolite that inhibits an enzyme important in the synthesis of the polyamine putrescine.
**(A)** Alpha-fluorodeoxyuridine
**(B)** Metronidazole
**(C)** Thiopurinol riboside
**(D)** Alpha-difluoromethylornithine (DFMO)
**(E)** Polymyxin

**6.** All of the following statements about the mechanisms of action of antiparasitic drugs are accurate EXCEPT:
**(A)** 4-Hydroxyquinolines inhibit phospholipase C
**(B)** Metronidazole is bioactivated to a cytotoxic product
**(C)** Salicylhydroxamic acid is an inhibitor of glycerol-3-phosphate oxidase
**(D)** Mebendazole binds to tubulins to change transport functions of microtubules

7. Enzymes unique to parasites include all of the following EXCEPT
   (A) trypanothione reductase
   (B) dihydropteridine pyrophosphokinase
   (C) hypoxanthine-guanine phosphoribosyltransferase
   (D) purine nucleoside phosphotransferase

8. All of the following statements about specific antiparasitic drugs are accurate EXCEPT:
   (A) Sulfadoxine is an inhibitor of dihydropteroate synthetase in the malarial parasite
   (B) Allopurinol riboside is a potent inhibitor of mitochondrial electron transfer
   (C) Amprolium is an inhibitor of thiamine transport in *Eimeria* spp
   (D) Suramin binds to glycolytic enzymes, preventing their incorporation into glycosomes

## ANSWERS

1. Certain anaerobic protozoan parasites lack mitochondria and possess ferredoxinlike electron transport proteins to convert pyruvate to acetyl-CoA. In *Trichomonas vaginalis* this process takes place in the hydrogenosome, a membrane-limited organelle, via the actions of pyruvate:ferredoxin oxidoreductase. The answer is **(C)**.

2. Allopurinol is a good substrate for HGPRTase in trypanosomes but not mammals. Recall that it is also an inhibitor of xanthine oxidase, used in gout and as an adjunct in cancer chemotherapy. The answer is **(C)**.

3. African trypanosomes lack mitochondrial cytochromes and functional Krebs cycle enzymes and are entirely dependent on glycolysis for ATP production. Glycolytic enzyme inhibitors, such as SHAM, which inhibits glycerol-3-phosphate oxidase, may be selectively toxic to such parasites. The answer is **(D)**.

4. Several antiparasitic drugs, including piperazine, milbemycins, and avermectins, enhance GABA neurotransmission in nematodes and arthropods, leading to muscle paralysis. The answer is **(B)**.

5. DFMO is a suicidal inhibitor of ornithine decarboxylase. Although it also inhibits mammalian ornithine decarboxylase, it is less toxic to the host because of more rapid turnover and replacement of the irreversibly inhibited enzyme in the host than in parasites. The answer is **(D)**.

6. The anticoccidial 4-aminoquinolones inhibit mitochondrial respiration in *Eimeria* spp, probably through interaction with a component between NADH oxidase and cytochrome b in the electron transport chain. The answer is **(A)**.

7. HGPRTase, an enzyme involved in purine salvage, is present in parasite and mammalian species. However, the enzyme is more important in protozoans and trematodes because of the absence of *de novo* purine nucleotide synthesis. The answer is **(C)**.

8. *Leishmania* species possess the unique salvage enzyme purine nucleoside phosphotransferase. This enzyme phosphorylates allopurinol riboside to form the corresponding nucleotide, which interferes with purine and nucleic acid metabolism. The answer is **(B)**.

# Antiprotozoal Drugs

# 54

## OBJECTIVES

**Define the following terms:**

- Amebicide
- Schizonticide
- Hypnozoite
- Gametocide
- Sporonticide
- Antifol

**You should be able to:**

- List the major groups of antiprotozoal drugs.
- Describe the main pharmacodynamic and pharmacokinetic properties of the antimalarial drugs (chloroquine, quinine, primaquine, and the antifolate agents).
- Describe the main pharmacodynamic and pharmacokinetic properties of the amebicides (diloxanide, emetine, iodoquinol, and metronidazole). List other clinical applications of nitroimidazoles.
- Identify the main trypanosomicidal drugs and list their toxic effects.

## CONCEPTS

### DRUGS FOR MALARIA

Malaria parasites have a complex life cycle that permits drug action at several different points. *Plasmodium* species that infect humans *(P falciparum, P malariae, P ovale, P vivax)* are spread by the female *Anopheles* mosquito and, after inoculation into the human host, undergo a primary developmental stage in the liver (primary tissue phase). They then enter the blood and parasitize erythrocytes (erythrocytic phase). *P falciparum* and *P malariae* have only one cycle of liver cell invasion, and thereafter, multiplication is confined to erythrocytes. The other species have a dormant hepatic stage (in which they become **hypnozoites**) that is responsible for recurrent infections and relapses after apparent recovery from initial infection.

Primary tissue **schizonticides** (eg, primaquine) kill schizonts in the liver soon after infection, whereas blood schizonticides (eg, chloroquine, quinine) kill these parasitic forms only in the erythrocyte. Antimalarial drugs may exert multiple actions. Primaquine is **gametocidal,** since it kills gametes in the blood; it also destroys the secondary exoerythrocytic (liver) schizonts that cause the relapsing fevers of malaria. **Sporonticides** (proguanil, pyrimethamine) prevent sporogony and multiplication in the mosquito.

#### A. Chloroquine:

1. **Mechanism of action.** This drug is a 4-aminoquinoline derivative. It forms a complex with hemin that has deleterious effects on cellular membranes. Because it is a weak base, it may also act to buffer the cellular pH, decreasing cellular invasion by parasitic organisms. Its selective toxicity is due to an energy-dependent carrier mechanism in parasitized cells. Resistance occurs in *P falciparum* because of decreased drug accumulation.
2. **Clinical use.** Chloroquine is used for acute attacks of malaria and as a chemosuppressant, except in regions where *P falciparum* is resistant. It is solely a blood schizonticide and will not eradicate secondary tissue schizonts. Chloroquine is also used in amebic liver disease and in autoimmune disorders.
3. **Pharmacokinetics.** Chloroquine is rapidly absorbed when given orally, widely distributed to tissues, and has a large volume of distribution. It is excreted largely unchanged in the urine.
4. **Toxicity.** At low doses, toxic effects include gastrointestinal irritation, skin rashes, and headaches. High doses may cause severe skin lesions, peripheral neuropathies, myocardial depression, retinal damage, auditory impairment, and toxic psychosis. Chloroquine may precipitate porphyria attacks.

**B. Quinine & Mefloquine:**

1. **Mechanism of action.** Quinine complexes with double-stranded DNA to prevent strand separation, resulting in block of DNA replication and transcription to RNA. The mechanism of action of mefloquine, a synthetic agent similar to quinine, is unknown but does not appear to involve binding to DNA. Quinine and mefloquine are blood schizonticides and have no effect on liver stages of the malaria parasite.
2. **Clinical use.** The main use of these drugs is in *P falciparum* infections resistant to chloroquine. To delay the emergence of resistance, the drugs should not be used routinely for prophylaxis.
3. **Pharmacokinetics.** Quinine is rapidly absorbed orally and is metabolized before renal excretion. It may be given intravenously in severe infections. Mefloquine can be given only orally (variable absorption) because of local reactions. It binds to plasma and tissue proteins and has a long plasma half-life (>6 days).
4. **Toxicity.** Quinine commonly causes **cinchonism,** whose symptoms include gastrointestinal distress, headache, vertigo, blurred vision, tinnitus, and, when severe, disturbances in cardiac conduction. Hematotoxic effects occur, including hemolysis in glucose-6-phosphate dehydrogenase-deficient patients. **Blackwater fever** (intravascular hemolysis) is a rare and possibly fatal complication in quinine-sensitized persons. Mefloquine is less toxic than quinine; its adverse effects include gastrointestinal distress, skin rashes, headache, and dizziness. At high doses it may cause neurologic symptoms and seizures.

**C. Primaquine:**

1. **Mechanism of action.** Primaquine is an 8-aminoquinoline that forms quinoline-quinone metabolites, which are electron-transferring redox compounds that act as cellular oxidants. The drug is a tissue schizonticide and also limits malaria transmission by acting as a gametocide.
2. **Clinical use.** Primaquine is not effective in acute attacks but is used to eradicate liver stages of *P vivax* and *P ovale*. It should be used in conjunction with a blood schizonticide.
3. **Pharmacokinetics.** Absorption is complete after oral administration and is followed by extensive metabolism, involving demethylation and oxidation.
4. **Toxicity.** Primaquine is usually well tolerated but may cause gastrointestinal distress, pruritus, headaches, and methemoglobinemia. More serious toxicity involves hemolysis in glucose-6-phosphate dehydrogenase-deficient patients; this is thought to be a result of the formation of redox intermediates.

**D. Antifolate Drugs (Antifols):**

1. **Mechanism of action.** Sulfonamides, acting as antimetabolites of PABA, block folic acid synthesis in certain protozoans by inhibiting dihydropteroate synthetase. Pyrimethamine and proguanil (chloroguanide), which is bioactivated to cycloguanil, are selective inhibitors of protozoan dihydrofolate reductases, preventing the formation of tetrahydrofolate. The combination of pyrimethamine with sulfadoxine may have synergistic antimalarial effects through the **sequential blockade** of 2 steps in folic acid synthesis. Other combinations include sulfadiazine or dapsone with pyrimethamine.
2. **Clinical use.** The antifols are blood schizonticides that act mainly against *P falciparum* and are used in the prophylaxis and treatment of 4-aminoquinoline-resistant forms of this species, although the onset of activity is slow. Many strains of *P falciparum* are now resistant to antifols.
3. **Pharmacokinetics.** All antifols are effective orally and are excreted in the urine in partly unchanged form. Proguanil has a shorter half-life than do the other drugs in this subclass. Sulfonamides share plasma protein sites with many drugs and may be responsible for drug interactions.
4. **Toxicity.** The toxic effects of sulfonamides include skin rashes, gastrointestinal distress, hemolysis, and kidney damage. Pyrimethamine may cause folic acid deficiency when used in high doses.

## DRUGS FOR AMEBIASIS

**Tissue amebicides** (chloroquine, emetines, metronidazole) act on organisms in the bowel wall and the liver; **luminal amebicides** (diloxanide furoate, iodoquinol, paromomycin) act only in the lumen of the bowel. The choice of a drug depends on the form of amebiasis. For asymptomatic disease, diloxanide furoate is the choice. For mild to severe intestinal infection, metronidazole is used with diloxanide furoate or iodoquinol. The latter regimen, plus chloroquine, is recommended in liver abscess. The mechanisms of amebicidal action of many drugs in this subclass are unknown.

**A. Diloxanide Furoate:** This drug is used extensively for intestinal amebiasis outside the USA. It is converted in the gut to the diloxanide free-base form, which is the active amebicide. Toxic effects are mild and are usually restricted to gastrointestinal symptoms.

**B. Emetines:** Emetine and dehydroemetine inhibit protein synthesis by blocking ribosomal movement along RNA. These alkaloids are used as back-up drugs for treatment of severe intestinal or hepatic amebiasis in hospitalized patients. They are given parenterally, widely distributed to tissues, and excreted slowly by the kidneys. The drugs have limited selective toxicity and cause severe adverse effects, including gastrointestinal distress, muscle weakness, and cardiovascular dysfunction (tachycardia and congestive heart failure).

**C. Iodoquinol:** Iodoquinol is a halogenated hydroxyquinoline drug with an unknown mechanism of action. It is an orally active luminal amebicide that is used as an alternative drug for mild to severe intestinal infections. Adverse gastrointestinal effects are common but usually mild. Systemic absorption after high doses may lead to thyroid enlargement and neurotoxic effects, including peripheral neuropathy and visual dysfunction.

**D. Metronidazole:**

1. **Mechanism of action.** This nitroimidazole drug undergoes a reductive bioactivation of its nitro group by ferredoxin (present in anaerobic parasites) to form reactive cytotoxic products.
2. **Clinical use.** Metronidazole is the drug of choice in severe intestinal wall disease and in hepatic abscess and other extraintestinal amebic disease. It is always used with a luminal amebicide. Other important clinical uses of metronidazole include treatment of trichomoniasis *(Trichomonas vaginalis,)* giardiasis, and infections caused by *Gardnerella vaginalis* and anaerobic bacteria.
3. **Pharmacokinetics.** The drug is effective orally and is distributed widely to tissues. Its elimination involves hepatic metabolism.
4. **Toxicity.** Adverse effects include gastrointestinal irritation, headache, and discoloration of urine. More serious toxicity includes leukopenia, dizziness, and ataxia. Drug interactions with metronidazole include a disulfiramlike reaction with ethanol and potentiation of coumarin anticoagulant effects. Because of its possible teratogenicity, the drug should be avoided by pregnant women and nursing mothers.

**E. Paromomycin:** This is an aminoglycoside antibiotic used as a back-up luminal amebicide. Adverse gastrointestinal effects are common, and systemic absorption may lead to headaches, dizziness, rashes, and arthralgia. Tetracyclines (eg, doxycycline) are sometimes used with a luminal amebicide in mild intestinal disease.

## DRUGS FOR TRYPANOSOMIASIS

**A. Pentamidine:**

1. **Mechanism of action.** The precise mechanism of action is unknown but may involve inhibition of glycolysis and possibly interference with nucleic acid metabolism of trypanosomes. Preferential accumulation of the drug by the parasite may account for its selective toxicity.
2. **Clinical use.** It is commonly used in the hemolymphatic stages of disease caused by the trypanosomes *T gambiense* and *T rhodesiense*. Because it does not cross the blood-brain barrier, it is not used in later stages of trypanosomiasis. Other clinical uses include the prophylaxis and therapy of *Pneumocystis carinii* infections (eg, in AIDS patients) and treatment of the kala azar form of leishmaniasis.
3. **Pharmacokinetics.** The drug is administered parenterally and is strongly bound to tissues. It has a long half-life (2–4 weeks) and is excreted unchanged in the urine.
4. **Toxicity.** Adverse effects include respiratory stimulation followed by depression, hypoten-

sion due to peripheral vasodilation, nephrotoxicity, and pancreatic B cell dysfunction. Systemic toxicity in AIDS patients is reduced by aerosol inhalation.

**B. Other Trypanosomicidal Agents:**

1. **Melarsoprol** is an organic arsenical that inhibits enzyme sulfhydryl groups. Because it enters the CNS, it is the drug of choice in African sleeping sickness. It is given parenterally because it causes gastrointestinal irritation; it has caused a reactive encephalopathy that may be fatal.
2. **Nifurtimox** is a nitrofurazone derivative that inhibits the unique enzyme trypanothione reductase. It is the drug of choice in American trypanosomiasis and has also been effective in mucocutaneous leishmaniasis. It causes severe toxicity, including allergies, gastrointestinal irritation, and CNS effects.
3. **Suramin** is a polyanionic drug that has been used for early stages of African trypanosomiasis (before CNS involvement). It is used parenterally and causes skin rashes, gastrointestinal distress, and neurologic complications.

## DRUGS FOR LEISHMANIASIS

The leishmaniae, parasitic protozoa transmitted by flesh-eating flies, cause various diseases ranging from cutaneous or mucocutaneous lesions to splenic and hepatic enlargement with fever. **Sodium stibogluconate** (pentavalent antimony) is the primary drug in all forms of the disease and appears to kill the parasite by inhibition of glycolysis or effects on nucleic acid metabolism. Back-up agents include pentamidine (for visceral leishmaniasis), metronidazole (for cutaneous lesions), and amphotericin B (for mucocutaneous leishmaniasis).

# DRUG LIST

The following drugs are important members of the group discussed in this chapter. Prototype agents should be learned in detail; the major variants and other significant agents should be identifiable.

| Subclass | Prototype | Major Variants | Other Significant Agents |
|---|---|---|---|
| Drugs for malaria<br>Alkaloids | Quinine | Mefloquine | |
| Aminoquinolines | Chloroquine | Amodiaquine | Primaquine |
| Acridines | Quinacrine | | |
| Antifolates | Chloroguanide | | Pyrimethamine |
| Drugs for amebiasis<br>Alkaloids | Emetine | Dehydroemetine | |
| Dichloroacetamides | Diloxanide furoate | | |
| Hydroxyquinolines | Iodoquinol | Clioquinol | |
| Nitroimidazoles | Metronidazole | Tinidazole | |
| Antibiotics | Paromomycin | | Tetracyclines |
| Drugs for leishmaniasis<br>Pentavalent antimony | Sodium stibogluconate | | Metronidazole, allopurinol, amphotericin B, nifurtimox |
| Drugs for trypanosomiasis<br>Aromatic diamidines | Pentamidine | Stilbamidine, propamidine | |
| Organic arsenicals | Melarsoprol | | Nifurtimox, suramin |
| Drugs for trichomoniasis and giardiasis<br>Nitroimidazoles | Metronidazole | Tinidazole | |

## QUESTIONS

**DIRECTIONS (items 1–10):** Each numbered item or incomplete statement in this section is followed by answers or by completions of the statement. Select the ONE lettered answer or completion that is BEST in each case.

**1.** All of the following statements about antimalarial drugs are accurate EXCEPT:
**(A)** Chloroquine is a blood schizonticide but does not affect secondary tissue schizonts
**(B)** Proguanil is converted to a reactive metabolite that is sporonticidal
**(C)** Primaquine acts primarily on exoerythrocytic stages of the malarial life cycle
**(D)** Mefloquine destroys secondary exoerythrocytic schizonts

**2.** This antimalarial drug causes a dose-dependent toxic state that includes a flushed and sweaty skin, dizziness, nausea, diarrhea, tinnitus, blurred vision, and impaired hearing.
**(A)** Amodiaquine
**(B)** Primaquine
**(C)** Quinine
**(D)** Pyrimethamine

**3.** Plasmodial resistance to chloroquine is due to
**(A)** induction of inactivating enzymes
**(B)** change in receptor structure
**(C)** increase in the activity of DNA repair mechanisms
**(D)** decreased carrier-mediated drug transport

**4.** The antimalarial drug to avoid in G6PDH deficiency is
**(A)** proguanil
**(B)** primaquine
**(C)** chloroquine
**(D)** mefloquine

**5.** All of the following statements about amebicides are accurate EXCEPT:
**(A)** Paromomycin is effective in extraintestinal amebiasis
**(B)** Diloxanide furoate is a luminal amebicide
**(C)** Metronidazole has little activity in the gut lumen
**(D)** Systemic use of iodoquinol may cause thyroid enlargement and peripheral neuropathy

**6.** Which of the following toxic effects is characteristic of emetine?
**(A)** Acute hemolytic anemia
**(B)** Methemoglobinemia
**(C)** Myelo-optic neuropathy
**(D)** Atrial and ventricular arrhythmias

**7.** This drug can clear trypanosomes from the blood and lymph nodes and is active in the late CNS stages of African sleeping sickness.
**(A)** Pyrimethamine
**(B)** Melarsoprol
**(C)** Pentamidine
**(D)** Metronidazole

**8.** This drug is bioactivated to cytotoxic products by pyruvate:ferredoxin oxidoreductases in anaerobic organisms, including bacteria and protozoa. Its clinical uses include the treatment of amebiasis, trichomoniasis, giardiasis, and infections caused by anaerobic bacteria.
**(A)** Emetine
**(B)** Iodoquinol
**(C)** Metronidazole
**(D)** Diloxanide furoate

9. All of the following statements about antiprotozoal drugs are accurate EXCEPT:
   (A) Nifurtimox is selectively toxic to some protozoans because it inhibits trypanothione reductase
   (B) Pyrimethamine is synergistic with sulfadoxine against malarial parasites ("sequential blockade")
   (C) Blackwater fever occurs in patients sensitized to chloroquine
   (D) Intravenous injection of pentamidine produces a sharp fall in blood pressure only partially blocked by atropine

10. All of the following statements concerning adverse effects of antiprotozoal drugs are correct EXCEPT:
   (A) Metronidazole may have a disulfiramlike effect with ethanol
   (B) Irreversible retinopathy and ototoxicity are possible adverse effects of long-term use of chloroquine
   (C) Toxic effects on pancreatic B cells have been associated with pentamidine use
   (D) Parenteral sodium stibogluconate may cause fatal reactive encephalopathy

## ANSWERS

1. Mefloquine has many properties similar to those of quinine. Both drugs are effective blood schizonticides. They have minimal effect on the secondary exoerythrocytic (liver) schizonts that cause the relapsing fevers of malaria. The answer is **(D)**.

2. These dose-related symptoms are characteristic adverse effects of cinchona alkaloids (quinine, quinidine). The early signs are tinnitus, headache, nausea, and disturbed vision. Gastrointestinal distress, rashes, angioedema, hypotension, and CNS dysfunction occur in more severe forms of cinchonism. The answer is **(C)**.

3. The selective toxicity of chloroquine depends on its intracellular accumulation in plasmodia. This is effected by a carrier-mediated transport system in the cellular membrane of the organism. Concentrations of chloroquine in parasite-infected erythrocytes may be 25 times those in normal red blood cells! Resistance occurs through decreases in the activity of this transport system. The answer is **(D)**.

4. Too easy? Primaquine is the prototype of drugs that induce hemolysis in persons deficient in glucose-6-phosphate dehydrogenase. The answer is **(B)**.

5. Paromomycin is an aminoglycoside antibiotic used as a back-up drug in the treatment of amebiasis. It acts only on organisms in the lumen of the bowel. You may recall that because they are highly polar compounds, the aminoglycosides are not absorbed into the systemic circulation when used orally. The answer is **(A)**.

6. Used in the treatment of severe amebiasis, emetine should be administered only to closely monitored hospitalized patients. The drug has limited selective toxicity and causes severe side effects including congestive heart failure, hypertension, and cardiac arrhythmias. The answer is **(D)**.

7. Melarsoprol and pentamidine are both used in the treatment of trypanosomiasis. Melarsoprol is the drug of choice in African sleeping sickness because, unlike pentamidine, it effectively enters the CNS. The answer is **(B)**.

8. Of the drugs listed, only metronidazole has both antiprotozoal activity and clinically useful activity in bacterial infections. The answer is **(C)**.

9. Massive intravascular hemolysis (blackwater fever) is now a rare complication of the treatment

of malaria with quinine. It does not occur in the few patients who may be sensitive to chloroquine. The answer is **(C)**.

**10.** Sodium stibogluconate is a pentavalent antimonial, the drug of choice in leishmaniasis. It is painful on injection and causes gastrointestinal distress, myalgia, and arthralgia, but is not neurotoxic. Reactive encephalopathy is associated with use of the trypanosomicidal drug melarsoprol. The answer is **(D)**.

# Clinical Pharmacology of the Anthelmintic Drugs 55

## OBJECTIVES

**You should be able to:**

- Identify the drugs of choice for treatment of common infections caused by nematodes, trematodes, and cestodes.
- Describe the mechanisms of action (if known), important pharmacokinetic features, and major toxic effects of these drugs.
- Describe the main features of important back-up anthelmintics.

## CONCEPTS

This chapter describes the pharmacology of many anthelmintic drugs that have diverse chemical structures, mechanisms of action, and properties. Most were discovered by empiric screening methods; many act against specific parasites; and few are devoid of significant toxicity to host cells.

### DRUGS THAT ACT AGAINST NEMATODES (ROUNDWORMS)

**A. Mebendazole:** The mechanism of action of this benzimidazole is inhibition of microtubule synthesis. It is the drug of choice for pinworm and whipworm infections, for combined infections with ascarids and hookworm, and for treatment of hydatid disease. It is also a back-up drug in specific cestode and trematode infections. Less than 10% of the drug is absorbed systemically after oral use, and this portion is metabolized rapidly. The drug has a high therapeutic index, and its toxic effects are limited to gastrointestinal irritation. It is contraindicated in pregnancy because of possible embryotoxicity.

**B. Thiabendazole:** A structural congener of mebendazole, this agent has a similar mechanism of action on microtubules. It is the drug of choice for treatment of threadworm infections, trichinosis, and cutaneous and visceral forms of larva migrans. Thiabendazole is rapidly absorbed from the gut and is metabolized by liver enzymes. The drug has anti-inflammatory and immunorestorative actions on the host. Toxic effects include gastrointestinal irritation, headache, dizziness, leukopenia, hematuria, and allergic reactions, including intrahepatic cholestasis. Reactions caused by dying parasites include fever, chills, lymphadenopathy, and skin rashes.

**C. Diethylcarbamazine:** This piperazine derivative has an unknown mechanism of action. It is the drug of choice for filariasis and an alternative drug for onchocerciasis (in combination with suramin). Microfilariae are killed more readily than adult worms. The drug is rapidly absorbed from the gut and is excreted partly unchanged in the urine. Toxic effects include headache, malaise, weakness, and anorexia. Reactions to proteins released by dying filariae include fever, rashes, ocular damage, joint and muscle pain, and lymphangitis. In onchocerciasis, the **Mazzotti reaction** includes most of these symptoms as well as hypotension, pyrexia, respiratory distress, and prostration.

**D. Ivermectin:** This drug is a macrocyclic lactone. It intensifies GABA-mediated neurotransmission in nematodes and causes immobilization of parasites, facilitating their removal by the reticuloendothelial system. Selective toxicity results because GABA is a neurotransmitter in humans only in the CNS and ivermectin does not cross the blood-brain barrier. Ivermectin is the drug of choice for onchocerciasis, acting more slowly than diethylcarbamazine and causing fewer systemic and ocular reactions. Other potential uses include treatment of filariasis and strongyloidiasis. Single-dose oral treatment in onchocerciasis results in multiple reactions, including fever, headache, dizziness, rashes, pruritus, tachycardia, hypotension, and pain in joints, muscles, and lymph glands. Such symptoms are usually of short duration, and most can be controlled with antihistamines and nonsteroidal anti-inflammatory drugs (NSAIDs).

**E. Pyrantel Pamoate:** A tetrahydropyrimidine derivative, this agent and its congener, **oxantel pamoate,** cause neuromuscular blockade by interaction with nicotinic receptors, and this blockade leads to paralysis of parasites. Pyrantel pamoate is the drug of choice in *Ascaris* infections and is equivalent to mebendazole for hookworm and *Trichostrongylus* infections. Both drugs are poorly absorbed from the gut when given orally. Toxic effects are minor but include gastrointestinal distress, headache, and weakness.

**F. Levamisole:** This agent causes a depolarizing neuromuscular blockade by stimulating nicotinic receptors. It is the drug of choice for infections caused by *Angiostrongylus cantonensis* and an alternative agent in *Ascaris* and hookworm diseases. The drug affects host defenses by promoting cell-mediated immune responses, including macrophage and T cell functions. Toxic effects are limited to gastrointestinal irritation.

**G. Albendazole:** The mechanism of action of albendazole is unclear. The drug blocks glucose uptake in both larval and adult parasites, which leads to decreased formation of ATP and subsequent parasite immobilization. Its actions may also include inhibition of microtubule assembly, as has been described for other benzimidazoles. Albendazole has a wide anthelmintic spectrum and is an important alternative drug for hookworm and pinworm infections and for the treatment of ascariasis, strongyloidiasis, trichuriasis, and hydatid diseases. The drug is effective orally and is metabolized by the liver mainly to the sulfoxide, which is excreted in the urine. Toxic effects during short courses of therapy are minimal. Reversible leukopenia, alopecia, and changes in liver enzymes may occur with prolonged use. Long-term animal toxicity studies report bone marrow suppression and fetal toxicity.

## DRUGS THAT ACT AGAINST TREMATODES (FLUKES)

**A. Praziquantel:** This drug is an isoquinoline-pyrazine derivative that increases membrane permeability to calcium. This action causes contraction and paralysis of trematode muscles, followed by vacuolization and parasite death. Praziquantel is the drug of choice for schistosomiasis (as caused by all species), for infections due to *Paragonimus westermani,* and for specific tapeworm infections (cysticercosis, that caused by *Hymenolepis nana*). It is active against immature and adult schistosomal forms. Absorption from the gut is rapid, and the drug is metabolized to inactive products. Common adverse effects include headache, dizziness, malaise, and, less frequently, gastrointestinal irritation, skin rashes, and fever. Increased rates of abortion with praziquantel therapy preclude its use in pregnancy.

**B. Bithionol:** Although little information is available on its efficacy, bithionol is regarded as the drug of choice in infections due to *Fasciola hepatica* and is an alternative drug for paragonimiasis. Its mechanism of action is unknown. Toxic effects, which occur in up to 40% of patients, include gastrointestinal irritation, dizziness, headache, tinnitus, pruritus, skin rashes, and leukopenia.

**C. Alternative Agents:**

1. **Metrifonate** acts solely against *Schistosoma haematobium mansoni* (the agent of bilharziasis). It is an organophosphate pro-drug that forms the cholinesterase inhibitor dichlorvos. Toxic effects occur because of excess cholinergic stimulation.
2. **Oxamniquine** is effective solely in *Schistosoma mansoni* infections, acting on male immature forms and adult schistosomal forms. Dizziness is a common adverse effect; headache, gastrointestinal irritation, and pruritus may also occur. Reactions to dying parasites include eosinophilia, urticaria, and pulmonary infiltrates.
3. **Niridazole** is an alternative drug for schistosomiasis. It concentrates in adult worms and causes glycogen depletion. Its actions on the host include immunosuppression and anti-inflammatory effects. Toxic effects may be severe and can include gastrointestinal irritation, dizziness, fatigue, arthralgia, eosinophilia, pulmonary infiltration, and hemolysis in cases of glucose-6-phosphate dehydrogenase deficiency. Neuropsychiatric symptoms may occur. Spermatogenesis is inhibited, and the agent is both mutagenic and carcinogenic.

## DRUGS THAT ACT AGAINST CESTODES (TAPEWORMS)

**A. Niclosamide:** This is the most important drug in the subclass that acts against cestodes. It is a salicylamide derivative that may act by uncoupling oxidative phosphorylation or by activating ATPases. It is the drug of choice for all tapeworm infections except cysticercosis (for which praziquantel is used) and those caused by *Echinococcus granulosus* (for which mebendazole is used). Scoleces and cestode segments are killed, but ova are not. The drug is minimally absorbed from the gut. Its toxic effects are mild and include gastrointestinal distress, headache, rashes, and fever, which may result from systemic absorption of antigens from disintegrating parasites.

## DRUG LIST

Drugs of choice and alternative (back-up) agents for selected important helminthic infections are listed.

| Infecting Organism | Drug of Choice | Alternative Drugs |
|---|---|---|
| Nematodes | | |
| *Ascaris lumbricoides* (roundworm) | Pyrantel pamoate | Levamisole, mebendazole |
| *Necator americanus* *Ancylostoma duodenale* (hookworm) | Pyrantel pamoate, mebendazole | Albendazole, levamisole |
| *Trichuris trichiura* (whipworm) | Mebendazole | Albendazole, pyrantel pamoate |
| *Strongyloides stercoralis* (threadworm) | Thiabendazole | Albendazole, mebendazole |
| *Enterobius vermicularis* (pinworm) | Mebendazole, pyrantel pamoate | Albendazole |
| Larva migrans | Thiabendazole | Albendazole, diethylcarbamazine |
| *Wuchereria bancrofti* *Brugia malayi* | Diethylcarbamazine | |
| *Onchocerca volvulus* | Ivermectin | Diethylcarbamazine plus suramin |
| Trematodes (flukes) | | |
| *Schistosoma haematobium* | Praziquantel | Metrifonate |
| *Schistosoma mansoni* | Praziquantel | Oxamniquine |
| *Schistosoma japonicum* | Praziquantel | Niridazole |
| *Paragonimus westermani* | Praziquantel | Bithionol |
| *Fasciola hepatica* | Bithionol | Dehydroemetine, praziquantel |
| Cestodes (tapeworms) | | |
| *Taenia saginata* | Niclosamide | Praziquantel, mebendazole |
| *Taenia solium* | Niclosamide | Praziquantel, mebendazole |
| *Diphylobothrium latum* | Niclosamide | Praziquantel |
| Cysticercosis | Praziquantel | |
| Hydatid disease | Mebendazole | Albendazole |

## QUESTIONS

**DIRECTIONS (items 1–10):** Each numbered item or incomplete statement in this section is followed by answers or by completions of the statement. Select the ONE lettered answer or completion that is BEST in each case.

**1.** This drug is currently an alternative agent in onchocerciasis, and its use is associated with severe reactions from dying parasites, called the Mazzotti reaction.
**(A)** Albendazole
**(B)** Pyrantel pamoate
**(C)** Diethylcarbamazine
**(D)** Mebendazole

**2.** Each of the following statements concerning niclosamide is accurate EXCEPT:
**(A)** It is effective in many tapeworm infections
**(B)** It kills parasitic ova
**(C)** Its effects include inhibition or uncoupling of oxidative phosphorylation
**(D)** It is a salicylamide derivative

**3.** The mechanism of antiparasitic action of mebendazole and thiabendazole is thought to involve
**(A)** stimulation of acetylcholine receptors at neuromuscular junctions
**(B)** inhibition of dihydrofolate reductase
**(C)** interference with microtubule synthesis and assembly
**(D)** block of thiamine transport

**4.** All of the following statements about pyrantel pamoate are accurate EXCEPT:
**(A)** It is effective in *Ascaris* infections
**(B)** It blocks nicotinic receptors, leading to muscle paralysis in parasites
**(C)** Since only a small fraction of an oral dose is absorbed systemically, toxic effects mainly concern the gastrointestinal tract
**(D)** It is equivalent to niclosamide in the treatment of tapeworm infections

**5.** This drug is reserved as an alternative agent in schistosomiasis, partly because of the high incidence of severe toxic effects.
**(A)** Niridazole
**(B)** Diethylcarbamazine
**(C)** Niclosamide
**(D)** Ivermectin

**6.** All of the following statements about ivermectin are accurate EXCEPT:
**(A)** It is the drug of choice in onchocerciasis
**(B)** Fever, rash, pruritus and joint pain may occur during treatment of onchocerciasis
**(C)** It enhances the actions of GABA in neurotransmission
**(D)** It crosses the blood-brain barrier

**7.** All of the following statements about mebendazole are accurate EXCEPT:
**(A)** It is the drug of choice in mixed infections with ascarids and hookworms
**(B)** It has a high therapeutic index
**(C)** It is safe to use during pregnancy
**(D)** Fat-containing foods increase its oral absorption

**8.** Which of the following is an alternative drug for nematode infections, including those caused by hookworm, pinworm and ascarids? Long-term use may cause alopecia, changes in liver enzymes, and reversible leukopenia.
**(A)** Albendazole
**(B)** Oxantel pamoate
**(C)** Diethylcarbamazine
**(D)** Levamisole

**9.** All of the following statements about praziquantel are accurate EXCEPT:
**(A)** It is effective in the treatment of trichinosis
**(B)** It causes muscle paralysis in parasites by increasing membrane permeability to calcium
**(C)** Malaise, headache, anorexia, and gastrointestinal distress are less common adverse effects in children than in adults
**(D)** It is the drug of choice for schistosomiasis

**10.** Which of the following is thought to promote host defense mechanisms by increasing cell-mediated immune responses?
**(A)** Niridazole
**(B)** Metrifonate
**(C)** Levamisole
**(D)** Albendazole

## ANSWERS

1. Symptoms of the Mazzotti reaction can include rashes, pyrexia, respiratory distress, hypotension, and prostration and may require hospitalization during therapy of onchocerciasis. The reaction results from the rapid killing of parasites by diethylcarbamazine. The answer is **(C)**.

2. Niclosamide is the major drug for treatment of cestode infections. Scoleces and cestode segments are killed, but ova are not. The answer is **(B)**.

3. Mebendazole and thiabendazole bind to tubulin and cause a selective loss of cytoplasmic microtubules in affected worms. The answer is **(C)**.

4. Pyrantel pamoate is not equivalent to niclosamide in the treatment of infections caused by cestodes. Niclosamide is the drug of choice in most tapeworm infections. Its toxic effects are mild, and fasting is not required during treatment. The answer is **(D)**.

5. The toxic effects of niridazole include gastrointestinal distress, arthralgia, eosinophilia, immunosuppression, pulmonary infiltration, and hemolysis in glucose-6-phosphate dehydrogenase deficiency. The drug is both mutagenic and carcinogenic. The answer is **(A)**.

6. Ivermectin intensifies the actions of GABA in nematodes, but since the drug not penetrate the blood-brain barrier it does not increase GABA-mediated neurotransmission in the CNS of the host. The answer is **(D)**.

7. Mebendazole has embryotoxic potential and is contraindicated in pregnancy. The answer is **(C)**.

8. Albendazole has a wide anthelmintic spectrum and is an important back-up drug in the treatment of nematode infections. Toxic effects during short courses of therapy are minor. Bone marrow suppression and embryotoxicity have been reported in long-term animal studies. The answer is **(A)**.

9. The antiparasitic activity of praziquantel is restricted to trematodes (flukes). In trichinosis mebendazole is the drug of choice. The answer is **(A)**.

10. In the USA levamisole is currently approved only for treatment of colon cancer. However, it is useful in hookworm infections and is the drug of choice for treatment of *Angiostrongylus cantonensis*. Its properties include stimulation of macrophage and T cell functions. The answer is **(C)**.

# Cancer Chemotherapy 56

## OBJECTIVES

**Define the following terms:**

- Cell cycle kinetics
- Cell cycle-specific (CCS)
- Cell cycle-nonspecific (CCNS)
- Growth fraction
- Log kill hypothesis
- Pulse therapy
- Rescue therapy

**You should be able to:**

- Describe the relevance of cell cycle kinetics to the mode of action and clinical use of anticancer drugs.
- Identify the major subclasses of anticancer drugs and describe the mechanisms of action of the main drugs in each subclass.
- Identify the drugs of choice for the more important neoplastic diseases and describe their pharmacokinetics and their toxic effects.
- Understand the strategies of combination chemotherapy and pulse, recruitment, and rescue therapies.

## CONCEPTS

### CANCER CELL CYCLE KINETICS

A knowledge of cancer cell cycle and population kinetics is important for an understanding of the modes of action of anticancer drugs and their clinical pharmacologic characteristics. Anticancer drugs that act specifically on cells undergoing cycling are called **cell cycle-specific (CCS)** drugs. Less specific drugs that kill tumor cells in both cycling and resting states are called **cell cycle-nonspecific (CCNS)** drugs. CCS drugs may be more active in a specific phase of the cell cycle—and, in general, they are particularly effective when a large proportion of cells proliferate (ie, when the **growth fraction** is high).

Cytotoxic drugs act via first-order kinetics, killing a constant proportion of a cell population rather than a constant number of cells. The **"log kill" hypothesis** describes tumor cell kill by anticancer drugs. For example, a 3-log kill by a drug or by a combination of drugs would reduce cancer cell populations of $10^{12}$ and $10^{6}$ cells to $10^{9}$ and $10^{3}$ cells, respectively. Since individual drugs often exhibit a limited log kill, combinations of anticancer drugs that have different mechanisms of action and different toxic effects are frequently used. This can result in additive or synergistic cytotoxic effects on cancer cells.

Resistance is a major problem in cancer chemotherapy. It commonly involves changes in gene expression that can lead to resistance of neoplastic cells to either an individual drug or multiple anticancer drugs. Mechanisms of resistance include an increased rate of DNA repair, changes in drug sensitivity of receptors or target enzymes, the production of drug-trapping reagents, an increased formation of competing metabolites, an increased activity of drug-inactivating enzymes, and the accelerated efflux of drugs as a result of increased activity of membrane drug transporters.

### ANTICANCER DRUGS

#### A. Alkylating Agents:

1. **Chemistry.** The alkylating agents are a large group that includes nitrogen mustards (**mechlorethamine, cyclophosphamide**), nitrosoureas (**carmustine [BCNU], lomustine [CCNU]**), and alkylsulfonates (**busulfan**).
2. **Mechanisms of action.** These CCNS drugs are cytotoxic via the formation of reactive imo-

nium or carbonium intermediates that alkylate nucleophilic groups on DNA bases, particularly purines. The N-7 position of guanine is a major target. This leads to cross-linking of bases, abnormal base-pairing, or DNA strand breakage. Resistance occurs through increased DNA repair, decreased drug permeability, or the production of trapping agents such as thiols.

3. **Pharmacokinetics.** The features of interest include the direct cytotoxicity of mechlorethamine, a requirement for cytochrome P-450-mediated biotransformation of cyclophosphamide for antitumor activity, and the high lipophilicity of the nitrosoureas, which is important for their use in brain tumors.
4. **Clinical use.** The alkylating agents (especially cyclophosphamide) are important in combination regimens for the therapy of lymphomas, leukemias, and myelomas (see Table 56–1).
5. **Toxicity.** Common toxic effects of alkylating agents include bone marrow suppression, gastrointestinal irritation, and changes in gonadal function. Busulfan causes adrenal insufficiency, pulmonary fibrosis, and increased skin pigmentation.

### B. Antimetabolites:

1. **Chemistry.** The antimetabolites are structurally similar to endogenous compounds and are antagonists of folic acid **(methotrexate),** purines **(mercaptopurine, thioguanine),** or pyrimidines **(fluorouracil, cytarabine).**
2. **Mechanisms of action:** The sites of action of the antimetabolites are shown in Fig 56–1.
   a. **Methotrexate** inhibits dihydrofolate reductase, leading to decreased synthesis of thymidylate, purine nucleotides, and amino acids and thus interfering with nucleic acid and protein metabolism. Tumor resistance mechanisms include decreased drug accumulation and changes in the activity of dihydrofolate reductase.
   b. **Mercaptopurine** and **thioguanine** are converted to nucleotide forms by hypoxanthine-guanine phosphoribosyltransferases (HGPRTase) that inhibit several enzymes involved in purine metabolism. Resistance can involve decreased transferase activity or increased production of alkaline phosphatases that inactivate the toxic nucleotides.
   c. **Fluorouracil** (5FU) is biotransformed to 5-fluoro-2′-deoxyuridine-5′-monophosphate (5-FdUMP), which inhibits thymidylate synthase, leading to "thymineless death" of cells. Resistance mechanisms include decreased bioactivation of 5FU, increased thymidylate synthase, and altered drug sensitivity of this enzyme.
   d. **Cytarabine** (cytosine arabinoside, AraC), is activated by kinases to AraCTP, an inhibitor of DNA polymerases that is specific for the S phase of the cell cycle. Resistance occurs through decreased uptake of AraC or decreased conversion to AraCTP.

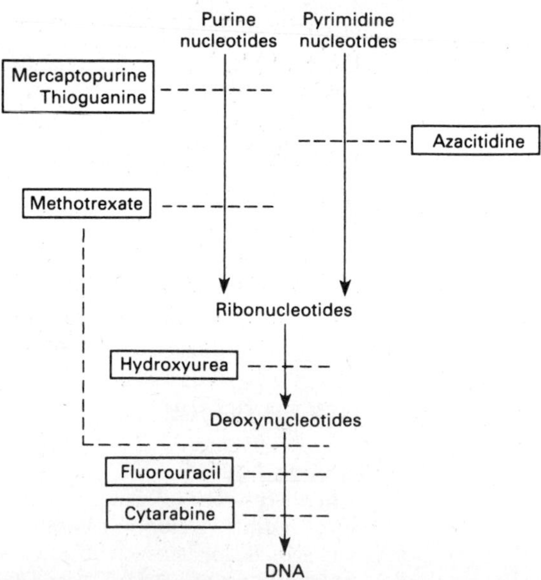


**Figure 56–1.** Sites of action of antimetabolites on DNA synthetic pathways.

**Table 56–1.** Selected examples of cancer chemotherapy.[1]

| Diagnosis | Current Drug Therapy of Choice |
|---|---|
| Acute lymphocytic leukemia | Induction: vincristine plus prednisone. Maintenance: mercaptopurine, methotrexate, and cyclophosphamide in various combinations. |
| Acute myelocytic and myelomonocytic leukemia | (A) Cytarabine and daunorubicin.<br>(B) Combination of above drugs and thioguanine, mitoxantrone, prednisone, and vincristine |
| Hodgkin's disease | (A) Mechlorethamine, vincristine, procarbazine and prednisone.<br>(B) Doxorubicin, bleomycin, vinblastine, and dacarbazine. |
| Non-Hodgkin's lymphoma | Cyclophosphamide, vincristine, prednisone, and doxorubicin. |
| Breast carcinoma (adjuvant) | Cyclophosphamide, methotrexate, and fluorouracil plus tamoxifen if lymph nodes are positive. Glutethimide may be useful in hormone-positive cancers. |
| Carcinoma of the ovary | Cyclophosphamide and cisplatin. |
| Cervical carcinoma | Mitomycin plus bleomycin, vincristine, and cisplatin. |
| Testicular carcinoma | Vinblastine, bleomycin, and cisplatin are standard. Replacement of vinblastine with etoposide is equally effective and appears to be less toxic. |
| Prostate carcinoma | Estrogens or leuprolide. |
| Lung cancer (oat cell) | Etoposide plus cisplatin or combinations including doxorubicin, cyclosphosphamide, and *Vinca* alkaloids. |

[1]Adapted from Katzung BG (editor): *Basic & Clinical Pharmacology,* 5th ed. Appleton & Lange, 1992.

3. **Pharmacokinetics.** Important biodisposition features include the dependence of methotrexate on renal function for its elimination and allopurinol inhibition of xanthine oxidase, which metabolizes mercaptopurine, leading to toxic levels of the antimetabolite.
4. **Clinical uses.** Antimetabolites are used in combination regimens for acute leukemias, choriocarcinoma, and carcinoma of the head and neck, the lungs, and the intestine (see Table 56–1).
5. **Toxicity.** Common adverse effects include bone marrow suppression and toxic effects on the skin and gastrointestinal mucosa. The toxic effects of methotrexate on normal cells may be reduced by administration of folinic acid; this strategy is called **"leucovorin rescue."**

**C. Plant Alkaloids:**

1. **Chemistry.** This subclass includes the *Vinca* alkaloids (**vinblastine, vincristine**) and the podophyllotoxins (**etoposide**).
2. **Mechanisms of action.** Vinblastine and vincristine interact with tubulin to block the assembly of the mitotic spindle and are thus called **"spindle poisons."** They are CCS drugs that act primarily in the M phase of the cancer cell cycle. Etoposide increases degradation of DNA, possibly via activation of topoisomerase II, and also inhibits mitochondrial electron transport. It acts in the late S to early $G_2$ phases of the cell cycle. Resistance to the plant alkaloids may occur from increased efflux via the membrane drug transporter.
3. **Clinical use.** Vincristine is a component of the MOPP and COP regimens* used in lymphomas and is also used in Wilms' tumor and choriocarcinoma. Vinblastine is a component of the ABVD regimen for Hodgkin's disease and the VBC regimen for testicular carcinoma.* Etoposide is used for therapy of lung (oat cell), prostate, and testicular carcinoma.
4. **Toxicity.** Vinblastine causes nausea, alopecia, and bone marrow suppression; vincristine causes neurotoxicity (areflexia, peripheral neuritis) and paralytic ileus; etoposide is a gastrointestinal irritant and causes alopecia and bone marrow suppression.

**D. Antibiotics:**

1. **Chemistry.** This subclass is made up of several structurally dissimilar drugs, including the anthracyclines (**doxorubicin, daunorubicin**), **bleomycin, dactinomycin, mitomycin,** and **mithramycin.**
2. **Mechanisms of action:**
   a. **Anthracyclines** are CCNS drugs that can intercalate between base pairs to block DNA and

*Combination drug chemotherapy regimens. See p 299.

RNA synthesis, but they also cause membrane disruption and generate free radicals that lead to cardiotoxicity.

b. **Bleomycin** is a mixture of glycopeptides that bind to DNA and generate free radicals, which cause strand breaks and inhibit DNA synthesis. They are CCS drugs that act mainly in the $G_2$ phase of the cell cycle.

c. **Dactinomycin** is a CCNS drug that binds to double-stranded DNA to inhibit DNA-dependent RNA synthesis.

d. **Mitomycin** is a CCNS drug that is metabolized by liver enzymes to form an alkylating agent that cross-links DNA.

e. **Mithramycin** (plicamycin) interferes with DNA metabolism, but its major use is to lower calcium levels in hypercalcemia associated with malignant disease.

3. **Pharmacokinetics.** Important biodisposition features include the following:

a. Metabolism of anthracyclines by liver enzymes to form both active and inactive metabolites that are excreted in the bile.

b. Inactivation of bleomycins by tissue aminopeptidases but some renal clearance of intact drug.

c. Short half-life of dactinomycin, with intact drug excreted in the bile.

4. **Clinical use.** Doxorubicin is a component of the ABVD regimen and is used in therapy of myelomas and sarcomas. The main use of daunorubicin is the treatment of acute leukemias. Bleomycin is a component of the VBC regimen for testicular carcinoma. Dactinomycin is used in melanomas and Wilms' tumor. Mitomycin acts against hypoxic tumor cells and is used for cervical carcinoma. Other clinical uses are indicated in Table 56–1.

5. **Toxicity:**

a. **Anthracyclines:** Bone marrow suppression, marked alopecia, and **cardiotoxicity,** including congestive heart failure.

b. **Bleomycins:** Anorexia, hyperkeratosis, fever, and pulmonary fibrosis.

c. **Dactinomycin:** Bone marrow suppression, skin reactions, and gastrointestinal irritation.

d. **Mitomycin:** Severe myelosuppression, nephrotoxicity, and interstitial pneumonia.

### E. Hormones & Hormone Antagonists:

1. **Prednisone** is the most commonly used glucocorticoid in cancer chemotherapy. It has applications in drug regimens for chronic lymphocytic leukemia, Hodgkin's disease, and other lymphomas.
2. **Sex hormones** (estrogens, progestins, androgens) are used in hormone-dependent cancers to change the hormone balance.
3. **Tamoxifen** (an estrogen receptor antagonist) blocks the binding of estrogen to receptors of estrogen-sensitive cancer cells. It is used in therapy of breast cancer and also acts against progestin-resistant endometrial carcinoma.
4. **Leuprolide** and **nafarelin** are gonadotropin-releasing hormone agonists. They are as active as diethylstilbestrol in prostatic carcinoma but cause fewer toxic effects.
5. **Aminoglutethimide** is an aromatase inhibitor that decreases estrone formation and is used in drug regimens for metastatic breast cancer.

### F. Possible Alkylating Agents:

1. **Procarbazine.** This reactive agent forms hydrogen peroxide, which generates free radicals that affect DNA strand scission. Several of its metabolites are cytotoxic, and one is a monoamine oxidase inhibitor. The drug is a component of the MOPP regimen and has many toxic effects, including myelosuppression, CNS disturbances, disulfiramlike reactions with ethanol, and pulmonary dysfunction.
2. **Dacarbazine.** This drug is bioactivated by liver enzymes to form methylcarbonium species that act as alkylating agents and interfere with nucleic acid metabolism. When used in Hodgkin's disease (as part of the ABVD regimen), it causes marked myelosuppression and gastrointestinal distress.
3. **Cisplatin.** Cisplatin is a CCNS drug that binds to DNA to alter its structure and inhibit nucleic acid synthesis. It is used in combination for treatment of testicular and lung carcinomas. It causes nephrotoxicity and acoustic nerve damage. Renal damage may be reduced by use of mannitol with adequate hydration.

## STRATEGIES IN CANCER CHEMOTHERAPY

**A. Principles of Combination Therapy:** Chemotherapy with combinations of anticancer drugs usually increases the log kill markedly, and in some cases synergistic effects are achieved (see section B, below). Combinations are often cytotoxic to a heterogeneous population of cancer cells and may prevent the development of resistant clones. Drug combinations using CCS and CCNS drugs may be cytotoxic to both dividing and resting cancer cells. The following principles are important for selecting appropriate drugs to be used in combination chemotherapy.

1. Each drug should be active against the particular cancer.
2. The drugs should have different mechanisms of action.
3. Cross-resistance between drugs should be minimal.
4. The drugs should have different toxic effects.

**B. Examples of Combination Chemotherapy:**

1. **Hodgkin's disease:**
   a. **MOPP regimen:** *M*echlorethamine, *O*ncovin (vincristine), *p*rocarbazine, and *p*rednisone.
   b. **ABVD regimen:** *A*driamycin (doxorubicin), *b*leomycin, *v*inblastine, and *d*acarbazine.
2. **Non-Hodgkin's lymphomas:** COP regimen: *c*yclophosphamide, *O*ncovin (vincristine), and *p*rednisone, with or without doxorubicin.
3. **Testicular carcinoma:**
   a. Vinblastine, bleomycin and cisplatin.
   b. Etoposide, bleomycin and vinblastine.
4. **Breast carcinoma:** CMF regimen: *c*yclophosphamide, *m*ethotrexate and *f*luorouracil, with or without tamoxifen.

**C. Additional Strategies:**

1. **Pulse therapy.** Intermittent, or **"pulse,"** treatment with high doses of an anticancer drug has been used as an alternative to continuous daily therapy. Intensive drug treatment every 3–4 weeks allows for maximum effects on neoplastic cells, with hematologic and immunologic recovery between courses. This type of regimen is used successfully in therapy of acute leukemias, testicular carcinomas, and Wilms' tumor.
2. **Recruitment and synchrony.** The strategy of **recruitment** involves the initial use of a CCNS drug to achieve a significant log kill, which results in the recruitment into cell division of resting cells in the $G_0$ phase. With subsequent administration of a CCS drug active against dividing cells, maximal cell death may be achieved. A similar approach involves **synchrony,** one example being the use of **Vinca** alkaloids to hold cancer cells in the M phase. Subsequent treatment with another CCS drug, such as the S phase-specific agent cytarabine, may result in a greater killing effect on the neoplastic cell population.
3. **Rescue therapy.** Toxic effects of anticancer drugs can sometimes be alleviated by **rescue** strategy. For example, high doses of methotrexate may be given for 36–48 hours and terminated before severe toxicity to cells of the gastrointestinal tract and blood can occur. **Leucovorin** (formyl tetrahydrofolate) is then administered and is accumulated more readily by normal than by neoplastic cells. This results in "rescue" of the normal cells, since leucovorin bypasses the dihydrofolate reductase step in folic acid synthesis.

## DRUG LIST

The following drugs are important members of the group discussed in this chapter. Prototype agents should be learned in detail; the major variants should be known well enough to list the factors that distinguish them from the prototypes and from each other; and the other significant agents should be recognized as belonging to a specific subclass.

| Subclass | Prototype | Major Variants | Other Significant Agents |
|---|---|---|---|
| Alkylating agents | | | |
| Nitrogen mustards | Mechlorethamine | | Cyclophosphamide, chlorambucil |
| Nitrosureas | Carmustine | Lomustine | Semustine |
| Alkylsulfonates | Busulfan | | |
| Platinum complex | Cisplatin | | |
| Triazenes | Dacarbazine | | |
| Hydrazines | Procarbazine | | |
| Antimetabolites | | | |
| Folate analogs | Methotrexate | | |
| Purine analogs | Mercaptopurine | | Thioguanine |
| Pyrimidine analogs | Fluorouracil | | Cytarabine |
| Plant alkaloids | | | |
| *Vinca* agents | Vinblastine | Vincristine | |
| Podophyllotoxins | Etoposide | | |
| Antibiotics | | | |
| Anthracyclines | Doxorubicin | Daunorubicin | |
| Bleomycins | Bleomycin | | |
| Actinomycins | Dactinomycin | | |
| Mitomycins | Mitomycin | | |
| Chromomycins | Mithramycin | | |
| Hormones | | | |
| Adrenocorticoids | Prednisone | Hydrocortisone | |
| Androgens | Testosterone | Fluoxymesterone | |
| Estrogens | Diethylstilbestrol | Ethinyl estradiol | |
| Progestins | Hydroxyprogesterone | Medroxyprogesterone | |
| Antiestrogens | Tamoxifen | | |
| Gonadotropin-releasing hormone agonists | Leuprolide | | |

## QUESTIONS

**DIRECTIONS (items 1–8):** Each numbered item or incomplete statement in this section is followed by answers or by completions of the statement. Select the ONE lettered answer or completion that is BEST in each case.

**1.** This drug is a nitrogen mustard that must be bioactivated by liver enzymes to become an alkylating agent. Its adverse effects include bone marrow depression, gastrointestinal distress, and amenorrhea.
**(A)** Cytarabine
**(B)** Cyclophosphamide
**(C)** Carmustine
**(D)** Methotrexate

**2.** This drug is an antimetabolite that is used in acute myelogenous leukemia. It is phosphorylated to form a nucleotide inhibitor of DNA polymerases. Its major toxic effect is myelosuppression.
**(A)** Mechlorethamine
**(B)** Vincristine
**(C)** Prednisone
**(D)** Cytarabine

**3.** This antibiotic is used in the drug treatment of testicular carcinoma. Its adverse effects include hyperpigmentation and distinctive pulmonary toxicity.
**(A)** Bleomycin
**(B)** Mithramycin
**(C)** Dactinomycin
**(D)** Doxorubicin

**4.** This drug is an antimetabolite that inhibits dihydrofolate reductase and is used in certain leukemias and lymphomas. Its myelosuppressant and gastrointestinal effects can be reduced by "leucovorin rescue."
**(A)** Semustine (methyl-CCNU)
**(B)** Thioguanine
**(C)** Methotrexate
**(D)** Fluorouracil

**5.** Concerning mechanisms of action of anticancer drugs, all of the following statements are accurate EXCEPT.
**(A)** Alkylating agents commonly attack the nucleophilic N–7 position in guanine
**(B)** Fluorouracil can cause "thymineless death" of cancer cells
**(C)** Anthracyclines intercalate with base pairs to block nucleic acid synthesis
**(D)** Mercaptopurine is an irreversible inhibitor of HGPRTase

**6.** Mechanisms of cancer cell resistance to drugs include all of the following EXCEPT
**(A)** increase in DNA repair
**(B)** increase in cytochrome P-450 activity
**(C)** increase in production of drug-trapping reagents
**(D)** change in properties of a target enzyme

**7.** Characteristic toxic effects of anticancer drugs include all of the following EXCEPT
**(A)** myelosuppression with vincristine
**(B)** cardiotoxicity with doxorubicin
**(C)** renal dysfunction with cisplatin
**(D)** pulmonary dysfunction with procarbazine

**8.** Which ONE of the following anticancer drugs is cell cycle nonspecific?
**(A)** Vinblastine
**(B)** Etoposide
**(C)** Cytarabine
**(D)** Daunorubicin

**DIRECTIONS (items 9–12):** Items 9–12 consist of lettered headings followed by a set of numbered phrases. For each numbered phrase, select the ONE lettered heading that is most closely associated with it. Each lettered heading may be selected once, more than once, or not at all.

**(A)** Mercaptopurine
**(B)** Vincristine
**(C)** Procarbazine
**(D)** Leuprolide
**(E)** Cisplatin

**9.** A component of the COP regimen used in therapy of non-Hodgkin's lymphomas

**10.** A gonadotropin-releasing hormone agonist used in prostatic carcinoma

**11.** An anticancer drug that may be mutagenic and carcinogenic

**12.** A drug whose metabolism is inhibited by allopurinol

## ANSWERS

**1.** Only 2 of the drugs listed are alkylating agents. Carmustine (BCNU) is a nitrosourea that decomposes spontaneously in aqueous environments to form reactive products. Cyclophosphamide is a nitrogen mustard pro-drug that is bioactivated by hepatic cytochrome P-450 to form reactive metabolites. The answer is **(B)**.

**2.** Antimetabolites are almost always structurally similar to endogenous molecules. Two of the agents listed are possibilities: prednisone, which has corticosteroid actions (but is not an antimetabolite), and cytarabine (cytosine arabinoside), which undergoes phosphorylation to become an inhibitor of DNA polymerase. The answer is **(D)**.

**3.** All of the agents listed are antibiotics, but only one, bleomycin, is used in the treatment of testicular carcinoma. The drug causes distinctive pulmonary infiltrates and fibrosis as well as hyperkeratinization. The answer is **(A)**.

**4.** Methotrexate is structurally similar to dihydrofolic acid and inhibits its conversion to tetrahydrofolate via dihydrofolate reductase. A similar mechanism underlies both the antibacterial action of trimethoprim and the antimalarial action of pyrimethamine. The answer is **(C)**.

**5.** To exert anticancer activity, mercaptopurine (and thioguanine) must first be bioactivated to nucleotides by HGPRTase. If mercaptopurine were an irreversible inhibitor of this enzyme, this bioactivation process could not take place. The answer is **(D)**.

**6.** Increases in the activity of cytochrome P-450 have not been reported as a mechanism of resistance to anticancer drugs. In fact, one might predict enhanced cytotoxic effects of drugs that are bioactivated by this enzyme system, such as cyclophosphamide. Increased drug inactivation through increased production of alkaline phosphatases is a mechanism of resistance to purine antimetabolites. The answer is **(B)**.

**7.** Myelosuppression is a common toxic effect of anticancer drugs, particularly alkylating agents, antimetabolites, antibiotics, and plant alkaloids. However, vincristine is an exception! It causes characteristic neurotoxicity and, unlike vinblastine, has little effect on bone marrow. The other toxic effects listed are distinctive for the particular drugs. The answer is **(A)**.

**8.** Three of the drugs listed are CCS drugs. Vinblastine acts mainly in the M phase; etoposide in the late S to early G2 phases; and cytarabine mainly in the S phase. With the exception of bleomycin, none of the antibiotics (or alkylating agents) are CCS drugs. The answer is **(D)**.

**9.** The COP anticancer drug regimen combines cyclophosphamide, vincristine (Oncovin), and prednisone. We hope you didn't fall for cisplatin and procarbazine. The answer is **(B)**.

**10.** Leuprolide is a synthetic peptide that acts like gonadotropin-releasing hormone. It is as effective as diethylstilbestrol in therapy of prostatic carcinoma but is less likely to cause edema, gynecomastia, and thromboembolism. The answer is **(D)**.

**11.** Procarbazine is a highly reactive chemical that generates hydrogen peroxide and toxic free radicals. Its adverse effects include myelosuppression, gastrointestinal distress, disulfiramlike reactions with ethanol, and neurotoxicity. It is teratogenic and carcinogenic. Despite these problems, procarbazine is a component of the MOPP anticancer drug regimen used in Hodgkin's disease, the gains presumably outweighing the risks. The answer is **(C).**

12. Allopurinol, a xanthine oxidase inhibitor, is given adjunctively to control hyperuricemia that occurs in the drug therapy of malignant diseases. The antimetabolite 6-mercaptopurine is metabolized by xanthine oxidase, and, in the presence of an inhibitor of this enzyme, toxic levels of the drug may be reached rapidly. The answer is **(A).**

# Immunopharmacology 57

## OBJECTIVES

**Define the following terms:**

- B cell, T cell
- Cellular and serologic immunity
- Cytokines
- Interferons
- Interleukins
- Colony-stimulating factors

**You should be able to:**

- Describe cellular and serologic immunity.
- Identify the therapeutic similarities and the differences between immunosuppressant and anticancer drugs.
- Describe the mechanisms of action, clinical uses, and toxicities of glucocorticoids, cyclosporine, azathioprine, and cyclophosphamide.
- Describe the mechanisms of action, clinical uses, and toxicities of antibodies used as immunosuppressants.
- Identify the cytokines and other immunomodulating agents.
- List the different types of immunologic reactions to drugs.

## CONCEPTS

### IMMUNE MECHANISMS

A. **Development of Immunity:** The development of specific immunity requires the following steps (1) antigen recognition and processing; (2) proliferation of lymphoid cells; (3) differentiation of lymphoid cells; and (4) immune effects. The initial critical step (antigen recognition and processing) involves phagocytes that change antigens so that they become more recognizable to lymphoid cells. The **T (thymus) lymphoid cells** recognize and make contact with antigens; the resulting proliferation and differentiation of T cells leads to **cellular immunity.** The T cells, either by direct cytotoxic effects or by the release of lymphokines (endogenous immunomodulators), mediate delayed hypersensitivity reactions and are important in tissue graft rejection. The **B (bone marrow) lymphoid cells** respond to antigens by proliferation that is controlled by T helper or suppressor cells. B cells are responsible for **serologic immunity** via their differentiation into specific antibody-forming cells. Antibody-antigen interactions lead to precipitation of viruses, phagocytosis of bacteria, or lysis of red blood cells. Lymphoid cell proliferation may be modified by the secretion of inhibitors such as prostaglandins or by stimulants such as peptide growth factors. **Natural killer (NK) lymphoid cells,** which are of unknown origin, may also play an important role in immune defense mechanisms, including tumor rejection.

**B. Immunocompetence:** Techniques used to assess immunologic competence and its drug-induced suppression include the following:

1. Delayed hypersensitivity testing with skin test antigens
2. Assays of serum immunoglobulins, complement, and specific antibodies
3. Measurement of antibody response to primary or secondary immunization
4. Absolute circulating-lymphocyte count
5. Differential lymphocyte count

**C. Sites of Action of Immunosuppressant Agents:** The possible sites of action of immunosuppressive agents are shown in Fig 57–1. Agents that act at the step of antigen recognition are antibodies and include $Rh_0$(D) immune globulin, antilymphocyte globulin (ALG), and a monoclonal antibody, OKT-3. Lymphoid cell proliferation is a primary site of action of the cytotoxic drugs and is also inhibited by cyclosporine, glucocorticoids, and ALG. The stages of differentiation of B and T cells are inhibited to some extent by cyclosporine, dactinomycin, and ALG. Corticosteroids also modify tissue injury from immune responses via their anti-inflammatory properties.

**D. Immunosuppressant Drugs Versus Cancer Chemotherapy:** Since most immune responses involve proliferating cells, there is a similarity between immunosuppressant agents and the drugs used in cancer chemotherapy. However, the therapeutic principles involved are not identical. In contrast to most neoplasms, immune cell proliferation is **synchronized.** This permits a greater selective toxicity of anti-immune cytotoxic drugs if they are given at the time of initial antigen exposure. In addition, immunosuppressant drugs are usually given in *low doses, continuously,* whereas anticancer drug therapy often follows *intermittent, high-dose* regimens.

## IMMUNOSUPPRESSANT DRUGS

**A. Corticosteroids:**

1. **Mechanism of action.** These hormone-related substances are cytotoxic to certain subsets of T cells. They suppress cellular immunity and antibody formation and inhibit the synthesis of prostaglandins and leukotrienes. Continuous therapy lowers immunoglobulin G (IgG) levels by increasing their catabolism.

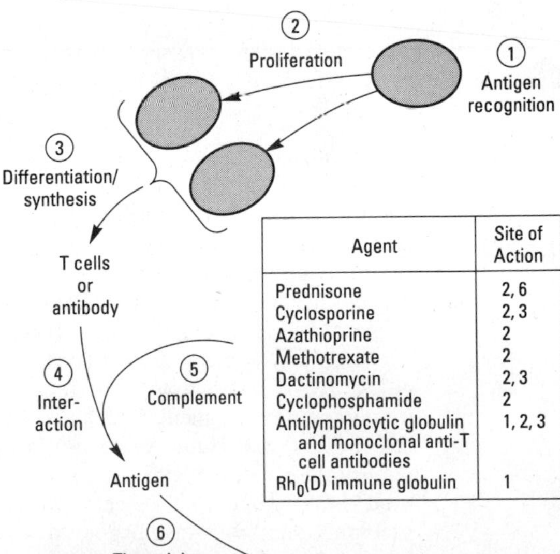


| Agent | Site of Action |
|---|---|
| Prednisone | 2, 6 |
| Cyclosporine | 2, 3 |
| Azathioprine | 2 |
| Methotrexate | 2 |
| Dactinomycin | 2, 3 |
| Cyclophosphamide | 2 |
| Antilymphocytic globulin and monoclonal anti-T cell antibodies | 1, 2, 3 |
| $Rh_0$(D) immune globulin | 1 |

**Figure 57–1.** The sites of action of immunosuppressive agents on the immune response. (Reproduced, with permission, from Katzung BG [editor]: *Basic & Clinical Pharmacology,* 5th ed. Appleton & Lange, 1992.)

2. **Clinical use.** Prednisone is the drug of choice in several autoimmune diseases, including idiopathic thrombocytopenic purpura, autoimmune hemolytic anemia, and acute glomerulonephritis. Corticosteroids are also used in combination with other agents for immunosuppression in organ transplantation.
3. **Toxicity.** Predictable adverse effects include adrenal suppression, growth inhibition, muscle wasting, osteoporosis, salt retention, diabetogenesis, and psychoses.

### B. Cyclosporine:

1. **Mechanism of action.** This peptide antibiotic inhibits early stages of the differentiation of T cells and blocks their activation. It inhibits the synthesis of factors that stimulate the growth of T cells but does not block the effects of such factors on primed T cells, nor does it block interaction with antigen.
2. **Clinical use.** The drug can be used orally and is metabolized slowly, with a long half-life. It is the drug of choice for immunosuppression in organ transplantation and is used in the graft-versus-host syndrome in bone marrow transplants. It has been used in combination with cytotoxic drugs but may be equally effective used alone. Cyclosporine may also be useful in the early treatment of type I diabetes.
3. **Toxicity.** Adverse effects include nephrotoxicity, transient liver dysfunction, an increase in viral infections, and possibly lymphomas. One virtue of cyclosporine is its low incidence of bone marrow toxicity.

### C. Azathioprine:

1. **Mechanism of action.** This pro-drug is biotransformed to the antimetabolite **mercaptopurine**, which, upon further metabolic conversion, inhibits enzymes involved in purine metabolism. It is cytotoxic to proliferating lymphoid cells.
2. **Clinical use.** Azathioprine is used in several autoimmune diseases and in renal homografts.
3. **Toxicity.** The major toxic effect is bone marrow suppression, but gastrointestinal irritation, skin rashes, and liver dysfunction also occur. The active compound, mercaptopurine, is metabolized by xanthine oxidase, and blood levels may be increased by allopurinol given for hyperuricemia.

### D. Cyclophosphamide:

1. **Mechanism of action.** This orally active drug is bioactivated by liver enzymes to form an alkylating agent that acts on proliferating lymphoid cells and is also antineoplastic. Other cytotoxic drugs that act similarly and are sometimes used as immunosuppressants include cytarabine, dactinomycin, methotrexate, and vincristine (see Chapter 56).
2. **Clinical use.** Cyclophosphamide is effective in autoimmune diseases (including hemolytic anemia), antibody-induced red cell aplasia, bone marrow transplants, and possibly other organ transplants It does not prevent the graft-versus-host reaction in bone marrow transplantation.
3. **Toxicity.** Large doses of the drug, which are usually needed in immunosuppression, cause pancytopenia and hemorrhagic cystitis.

## ANTIBODIES AS IMMUNOSUPPRESSANTS

### A. Antilymphocytic Globulin (ALG):

1. **Mechanism of action.** ALG can be produced by immunization of animals with human lymphoid cells or by production in hybridomas, using monoclonal antibody techniques. The latter method is potentially more specific. The antibodies bind to T cells involved in antigen recognition, initiating the destruction of the T cells by serum complement. ALG selectively blocks cellular immunity rather than antibody formation, which accounts for its clinical use to suppress organ graft rejection.
2. **Clinical use.** ALG is usually used in combination with cyclosporine or cytotoxic drugs (or both) in bone marrow, heart, and renal transplantations.
3. **Toxicity.** Since serologic immunity may remain intact, injection of ALG may cause hypersensitivity reactions, including serum sickness and anaphylaxis. Pain and erythema occur at injection sites, and histiocytic lymphoma has been noted as a late complication.

**B. Muromonab (OKT-3):**

1. **Mechanism of action.** OKT-3 is a murine monoclonal antibody directed against a molecule on the surface of human thymocytes and mature T cells. The antibody blocks the killing action of cytotoxic T cells and probably interferes with other T cell functions.
2. **Clinical use.** OKT-3 is used in the treatment of renal allograft rejection crisis.
3. **Toxicity.** Hypersensitivity reactions may occur.

**C. $Rh_0$(D)Immune Globulin ($Rh_0$GAM):**

1. **Mechanism of action.** $Rh_0$GAM is a human IgG preparation that contains antibodies against red cell $Rh_0$(D) antigens. Administration of this antibody to $Rh_0$(D)-negative, $D^u$-negative mothers at time of antigen exposure (ie, birth of $Rh_0$(D)-positive, $D^u$-positive child) blocks the primary immune response to the foreign cells. The mechanism probably involves feedback immunosuppression.
2. **Clinical use.** $Rh_0$(D) is used for prevention of Rh hemolytic disease of the newborn. Maternal antibodies to Rh-positive cells are not produced in subsequent pregnancies, and hemolytic disease of the neonate is averted.

## IMMUNOMODULATING AGENTS

Agents that act as stimulators of immune responses represent a new area in immunopharmacology, with the potential for important therapeutic uses, including the treatment of immune-deficiency diseases, chronic infectious diseases, and cancer.

**A. Thymosin:** Thymosin is a protein hormone from the thymus that stimulates the maturation of pre-T cells and promotes the formation of T cells from ordinary lymphoid stem cells. It has been used in DiGeorge syndrome.

**B. Levamisole:** Levamisole is an antiparasitic drug that enhances T cell-mediated immune responses and delayed hypersensitivity. It promotes the oxidation of a precursor molecule to soluble immune response repressor substance (SIRS). The drug may be useful in rheumatoid arthritis and in the immunodeficiency of Hodgkin's disease.

**C. Bacille Calmette-Guérin (BCG):** BCG (bacille Calmette-Guérin) has been used for immunization against tuberculosis and as an immunostimulant in cancer therapy. BCG activates macrophages and may enhance immune responses in patients with superficial bladder cancer.

**D. Cytokines:** Cytokines are immunoregulatory proteins synthesized by lymphoreticular cells. These proteins appear to mediate their effects via interactions with cell surface components (receptors) of specific target cells. Cytokines include **interferons, colony-stimulating factors (CSFs), interleukins,** and **tumor necrosis factors (TNFs).** Potential clinical applications of cytokines include the use of interferons in leukemias and in hepatitis as well as the use of CSFs to reverse leukopenia during cancer chemotherapy and for supportive care of burn patients.

## MECHANISMS OF DRUG ALLERGY

**A. Type I (Immediate) Drug Allergy:** This form of drug allergy involves **IgE**-mediated reactions to stings as well as to drugs. Such reactions include anaphylaxis, urticaria, and angioedema. Small drug molecules can act as haptens when linked to carrier proteins, initiating B cell proliferation and IgE antibody formation. These antibodies bind to tissue mast cells and blood basophils, which become sensitized. On subsequent exposure, the antigenic drug is bound to antibodies, triggering release of mediators of vascular responses and tissue injury, including histamine, kinins, prostaglandins, and leukotrienes. Drugs that commonly cause type I reactions include penicillins and sulfonamides.

**B. Type II Drug Allergy:** This involves **IgG** or **IgM** antibodies, which bind to circulating blood cells. On reexposure to the antigen, complement-dependent cell lysis occurs. Type II reactions include autoimmune syndromes such as agranulocytosis (from several drugs) and systemic lupus erythematosus (from hydralazine or procainamide exposure).

**C. Type III Drug Allergy:** This complex reaction involves complement-fixing **IgM** or **IgG** antibodies and possibly **IgE** antibodies. Drug-induced serum sickness and vasculitis are examples, and Stevens-Johnson syndrome may also result from type III mechanisms.

**D. Type IV Drug Allergy:** This is a cell-mediated reaction and can occur from topical application of drugs. It results in contact dermatitis.

**E. Modification of Drug Allergies:** Some drugs that modify allergic responses to other pharmacologic agents (or to toxins) may act at several steps of the immune mechanism; eg, corticosteroids inhibit lymphoid cell proliferation and reduce tissue injury and edema. However, most drugs that are useful in type I reactions (eg, isoproterenol, theophylline, epinephrine) block mediator release or act as physiologic antagonists of the mediators.

## DRUG LIST

The following drugs are important members of the group discussed in this chapter. Prototype agents should be learned in detail; the major variant and other significant agents should be known well enough to distinguish them from the prototypes and from each other.

| Subclass | Prototype | Major Variants | Other Significant Agents |
|---|---|---|---|
| Steroids | Prednisone | | |
| Antibiotics | Cyclosporine | | Dactinomycin |
| Antimetabolites | Azathioprine | Mercaptopurine | Cytarabine, methotrexate |
| Alkylating agents | Cyclophosphamide | | Chlorambucil |
| Antibodies | Antilymphocytic globulin (ALG), Muromonab (OKT-3), $Rh_o$(D) immune globulin | | |

## QUESTIONS

**DIRECTIONS (items 1–10):** Each numbered item or incomplete statement in this section is followed by answers or by completions of the statement. Select the ONE lettered answer or completion that is BEST in each case.

**1.** Cyclosporine is effective in organ transplantation. Although its precise mechanism of action is unknown, cyclosporine
**(A)** interferes with antigen recognition
**(B)** blocks tissue responses to inflammatory mediators
**(C)** inhibits differentiation of T cells
**(D)** increases catabolism of IgG antibodies
**(E)** stimulates production of NK cells

**2.** Azathioprine
**(A)** is an inhibitor of dihydrofolate reductase
**(B)** is bioactivated to a cytotoxic intermediate by xanthine oxidase
**(C)** blocks both cellular and serologic immune mechanisms
**(D)** is not toxic to bone marrow cells
**(E)** prevents Rh hemolytic disease of the newborn

**3.** The immunosuppressive agent most likely to cause serum sickness and anaphylactic reaction is
**(A)** $Rh_o(D)$ immune globulin
**(B)** cyclophosphamide
**(C)** dactinomycin
**(D)** antilymphocytic globulin
**(E)** cyclosporine

**4.** This drug is a widely used agent that suppresses cellular immunity, inhibits prostaglandin and leukotriene synthesis, and increases the catabolism of IgG antibodies.
**(A)** Mercaptopurine
**(B)** Cyclophosphamide
**(C)** Prednisone
**(D)** $Rh_o(D)$ immune globulin
**(E)** Cyclosporine

**5.** This agent appears to confer T cell specificity on uncommitted lymphoid stem cells, inducing the maturation of pre-T cells.
**(A)** Interferon
**(B)** Bacille Calmette-Guérin
**(C)** Levamisole
**(D)** Thymosin
**(E)** Tumor necrosis factor

**6.** Functions of T cells include all of the following EXCEPT
**(A)** serologic immunity
**(B)** antigen recognition
**(C)** regulation of B cells
**(D)** production of cytokines

**7.** All of the following statements about the actions of antilymphocytic globulin are correct EXCEPT:
**(A)** It facilitates the complement-mediated destruction of T cells
**(B)** It stimulates the release of cytokines
**(C)** It blocks antigen recognition
**(D)** It may cause serum sickness

**8.** All of the following statements about cyclosporine are accurate EXCEPT:
**(A)** Mannitol diuresis decreases its nephrotoxic effects
**(B)** Viral infections can occur during treatment
**(C)** It causes severe myelosuppression
**(D)** It has good oral bioavailability

**9.** All of the following statements about type I drug allergies are accurate EXCEPT:
**(A)** Type I drug allergies involve IgE antibody binding to basophils and mast cells
**(B)** Anaphylaxis is a type I drug allergy
**(C)** Mediators of type I drug allergy include histamine, prostaglandins, and leukotrienes
**(D)** Type I drug allergies are responsible for drug-induced autoimmune syndromes

**10.** Which of the following is not a cytokine?
**(A)** OKT-3
**(B)** Alpha interferon
**(C)** Interleukin-2
**(D)** Tumor necrosis factor

## ANSWERS

1. Cyclosporine inhibits early stages in the differentiation of T cells and blocks their activation. It inhibits the synthesis of factors that stimulate T cell growth. The answer is **(C)**.

2. Azathioprine is a pro-drug metabolically activated to 6-mercaptopurine (but not via the action of xanthine oxidase, which inactivates mercaptopurine). It blocks both cellular and serologic immunity. The answer is **(C)**.

3. Antilymphocytic globulin (ALG) is produced mainly through the immunization of large animals. As a mixture of foreign proteins, ALG may cause hypersensitivity reactions, including serum sickness and anaphylaxis. The answer is **(D)**.

4. The corticosteroid prednisone is used extensively as an immunosuppressant in autoimmune diseases and organ transplantation. It has multiple actions, including those described in the question. The answer is **(C)**.

5. The peptide hormone thymosin, produced by the thymus gland, stimulates maturation of pre-T cells and promotes the formation of T cells from ordinary lymphoid cells. The answer is **(D)**.

6. Serologic immunity derives from B cells via their differentiation into antibody-forming cells. T cells are responsible for cellular immunity. The answer is **(A)**.

7. Since serologic immunity may remain intact, the injection of ALG may cause hypersensitivity reactions including serum sickness and anaphylaxis. ALG increases T cell destruction and blocks cellular immunity, but it does not stimulate the release of cytokines. The answer is **(B)**.

8. Cyclosporine is relatively free of bone marrow-suppressive effects. The answer is **(C)**.

9. Autoimmune syndromes that can be drug induced include agranulocytosis and systemic lupus erythematosus. They are type II reactions involving IgM and IgG antibodies that bind to circulating blood cells. The answer is **(D)**.

10. Cytokines are immunoregulatory proteins, synthesized by lymphoreticular cells, that usually exert their effects via interaction with cell surface receptors. This class of endogenous compounds includes interferons, interleukins, colony-stimulating factors, and tumor necrosis factors. OKT-3 is a murine monoclonal antibody directed against a surface component of human lymphocytes and mature T cells. The answer is **(A)**.

# Part IX. Toxicology

# Introduction to Toxicology — 58

## OBJECTIVES

**Define the following terms:**

- Bioaccumulation
- Biomagnification
- Ecotoxicology
- Generally recognized as safe (GRAS)
- Risk
- Threshold limit value (TLV)

**You should be able to:**

- List 4 major air pollutants and their clinical effects.
- List the major toxicities of benzene, chlorinated hydrocarbon insecticides, and organophosphate insecticides.
- List 2 important herbicides and their major toxicities.
- Describe the sources of dioxin exposure and of PCB exposure.

## DEFINITIONS

**A. Toxicology:** The area of pharmacology that deals with the untoward effects of chemicals on biologic systems.

**B. Occupational Toxicology:** Deals with the untoward effects of chemicals found in the workplace.

**C. Environmental Toxicology:** Deals with the effects of agents found in the environment (in air, water, etc).

**D. Ecotoxicology:** Deals with the untoward effects of agents in the environment on whole populations, as opposed to single individuals.

**E. Risk:** The expected frequency of occurrence of a particular untoward effect in response to a particular agent.

**F. Threshold Limit Value (TLV):** Denotes the amount of exposure to a given agent that is deemed safe for a stated period. It is higher for short periods than for longer periods.

**G. Bioaccumulation:** The increasing concentration of a substance in the environment as a result of environmental persistence and physicochemical properties (eg, lipid solubility) that permit it to accumulate in the tissues of organisms.

**H. Biomagnification:** The further concentration of chemicals within organisms that feed on other organisms and thereby concentrate the chemicals found in the tissues of the prey species.

**I. Generally recognized as safe (GRAS):** An official list of substances that through testing and experience do not appear to have significant toxicity.

## CONCEPTS

### AIR POLLUTANTS

**A. Classification & Prototypes:** The major air pollutants in industrialized countries include carbon monoxide (CO), sulfur oxides (particularly sulfur dioxide), nitrogen oxides, ozone, hydrocarbons, and particulate matter (eg, smoke particles).

**B. Carbon Monoxide:** CO is an odorless, colorless gas that competes avidly with oxygen for hemoglobin. Its affinity for hemoglobin is more than 200-fold greater than that of oxygen.

1. **Effects.** CO causes tissue hypoxia. Headache is one of the first symptoms, followed by confusion, loss of visual acuity, tachycardia, syncope, coma, convulsions, and death. Collapse and syncope occur at approximately 40% conversion of hemoglobin to carboxyhemoglobin.
2. **Treatment.** Removal of the source of carbon monoxide and breathing pure oxygen comprise the major treatment. Hyperbaric oxygen accelerates the clearance of carbon monoxide.

**C. Sulfur Dioxide:** Sulfur dioxide ($SO_2$) is a colorless irritating gas.

1. **Effects.** $SO_2$ forms sulfurous acid on contact with moist mucous membranes; this acid is responsible for most of the pathologic effects. Conjunctival and bronchial irritation are the primary signs of exposure. Five to ten parts per million (PPM) is a concentration high enough to cause severe bronchospasm.
2. **Treatment.** The major treatment consists of removal from exposure and treatment of irritation and inflammation.

**D. Nitrogen Oxides:** Nitrogen dioxide ($NO_2$) is the primary member of this group. It is formed in fires and in fresh silage on farms.

1. **Effects.** $NO_2$ causes deep lung irritation and pulmonary edema. Farmers exposed to high concentrations of the gas within enclosed silos may die of acute pulmonary edema very rapidly. Irritation of the eyes, nose, and throat is also common.
2. **Treatment.** No specific treatment is available; measures for reducing inflammation and pulmonary edema are important.

**E. Ozone:** Ozone ($O_3$) is a bluish irritant gas produced in air and water purification devices and in electrical fields.

1. **Effects.** Exposure to 0.1 PPM causes irritation and dryness of the mucous membranes. Pulmonary function may be impaired at higher concentrations. Chronic exposure leads to bronchitis, bronchiolitis, fibrosis, and emphysema.
2. **Treatment.** No specific treatment is available. Measures that reduce inflammation and pulmonary edema are emphasized.

**F. Hydrocarbons:** Solvents used in industry and in drycleaning of clothing are the major sources of hydrocarbons. Examples include carbon tetrachloride,trichlorocthylene, benzene, and toluene.

1. **Effects.** These agents are potent CNS depressants. The acute effects of excessive exposure are nausea, vertigo, locomotor disturbance, headache, and coma. Benzene is also a bone marrow suppressant. It may produce aplastic anemia, thrombocytopenia, or leukopenia.
2. **Treatment.** Removal from exposure is the only direct treatment available. Serious CNS depression is treated with support of vital signs, as described in Chapter 60.

### INSECTICIDES

**A. Classification & Prototypes:** The 3 major classes of insecticides are the chlorinated hydrocarbons (DDT and its analogues), acetylcholinesterase inhibitors (carbaryl, malathion, etc), and the botanical agents (nicotine, rotenone, pyrethrum alkaloids).

**B. Chlorinated Hydrocarbons:** DDT and its analogues are very stable chemicals that accumulate in body fat and thus are subject to both bioaccumulation and biomagnification. They are banned in many countries.

1. **Effects.** Chlorinated hydrocarbons have an acute effect on sodium channels in nerve membranes; this effect results in uncontrolled firing of action potentials. This is probably the mode of insecticidal action. In mammals, the same effect may occur with very high doses. Chronic exposure to lower concentrations leads to impaired egg survival in birds and, possibly, to increased tumorigenesis in mammals.
2. **Treatment.** No specific treatment is available, and the extremely long half-lives of these agents in the environment (years) required their removal from the market to prevent more severe environmental toxicity.

**C. Cholinesterase Inhibitors:** The carbamate and organophosphate inhibitors are effective insecticides and have much shorter environmental half-lives than do the chlorinated hydrocarbons. They are inexpensive and heavily used in agriculture.

1. **Effects.** As described in Chapter 7, these agents produce increased muscarinic and nicotinic stimulation: pinpoint pupils, sweating, salivation, bronchoconstriction, vomiting, diarrhea, CNS stimulation followed by depression, and muscle fasciculations, weakness, and paralysis. The most common cause of death in mammals is respiratory failure.
2. **Treatment.** Atropine is used in large doses to control muscarinic excess; pralidoxime is used to "regenerate" cholinesterase. Mechanical ventilation may be necessary.

**D. Botanical Insecticides:**

1. **Nicotine** has the same effects on nicotinic cholinoceptors in insects as in mammals and probably kills by the same mechanism. Effects include excitation followed by paralysis of ganglionic, CNS, and neuromuscular transmission. Treatment is supportive.
2. **Rotenone** is a strong local irritant when ingested or applied to the eyes. Treatment is symptomatic.
3. **Pyrethrum alkaloids** cause excitation of the CNS and peripheral nervous system, including convulsions. Treatment is symptomatic, with anticonvulsants if necessary.

## HERBICIDES

**A. Classification & Prototypes:** Paraquat and phenoxyacetic acids are the 2 major groups in this class.

**B. Paraquat:** Paraquat is used extensively and is relatively nontoxic unless ingested. If it is ingested, eg, in a suicide attempt, the initial effect is irritation with hematemesis and bloody stools. Within a few days, signs of pulmonary impairment occur and are usually progressive, resulting in severe pulmonary fibrosis and, often, death. No antidote is available; the best supportive treatment, including gastric lavage and dialysis, still results in less than 50% survival after ingestion of as little as 5 mL.

**C. Phenoxyacetic Acids:** 2,4-Dichlorophenoxyacetic acid (2,4-D) and 2,4,5-trichlorophenoxyacetic acid (2,4,5-T) are the 2 most important members of this group. During the manufacturing process, a contaminant, 2,3,7,8-tetrachlorodibenzo-*p*-dioxin (TCDD or dioxin) is produced. Acute exposure to TCDD causes teratogenic effects in some animals and dermatitis and chloracne in humans. No long-term toxic effects other than acne scarring have been documented in humans.

## POLYCHLORINATED BIPHENYLS

The polychlorinated biphenyls (PCBs) constitute a large group of related compounds. They are among the most stable organic compounds known and are poorly metabolized and lipophilic. They are therefore highly persistent in the environment and accumulate in the food chain. They were used extensively in manufacturing electrical equipment until their potential for environmental damage was recognized. The effects of PCBs are highly species-specific. In humans, the best documented effects involve the skin and include dermatitis and chloracne. Other effects include hepatic enzyme elevation and increased plasma triglycerides.

## QUESTIONS

**DIRECTIONS (items 1 and 2):** Each numbered item or incomplete statement in this section is followed by answers or by completions of the statement. Select the ONE lettered answer or completion that is BEST in each case.

**1.** All of the following are important air pollutants EXCEPT
**(A)** sulfur dioxide
**(B)** malathion
**(C)** ozone
**(D)** nitrogen dioxide
**(E)** carbon monoxide

**2.** Correct pairings of toxic agent with the best method of treatment include all of the following EXCEPT
**(A)** carbon monoxide: 100% or hyperbaric oxygen
**(B)** parathion: atropine and pralidoxime
**(C)** nitrogen dioxide: nonspecific treatment of noncardiogenic pulmonary edema
**(D)** carbon tetrachloride: support of vital signs
**(E)** paraquat: hemodialysis

**DIRECTIONS (items 3–5):** Items 3–5 consist of lettered headings followed by a set of numbered phrases. For each numbered phrase, select the ONE lettered heading that is most closely associated with it. Each lettered heading may be selected once, more than once, or not at all.

**(A)** Parathion
**(B)** Pyrethrum
**(C)** Dioxin
**(D)** Paraquat
**(E)** Polychlorinated biphenyl

**3.** Contaminant in the manufacture of a herbicide

**4.** Extremely stable compound previously used in the manufacture of electrical devices

**5.** Convulsant derived from a botanical source

## ANSWERS

**1.** Malathion is an organophosphate insecticide. It is not an air pollutant. The answer is **(B)**.

**2.** Hemodialysis is of no value in paraquat poisoning. The answer is **(E)**.

**3.** Dioxin is a contaminant in the manufacture of 2,4-D and 2,4,5-T. The answer is **(C)**.

**4.** The polychlorinated biphenyls are extremely stable lipid soluble organic insulators used in electrical transformers and switches. The answer is **(E)**.

**5.** Pyrethrum is a convulsant derived from plants. The answer is **(B)**.

# Chelators & Heavy Metals 59

## OBJECTIVES

**Define the following terms:**

- Chelator
- Erethism
- Minamata disease
- Pica
- Plumbism

**List or describe the following:**

- The general mechanism of metal chelation.
- Important chelator drugs.
- The major clinical features and treatment of acute and chronic lead poisoning.
- The major clinical features and treatment of arsenic poisoning.
- The major clinical features and treatment of inorganic and organic mercury poisoning.

## CONCEPTS

The metals of interest in this chapter are those that frequently cause significant toxicity in humans, especially lead, arsenic, and mercury. Chelators are organic compounds with 2 or more electronegative groups that can form stable covalent-coordinate bonds with cationic metal atoms. As emphasized in this chapter, these stable complexes are often readily excreted, thus reducing the toxicity of the metal.

### CHELATORS

The most useful chelators for clinical purposes are dimercaprol (BAL), penicillamine, edetate (EDTA), and deferoxamine.

**A. Dimercaprol:** Dimercaprol (2,3-dimercaptopropanol) is useful in **arsenic, lead, mercury,** and **cadmium** poisoning. It is a bidentate chelator; ie, it forms 2 bonds with the metal ion and permits its rapid excretion. Dimercaprol is an oily liquid that must be given parenterally. It causes a high incidence of minor to moderate adverse effects, possibly because it is very lipophilic and enters cells readily. These effects include transient hypertension and tachycardia, headache, nausea, vomiting, and paresthesias. Agents chemically similar to dimercaprol that are active by the oral route are being sought. The most promising dimercaprol analogue is 2,3-dimercaptosuccinic acid **(DMSA, dimercaprol succimer).** This agent appears to be more effective and less toxic than dimercaprol in mercury and arsenic poisoning, as well as lead intoxication.

**B. Penicillamine & N-Acetylpenicillamine:** Penicillamine (D-penicillamine) is a derivative of penicillin. It is water-soluble, well absorbed from the gastrointestinal tract, and excreted unchanged. It, too, is a bidentate chelator, forming 2 bonds with the metal ion. Its major use is in the treatment of copper poisoning and Wilson's disease. It is sometimes used as adjunctive therapy in **gold, arsenic,** and **lead** intoxication. Serious toxicity including aplastic anemia and lupus erythematosus has been reported. N-Acetylpenicillamine is more effective than penicillamine in **mercury** poisoning.

**C. Edetate:** Edetate is a very efficient polydentate chelator of many divalent and trivalent cations (including calcium). To prevent dangerous hypocalcemia, it is given as the calcium disodium salt. Because it is very polar, it is poorly absorbed and does not enter cells. Its primary use is in the treatment of **lead** poisoning. It may cause renal tubular necrosis and a variety of less important toxicities.

**D. Deferoxamine:** Deferoxamine is a polydentate bacterial product that has an extremely selective affinity for iron. Fortunately, it competes poorly for heme iron (in hemoglobin and cytochromes). It is useful in the treatment of acute iron intoxication. It has also been used investigationally for aluminum chelation. When given in high doses, it may cause cataracts and retinal degeneration.

## TOXICOLOGY OF THE HEAVY METALS

**A. Lead:** Lead damages the hematopoietic tissues and liver, the nervous system, the kidneys, the gastrointestinal tract, and the reproductive system (Table 59–1).

1. **Acute lead poisoning.** Acute inorganic lead poisoning is no longer common in the USA but may occur from industrial exposures and in children who have ingested a large quantity of lead-containing paint (paint ingestion is called pica). The primary signs of this syndrome are acute abdominal colic and CNS changes. In children, the latter may take the form of an acute encephalopathy. The mortality rate is high in lead encephalopathy, and prompt chelation therapy is mandatory.
2. **Chronic lead poisoning.** Chronic inorganic lead poisoning (plumbism) is much more common than the acute form. Signs include peripheral neuropathies (wrist drop is characteristic), anorexia, anemia, tremor, weight loss, and gastrointestinal symptoms. Treatment includes removal from the source of exposure and chelation therapy, usually with edetate (severe cases), dimercaprol, or penicillamine. In workers exposed to lead, prophylaxis by means of oral chelating agents is contraindicated, since some evidence suggests that lead absorption may be enhanced. However, high dietary calcium is indicated, since lead retention is reduced.
3. **Organic lead poisoning.** Poisoning by organic lead is usually due to tetraethyl or tetramethyl antiknock gasoline additives. This form of lead is readily absorbed through the skin and lungs. The primary signs of intoxication occur in the CNS and include hallucinations, headache, irritability, convulsions, and coma. Treatment consists of decontamination and seizure control.

**B. Arsenic:** This element is widely used in industrial processes and is also present in the natural environment. Although it exists in both trivalent and pentavalent forms, its toxicity is entirely due to the trivalent form.

1. **Acute arsenic poisoning.** Acute arsenic poisoning results in severe gastrointestinal discomfort, vomiting, "rice water" stools, and capillary damage with dehydration and shock (Table 59–1). Treatment involves supportive therapy to replace water and electrolytes and chelation with dimercaprol.
2. **Chronic arsenic poisoning.** Chronic arsenic intoxication is manifested by skin changes, hair loss, bone marrow depression and anemia, and chronic nausea and gastrointestinal disturbances. Dimercaprol therapy appears to be of value.
3. **Arsine gas.** Arsine gas ($AsH_3$) causes a unique form of toxicity characterized by massive hemolysis. Pigment overload from red cell breakdown may cause renal failure. Treatment is supportive.

**C. Mercury:**

1. **Acute mercury poisoning.** Acute mercury poisoning usually occurs through inhalation of inorganic elemental mercury. It causes chest pain, shortness of breath, nausea and vomiting, kidney damage, gastroenteritis, and CNS damage (Table 59–1). Chelation is achieved with dimercaprol.
2. **Chronic mercury poisoning.** Chronic mercury poisoning may occur with inorganic or organic mercury. Inorganic mercury poisoning in the chronic form usually presents as a diffuse set of symptoms involving the gums and teeth, gastrointestinal disturbances, and neurologic and behavioral changes. When mercury was used in the hat-making industry, the latter personality effects (erethism) were so common that they gave rise to the epithet "mad as a hatter." Chronic inorganic mercury intoxication has been treated with penicillamine as well as dimercaprol.
3. **Organic mercury poisoning.** Intoxication with organic mercury compounds was first recognized in connection with an epidemic of neurologic and psychiatric disease in the village of Minamata in Japan. The outbreak was found to be the result of consumption of fish containing

**Table 59–1.** Toxicology of lead, arsenic, and mercury.[1]

| | Form Entering Body | Route of Absorption | Distribution | Target Organs for Toxicity | Metabolism | Elimination |
|---|---|---|---|---|---|---|
| Lead | Inorganic lead oxides and salts | Gastrointestinal, respiratory, skin (minor) | Bone (90%), teeth, hair, blood (erythrocytes), liver, kidneys | Hematopoietic system, CNS, kidneys, neuromuscular junction | Dissociation and binding of lead to critical tissue sulfhydryl groups | Urine and feces (major); sweat (minor) |
| | Organic (tetraethyl lead) | Skin (major), gastrointestinal | Liver | CNS | Hepatic dealkylation (fast) → trialkylmetabolites (slow) → dissociation to lead | Urine and feces (major); sweat (minor) |
| Arsenic | Inorganic arsenic salts | Gastrointestinal, skin, respiratory (all mucous surfaces) | Red cells (95–99% bound to globin) (24 hours); then to liver, lungs, kidneys, wall of gastrointestinal tract, spleen, muscle, nerve tissue (2 weeks); then to skin, hair, and bone (years) | Increased vascular permeability leading to vasodilatation and vascular collapse; uncoupling of oxidative phosphorylation resulting in impaired cellular metabolism | Binds to cellular sulfhydryl groups of critical enzymes to form stable cyclic thioarsenicals; substitutes for inorganic phosphorus in synthesis of high-energy phosphates | Principally renal; sweat and feces minor |
| Mercury | Elemental mercury | Respiratory tract | CNS (where it is trapped as $Hg^{2+}$), kidneys (following conversion of elemental Hg to $Hg^{2+}$) | CNS (neuropsychiatric owing to elemental Hg and its $Hg^{2+}$ metabolite), kidneys (owing to conversion of elemental Hg to $Hg^{2+}$) | Elemental Hg converted to $Hg^{2+}$ | Urine (major); feces (minor) |
| | Inorganic $Hg^{+}$ (less toxic); $Hg^{2+}$ (more toxic) | Gastrointestinal, skin (minor) | Kidneys (predominant), blood, brain (minor) | Kidneys, gastrointestinal tract | $Hg^{2+}$ plus R–SH converted to $Hg^{+}$ –S–R, $Hg(S–R)_2$ | Urine |
| | Organic: alkyl, aryl, alkoxyalkyl | Gastrointestinal, skin | Kidneys, brain, blood | CNS | R–$Hg^{+}$ converted to $Hg^{2+}$ plus R (slow) | Urine |

[1]Modified and reproduced, with permission, from Katzung BG (editor): *Basic & Clinical Pharmacology,* 5th ed. Appleton & Lange, 1992.

a high content of methylmercury, which was produced in seawater from mercury in the effluent of a nearby vinyl plastics manufacturing plant. Similar epidemics have resulted from the consumption of grain intended for use as seed and treated with fungicidal organic mercury compounds. Treatment with chelators has been tried, but the benefits are uncertain.

## QUESTIONS

**DIRECTIONS (item 1):** The numbered incomplete statement in this section is followed by completions of the statement. Select the ONE lettered completion that is BEST.

**1.** Effects commonly associated with acute or subacute lead poisoning include all of the following EXCEPT
**(A)** abdominal pain
**(B)** headache
**(C)** lead "lines" (deposits) in the gums
**(D)** encephalopathy
**(E)** anemia

**DIRECTIONS: (items 2–5):** Items 2–5 consist of lettered headings followed by a set of numbered phrases. For each numbered phrase, select the ONE lettered heading that is most closely associated with it. Each lettered heading may be selected once, more than once, or not at all.

**(A)** Trivalent arsenic
**(B)** Methylmercury
**(C)** Dimercaprol
**(D)** Penicillamine
**(E)** Edetate calcium disodium

**2.** Produced in seawater by the action of bacteria and algae; synthesized for use as a fungicide

**3.** Used in the treatment of Wilson's disease and in copper, arsenic, and lead poisoning

**4.** Causes severe diarrhea, abdominal pain, and bone marrow depression

**5.** An oily chelator with high lipid solubility that readily enters cells

## ANSWERS

**1.** Lead lines are uncommon even in chronic lead poisoning. The answer is **(C).**

**2.** The answer is **(B),** methylmercury.

**3.** The answer is **(D),** penicillamine.

**4.** The answer is **(A),** trivalent arsenic.

**5.** The answer is **(C),** dimercaprol.

# Management of the Poisoned Patient

# 60

## OBJECTIVES

**Define the following terms:**

- Anion gap
- Hemodialysis
- Hemoperfusion
- Osmolar gap
- Specific antidote
- Toxicodynamics
- Toxicokinetics
- Universal antidote

**List or describe the following:**

- The most common causes of death in poisonings caused by sedative-hypnotics, narcotics, cocaine, paraquat, digitalis, and tricyclic antidepressants.
- Specific antidotes for heroin and other narcotics, acetaminophen, methanol and ethylene glycol, and parathion.
- The emergency treatment (before laboratory results are available) of a comatose patient.
- The contraindications to the use of emesis for treatment of a patient who has ingested a toxin.

## CONCEPTS

Most chemicals are capable of causing toxic effects. These agents include drugs usually used for therapeutic purposes as well as agricultural and industrial chemicals that have no medical applications. Many toxic effects of therapeutic agents have been discussed in previous chapters; the difference between obtaining a therapeutic action rather than a toxic one is usually a matter of dose. The nontherapeutic chemicals most commonly involved in poisonings are those readily accessible in the environment: solvents, corrosives, insecticides, drugs of abuse, and heavy metals. This chapter reviews the general pharmacology of such poisonings.

A. **General Principles:** The term **toxicokinetics** is sometimes applied to the pharmacokinetics of toxic doses of chemicals, because the toxic effects of an agent—on the heart, liver, or kidneys—may alter normal mechanisms of absorption, metabolism, or excretion of a foreign chemical. Similarly, the term **toxicodynamics** may be used to denote the altered pharmacodynamics of a drug when given in toxic dosage, since normal receptor and effector mechanisms may be altered.

B. **Cause of Death in Intoxicated Patients:** The most common causes of death from drug overdose in the USA reflect the drug groups most often selected for abuse or for suicide. Sedative-hypnotics and narcotics cause respiratory depression, coma, aspiration of gastric contents, and other respiratory malfunctions. Stimulants such as cocaine, phencyclidine (PCP), tricyclic antidepressants, and theophylline cause convulsions, which may lead to aspiration of gastric contents following vomiting, and postictal respiratory depression. Tricyclic antidepressants and cardiac glycosides cause dangerous and frequently lethal arrhythmias. Severe hypotension may occur with any of these drugs. A few intoxicants cause direct liver and kidney damage. These include acetaminophen and mushroom poisons of the *Amanita phalloides* type, certain inhalants, and some heavy metals. The metals are discussed in Chapter 59.

C. **Identification of Poisons:** Many intoxicants cause a characteristic syndrome of clinical and laboratory changes. A summary of some of these toxic syndromes is given in Table 60–1. When the chemical used in a case of poisoning cannot be directly examined and identified, the clinician must rely on indirect means of identifying the type of intoxication and the progress of therapy. In addition to the history and physical examination, certain laboratory examinations of blood may

**Table 60–1.** Toxic syndromes.[1]

**Acetaminophen**
Mild anorexia, nausea, vomiting, delayed jaundice, hepatic and renal failure

**Amphetamines**
Toxic psychosis, hyperthermia, flushing, increased blood pressure, dilated pupils, hallucinations, seizures, tachycardia, rhabdomyolysis

**Antifreeze (ethylene glycol)**
Renal failure, crystals in urine, anion and osmolar gap, initial CNS excitation, but eye examination normal

**Arsenic**
Early: garlic on breath, vomiting, profuse bloody diarrhea, burning tears; delayed: hair loss, lines on nails, neuropathy, increased skin pigmentation; arsine gas: hemolysis

**Botulism**
Dysphagia, dysarthria, ptosis, opthalmoplegia, muscle weakness; incubation period 12–36 h

**Bromide**
Increased pigmentation, acne, dementia, psychosis, hyperchloremia

**Cadmium**
Metallic taste, delayed pulmonary edema; late: kidney and lung disease

**Carbon monoxide**
Coma, metabolic acidosis, normal $PaO_2$, retinal hemorrhages

**Cocaine**
Perforated nasal septum, dilated pupils, psychosis, tachycardia, convulsions

**Cyanide**
Bitter-almond odor, convulsions, coma, abnormal ECG

**Gasoline**
Distinctive odor, coughing, pulmonary infiltrates

**Heroin**
Coma, decreased blood pressure, bradycardia, hypoventilation, miosis, needle marks, rapid response to naloxone

**Hydrocarbons**
Pneumonia, tinnitus, convulsions, ventricular fibrillation, unique odor

**Hydrogen sulfide**
Rotten egg smell, loss of sense of smell, sudden collapse and death

**Iron**
Bloody diarrhea, coma, radiopaque material in gut (seen on x-ray film), high leukocyte count, hyperglycemia

**Isopropyl alcohol**
Gastritis, ketonemia with normoglycemia, osmolar gap

**Lead**
Abdominal pain, increased blood pressure, convulsions, muscle weakness, metallic taste, anorexia, encephalopathy, delayed motor neuropathy, subtle changes in renal and reproductive function

**LSD**
Hallucinations, dilated pupils, hypertension

**Mercury**
Acute renal failure, tremor, salivation, gingivitis, colitis, erethism (fits of crying, irrational behavior), nephrotic syndrome

**Methyl alcohol (methanol)**
Rapid respirations, visual symptoms, osmolar gap, severe metabolic acidosis

**Methylene chloride**
History of paint-stripping exposure; confusion, increased carbon monoxide level

**Mushrooms**
Severe nausea and vomiting 8 hours after ingestion; delayed hepatic and renal failure with *Amanita phalloides*

**Nitrogen oxides**
History of silo or cave exposure; delayed pulmonary edema, chronic chemical pneumonitis

**Organophosphates or carbamates**
Miotic pupils, abdominal cramps, salivation, lacrimation, urination, increased bronchial secretions, muscle fasciculations, bradycardia

**Paraquat**
Oropharyngeal burning, headache, vomiting, delayed pulmonary fibrosis and death

**Phencyclidine (PCP)**
Coma with eyes open, hyperacusis, myoclonic jerks, vertical nystagmus, violent behavior

**Phosgene**
History of exposure to burning plastics; pulmonary edema

**Plants, poisonous**

**Nightshade family, Jimson weed**
Hallucinations, dilated pupils, seizures (contain atropinelike alkaloids)

**Oleander and foxglove**
Digitalislike poisoning

**Predatory bean (rosary pea)**
Delayed severe gastrointestinal distress, seizures, hemolytic anemia, death

**Strychnine**
Stiff neck, status epilepticus, hyperacusis

**Thallium (rat poison)**
Alopecia, gastrointestinal distress, motor and sensory neuropathy, hematologic examination normal

**Vacor (rat poison)**
Ketoacidosis, postural hypotension

**Vanadium**
Green tongue, severe pulmonary irritation

[1]Modified and reproduced, with permission, from Katzung BG (editor): *Basic & Clinical Pharmacology,* 3rd ed. Appleton & Lange, 1987.

be useful. A few intoxicants can be directly identified in the blood or urine, especially if there are reasons in the history for narrowing the search. In the more common situation (a comatose patient unable to provide a history), general tests for replacement of anions or osmotic equivalents in the blood (anion gap, osmolar gap) may be useful. A few intoxicants can be identified or strongly suspected on the basis of electrocardiographic or radiologic findings.

1. **Osmolar gap.** The osmolar gap is the difference between the measured osmolarity (measured by the freezing point depression method) and the predicted osmolarity:

$$\textbf{Gap} = \textbf{Osm (measured)} - [(2 \times Na^+ [meq/L]) + (Glucose [mg/dL] \div 18) + (BUN [mg/dL] \div 3)]$$

   This gap is normally zero. A significant gap is produced by high serum levels of low-molecular-weight intoxicants such as ethanol, methanol, and ethylene glycol.

2. **Anion gap.** The anion gap is the difference between the sum of the 2 primary cations, sodium and potassium, and the sum of the 2 primary anions, chloride and bicarbonate:

$$\textbf{Gap} = (Na^+ + K^+) - (HCO_3^- + Cl^-)$$

   This gap is normally 12–16 meq/L. A significant increase may be produced by diabetic ketoacidosis, renal failure, or drug-induced metabolic acidosis (from aspirin, methanol, ethylene glycol, isoniazid, and iron).

**D. Treatment of Poisoning:** Management of the poisoned patient consists of **maintenance of vital functions, decontamination, enhancement of elimination,** and, in a very few instances, the use of a **specific antidote.**

1. **Vital functions.** The most important aspect of treatment of a poisoned patient is maintenance of vital functions. Of these, the most commonly endangered or impaired is respiration. Therefore, an open and protected airway must be established first and effective ventilation ensured. The cardiac rhythm should be determined, and if ventricular fibrillation is present, it must be corrected at once. The blood pressure should be measured, but immediate treatment is rarely needed except in cases of traumatic hemorrhage. *Because of the danger of brain damage from hypoglycemia, intravenous glucose (50% solution) should be given to comatose patients immediately after blood has been drawn for laboratory tests and before laboratory results have been obtained.* Similarly, thiamine should be given to prevent Wernicke's syndrome in alcoholics.
2. **Decontamination.** Decontamination consists of removing any unabsorbed poison from the patient's body. In the case of ingested noncorrosive toxins, this may involve inducing vomiting (emesis) by means of **syrup of ipecac** if the patient is conscious. *Apomorphine and extract of ipecac are dangerous emetics and should not be used.* In unconscious patients, emesis will lead to aspiration into the respiratory tree and must be avoided. Gastric lavage with a large-bore tube may be used to remove noncorrosive drugs from the stomach of a comatose patient *if the airway has been protected with a cuffed endotracheal tube.* Corrosives (strong acids and bases) may cause severe esophageal damage if emesis is induced. These agents should be diluted (not neutralized) in the stomach. Activated charcoal, given orally or by stomach tube, may be very effective in adsorbing any remaining drug. Cathartics may be useful in enhancing the removal of unabsorbed drug from the intestine. In the case of topical exposure (insecticides, solvents), the clothing should be removed and the patient washed to remove any chemical still present on the skin. Medical personnel must be careful not to contaminate themselves during this procedure.
3. **Enhancement of elimination.** Enhancement of elimination is possible for a number of intoxicants. These methods include manipulation of urine pH to accelerate urinary excretion of weak acids and bases and hemodialysis or hemoperfusion to enhance the elimination of certain other compounds.
4. **Antidotes.** Specific antidotes exist for only a few poisons (Table 60–2). It must be remembered that the duration of action of most antidotes is shorter than that of the intoxicant and hence the antidotes may have to be given repeatedly. The use of chelating agents for metal poisoning is discussed in Chapter 59.

**E. Snake Bite:** The most common dangerous snake in the USA is the rattlesnake. Although bites are common, severe envenomation is infrequent.

**Table 60–2.** Specific antidotes.[1]

| Antidote | Poison(s) |
|---|---|
| Acetylcysteine | Acetaminophen |
| Atropine | Anticholinesterases |
| Deferoxamine | Iron salts |
| Ethanol | Methanol, ethylene glycol |
| Metal chelators<br>N-Acetylpenicillamine | Mercury |
| Calcium disodium edetate (CaEDTA) | Lead |
| Dimercaprol (BAL) | Arsenic, gold, mercury |
| Penicillamine | Copper, lead, gold |
| Naloxone | Narcotic drugs, propoxyphene, pentazocine, diphenoxylate |
| Physostigmine salicylate | May be considered for antimuscarinic anticholinergic agents |
| Pralidoxime (2-PAM) | Organophosphates |

[1]Modified and reproduced, with permission, from Katzung BG (editor): *Basic & Clinical Pharmacology,* 5th ed. Appleton & Lange, 1992.

1. **Effects.** Snake venom contains a large number of enzymes and tissue toxins. The most common effects of envenomation include local tissue necrosis, vascular damage, thrombosis, hemorrhage, and neural injury.
2. **Treatment.** It is well documented that once-popular remedies such as incision and suction, ice packs, and tourniquets are usually more dangerous than helpful. The most important prehospital therapy is to minimize movement of the bitten part to reduce the spread of the venom in the tissues. Effective therapy consists of an adequate dosage of **antivenin.** Since antivenins are prepared in horses, serum sickness frequently follows and may also require therapy.

## QUESTIONS

**DIRECTIONS (items 1–3):** Each numbered item or incomplete statement in this section is followed by answers or by completions of the statement. Select the ONE lettered answer or completion that is BEST in each case.

**1.** All of the following may cause an osmolar gap EXCEPT
  **(A)** ethylene glycol
  **(B)** ethanol
  **(C)** digoxin
  **(D)** methanol
  **(E)** isopropanol

**2.** Regarding snake bites,
  **(A)** rattlesnake bite is almost always associated with significant tissue injury
  **(B)** a snake bite should be treated in the field by incision, suction, and a tourniquet before the victim is moved
  **(C)** the most common manifestation of serious envenomation is convulsions
  **(D)** when a victim of serious envenomation reaches the hospital, the most effective therapy is prompt administration of snake antivenin
  **(E)** all of the above are correct

**3.** Intoxicants correctly associated with their effects include
   **(A)** carbon monoxide: carboxyhemoglobinemia
   **(B)** paraquat: pulmonary fibrosis
   **(C)** cyanide: cytochrome inactivation
   **(D)** sodium nitrite: methemoglobinemia
   **(E)** all of the above

**DIRECTIONS (items 4–8):** Items 4–8 consist of lettered headings followed by a set of numbered sentences. For each numbered sentence, select the ONE lettered heading that is most closely associated with it. Each lettered heading may be selected once, more than once, or not at all.

   **(A)** Heroin
   **(B)** Acetaminophen
   **(C)** Methanol
   **(D)** Parathion
   **(E)** Theophylline

**4.** The best antidote is atropine

**5.** The best antidote is an anticonvulsant but beta-blockers are sometimes appropriate

**6.** The best antidote is naloxone

**7.** The best antidote is ethanol

**8.** The best antidote is acetylcysteine

## ANSWERS

**1.** Digoxin is lethal at levels much too low to be detected by the osmolar gap method. This method is useful only for poisonings with relatively less potent substances of low molecular weight such as methanol and ethylene glycol. The answer is **(C).**

**2.** Only about 20% of rattlesnake bites involve significant envenomation. Incision, suction, and tourniquets are usually more damaging than helpful. Ice packs are contraindicated. Serious envenomation causes primarily local tissue damage. Antivenin is by far the most effective therapy for serious envenomation. The answer is **(D).**

**3.** All are correct. The answer is **(E).**

**4.** The answer is **(D),** parathion (see Table 60–2).

**5.** The most dangerous toxic effect of theophylline is convulsions. Cardiovascular toxicity (arrhythmias, hypotension) often responds to beta-blockers. The answer is **(E).**

**6.** The answer is **(A),** heroin (see Table 60–2).

**7.** The answer is **(C),** methanol (see Table 60–2).

**8.** The answer is **(B),** acetaminophen (see Table 60–2).

# Part X. Special Topics

# Drug Interactions 61

## OBJECTIVES

**Define the following terms:**

- Antagonism
- Enzyme induction
- Pharmacokinetic interaction
- Pharmacodynamic interaction
- Potentiation
- Synergism

**You should be able to:**

- Describe the mechanisms of the acute interaction between alcohol and barbiturates and between alcohol and disulfiram.
- Describe the mechanism of the interaction between barbiturates and warfarin.
- Describe the interaction between quinidine and digoxin.

## CONCEPTS

### A. Classification:

1. **Drug interactions.** These are actions of a drug in the body that are the result of, or affect the actions of, another drug. Usually such actions are quantitative—ie, an increase or a decrease in the size of an expected response. Interactions may be the result of pharmacokinetic alterations, pharmacodynamic changes, or a combination of both.
2. **Drug incompatibilities.** Interactions between drugs in vitro (eg, precipitation in intravenous administration solutions) are generally classified as incompatibilities.

### B. Pharmacokinetic Interactions:

1. **Absorption** from the gut may be influenced by agents that bind the drug (eg, resins, antacids, calcium-containing foods) and by agents that increase or decrease gastrointestinal motility (metoclopramide or antimuscarinics, respectively). Problems caused by slowed gastric emptying may not be expected, because the antimuscarinic action is often an unwanted effect of, eg, an antihistamine or antidepressant agent. Absorption from subcutaneous sites may be slowed predictably by vasoconstrictors given simultaneously (eg, local anesthetics and epinephrine).
2. **Distribution** and volume of distribution may be altered by drugs that compete for binding sites (eg, quinidine can displace digoxin) or alter the size of the physical compartment in which another drug distributes (eg, diuretics can reduce the total body water in which aminoglycosides distribute).
3. **Metabolism** may be increased by drugs (eg, barbiturates) that cause induction of hepatic drug-metabolizing enzymes or may be decreased by a variety of drugs (eg, cimetidine, monoamine oxidase [MAO] inhibitors) that inhibit enzymes.
4. **Excretion** of drugs by the kidneys may be changed by drugs that reduce renal blood flow (eg, beta-blockers) or inhibit specific renal transport mechanisms (eg, the action of probenicid on penicillin secretion).

### C. Pharmacodynamic Interactions:

1. **Antagonism,** the simplest type of drug interaction, is often predictable (eg, block of

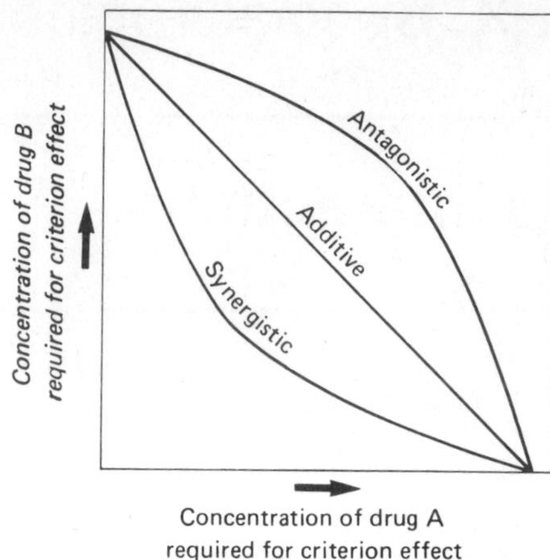


**Figure 61–1.** Isobologram showing possible interactions between 2 antimicrobials. The criterion effect is defined in setting up the assay and may be a specific bacteriostatic or bactericidal end point. The lines cross the ordinate at the concentration of drug *B* that is required to achieve the criterion effect when drug *B* is used alone. Similarly, the lines cross the abscissa at the concentration required for drug *A* alone to achieve the same effect. (Reproduced, with permission, from Katzung BG [editor]: *Basic & Clinical Pharmacology,* 5th ed. Appleton & Lange, 1992.)

$beta_2$-mediated bronchodilation by beta-blockers given for another condition). Antagonism by mixed agonist-antagonist drugs (eg, nalbuphine) or by partial agonists (eg, pindolol) is not as easily predicted but should be expected when such drugs are used with pure agonists. The interaction of a partial agonist with a pure agonist is described quantitatively by the antagonism curve in Fig 61–1.

2. **Additive interaction** describes the result of algebraic summing of the effects of 2 drugs. It is most often seen when 2 or more drugs that act on the same receptor are used (eg, 3 sulfonamides in triple sulfas) (Fig 61–1).
3. **Synergism** ("working together") is a term usually used to describe interactions that are more than additive (superadditive; Fig 61–1). Such interactions are more likely to result if the 2 drugs act on different receptors in a sequence or cascade (eg, sulfonamide and trimethoprim actions on folate synthesis in bacteria).
4. **Potentiation** is often confused with or used as a synonym for synergism. However, the term is probably best reserved for situations in which a drug that has no effect on a given variable greatly amplifies the response of that variable to another drug which normally has a much smaller effect on it.

**D. Clinical Importance of Drug Interactions:** Although many drug interactions have been documented, only a few are of clinical significance and require a change of drug. Some of these are listed in Table 61–1. Most often, a change in dosage is sufficient to correct any problems. In patients taking several drugs, the likelihood of significant drug interactions is high. This is especially true in elderly patients, because they often have age-related changes in drug clearance.

**Table 61–1.** Examples of drug interactions.

| Drug Causing the Interaction | Drugs Affected | Mechanism | Result of the Interaction |
|---|---|---|---|
| Alcohol | Other sedative-hypnotics | Pharmacodynamic | Additive sedation, ataxia, and depression |
| Antacids | Iron supplements, tetracyclines | Pharmacokinetic | Possible binding of drugs and prevention of their absorption |
| Antidepressants | Drugs with antimuscarinic effects | Pharmacodynamic | Additive antimuscarinic action, possibly leading to urinary retention, glaucoma, etc. |
| Antimuscarinics | Drugs absorbed from the small intestine | Pharmacokinetic | Slowed absorption because gastric emptying is delayed |
| Antihistamines ($H_1$ blockers) | Antimuscarinics | Pharmacodynamic | Additive block of muscarinic receptors |
| Barbiturates (especially phenobarbital) | Drugs metabolized by P-450-dependent liver enzymes | Pharmacokinetic | Increased metabolism because of enzyme induction |
| | Other sedative-hypnotics and antihistamines | Pharmacodynamic | Additive sedation, ataxia |
| Bile acid-binding resins | Digitalis, thyroid, acetaminophen | Pharmacokinetic | Binding of drug and reduced absorption |
| Carbamazepine | Doxycycline, estrogen | Pharmacokinetic | Increased metabolism because of enzyme induction |
| Cimetidine | Benzodiazepines, lidocaine, phenytoin, quinidine, theophylline, warfarin | Pharmacokinetic | Decreased metabolism because cimetidine inhibits hepatic enzymes |
| Disulfiram | Alcohol | Pharmacokinetic | Inhibition of degradation and resultant accumulation of acetaldehyde |
| Monoamine oxidase (MAO) inhibitors | Many amines, eg, phenylephrine | Pharmacokinetic | Decreased phenylephrine metabolism, prolonged action |
| | Indirect-acting sympathomimetics, including tyramine in foods | Pharmacodynamic | Increased hypertensive action because MAO inhibitors increase stores of norepinephrine |
| Nonsteroidal anti-inflammatory drugs (NSAIDs) | Anticoagulants | Pharmacodynamic | Increased risk of bleeding because NSAIDs interfere with platelet function |
| | Angiotensin-converting enzyme inhibitors | Pharmacodynamic | Decreased antihypertensive action |
| Phenytoin | Drugs metabolized in the liver | Pharmacokinetic | Increased metabolism because of enzyme induction |
| Quinidine | Digoxin | Pharmacokinetic | Displacement of digoxin from binding sites, with rise in digoxin plasma concentration |
| Rifampin | Drugs metabolized in the liver | Pharmacokinetic | Increased metabolism because of enzyme induction |
| Thiazides | Digitalis | Pharmacodynamic | Increased digitalis toxicity because of potassium loss |
| | Lithium | Pharmacokinetic | Reduced lithium clearance by the kidney |

## QUESTIONS

**DIRECTIONS (items 1–3):** Each numbered item or incomplete statement in this section is followed by answers or by completions of the statement. Select the ONE lettered answer or completion that is BEST in each case.

**1.** The risk of digitalis toxicity may be significantly increased by
(A) triamterene
(B) lidocaine
(C) captopril
(D) hydrochlorothiazide
(E) propranolol

**2.** Thiazides often reduce the excretion of
(A) phenothiazine antipsychotics
(B) tricyclic antidepressants
(C) second-generation antidepressants
(D) lithium
(E) potassium ion

**3.** Pharmacokinetic interactions include
(A) cimetidine interaction with phenytoin
(B) interaction of antidepressants with antimuscarinics
(C) interaction of aspirin with warfarin
(D) interaction of benzodiazepines with alcohol
(E) interaction of beta-blockers with aerosol antiasthmatic medications

**DIRECTIONS (items 4–8):** Items 4–8 consist of lettered headings followed by a set of numbered sentences. For each numbered sentence, select the ONE lettered heading that is most closely associated with it. Each lettered heading may be selected once, more than once, or not at all.

(A) Ibuprofen
(B) Heparin
(C) Tetracycline
(D) Trimethoprim
(E) Rifampin

**4.** This antibiotic is a potent inducer of hepatic drug-metabolizing enzymes

**5.** This drug interferes with the antihypertensive action of captopril and enalapril

**6.** This drug has a useful synergistic interaction with sulfonamides

**7.** This agent is absorbed poorly if given with antacids or dairy products

**8.** This drug has no effect on platelets but is most likely to cause bleeding in patients who are also taking aspirin

## ANSWERS

**1.** The risk of digitalis toxicity may be increased by quinidine because it displaces the glycoside from binding sites and reduces its clearance. Lidocaine has no such effect. The risk is also increased by thiazides because these diuretics reduce extracellular potassium. Triamterene and captopril both tend to increase potassium. Increased potassium tends to limit or prevent digitalis toxicity. The answer is **(D)**.

2. Thiazides reduce the clearance of lithium by about 25%. They do not interfere with the clearance of the other agents mentioned, except for potassium, whose clearance is increased. The answer is **(D)**.

3. Cimetidine inhibits the enzymatic clearance of phenytoin. The other interactions listed are pharmacodynamic interactions. The answer is **(A)**.

4. Rifampin is an effective inducer of hepatic P-450 isozymes. Tetracycline, the other antibiotic listed, has no such effect. The answer is **(E)**.

5. Nonsteroidal anti-inflammatory drugs (NSAIDs) interfere with the antihypertensive action of angiotensin-converting enzyme inhibitors. The answer is **(A)**.

6. In bacterial folate synthesis, trimethoprim inhibits dihydrofolate reductase, the enzyme that follows dihydropteroate synthetase, the step inhibited by sulfonamides. The answer is **(D)**.

7. Tetracyclines form insoluble complexes with calcium and other divalent and trivalent cations. The answer is **(C)**.

8. Heparin, the prototype parenteral anticoagulant, increases the risk of bleeding if given with any other drug that interferes with hemostasis. An interaction occurs with antiplatelet drugs such as aspirin. The answer is **(B)**.

# Vaccines, Immune Globulins, & Other Complex Biologic Products — 62

## OBJECTIVES

**Define the following terms:**

- Active immunization
- Passive immunization

**You should be able to:**

- Describe the principles of and the differences between active and passive immunization.
- List the types of materials available for passive immunization and the special uses of immune globulin (ISG).
- List the types of materials available for active immunization and describe the relative merits and disadvantages of live versus dead immunogens.

## CONCEPTS

**A. Passive Immunization:** In passive immunization, **preformed antibodies** of human or animal origin are used to transfer immunity to the host. Such materials, usually **immunoglobulins,** may contain high titers of specific antibodies or be relatively nonspecific (eg, **immune globulin, ISG**). Their clinical uses include prevention or amelioration of diseases after exposure (eg, hepatitis, measles, poliomyelitis), management of certain snake and insect bites, and treatment of hypogammaglobulinemias. The most commonly used preparation is ISG, a 25-fold concentration of gamma globulins (95% IgG) from human plasma, now available in formulations for intramuscular and intravenous use. Its biologic half-life is about 23 days, and hypersensitivity reactions are rare. ISG is used for passive immunization against hepatitis A, hypogammaglobulinemia, measles, poliomyelitis, and rubella. More specific products include diphtheria antitoxin, snake and spider antivenins, $Rh_0$(D) immune globulin, and immune globulins for hepatitis B, pertussis, rabies, tetanus, vaccinia, and varicella. Such antibodies usually have a half-life of only 5–7 days. Because animal antibodies can act as antigens in humans, allergic reactions to antibodies from nonhuman sources are more common and severe than those to antibodies from human sources.

**B. Active Immunization:** In active immunization, **antigens** are used to stimulate antibody formation and host cell-mediated immunity, giving protection against disease vectors. The major advantage of active over passive immunization is that it confers stronger host resistance by stimulating higher antibody levels. Immunization can be produced by live (attenuated) or dead (inactivated) immunogens. Live attenuated products stimulate natural resistance and confer longer-lasting immunity than dead immunogens; however, the risk of disease is greater. Examples of the use of live attenuated immunogens include the vaccines for measles, mumps, rubella, and polio. Materials containing dead immunogens include diphtheria and tetanus toxoids, rabies vaccine, and hepatitis B virus and surface antigen. Polysaccharide vaccines are also available for active immunization of selected patients at high risk of infection from *Haemophilus influenzae,* meningococci, and pneumococci. Recommended schedules for active immunization of children usually include DTP (toxins of diphtheria and tetanus with pertussis antigen), oral polio vaccine, and vaccines (separate or combined) for measles, mumps, and rubella.

## QUESTIONS

**DIRECTIONS (items 1–6):** Each numbered item or incomplete statement in this section is followed by answers or by completions of the statement. Select the ONE lettered answer or completion that is BEST in each case.

**1.** All of the following statements about immunization are accurate EXCEPT:
**(A)** Passive immunization involves the use of preformed antibodies such as human gamma globulin
**(B)** Immune globulin is not usually effective in preventing viral upper respiratory tract infections
**(C)** The use of black widow spider antivenin should be restricted to children, the only group with significant morbidity or mortality
**(D)** Antibodies from human serum have a much shorter half-life than those of animal origin

**2.** All of the following statements about active immunization are accurate EXCEPT:
**(A)** Immunization against hepatitis B involves the use of a purified and inactivated virus coat protein
**(B)** Polio vaccine containing live virus types can be administered orally
**(C)** Active immunization results in permanent protection
**(D)** Protective factors may not be stimulated by inactivated (killed) products

**3.** All of the following statements about passive immunization are accurate EXCEPT:
**(A)** Patients with IgA deficiency may develop hypersensitivity reactions to ISG
**(B)** Rabies immune globulin is recommended only in patients who demonstrate an antibody response from preexposure prophylaxis
**(C)** Equine-derived antivenins are used in the treatment of snake bite
**(D)** It is useful in the treatment of certain diseases normally prevented by active immunization (eg, tetanus)

**4.** Which of the following is used in active immunization of children, and combines bacterial toxoids with a bacterial antigen?
**(A)** BCG
**(B)** ISG
**(C)** DTP
**(D)** $Rh_o$(D)

**5.** Which of the following is a polysaccharide used for active immunization in patients with chronic cardiorespiratory ailments?
**(A)** Mumps virus vaccine
**(B)** BCG vaccine
**(C)** Pertussis immune globulin
**(D)** Pneumococcal vaccine
**(E)** Antilymphocyte immune serum

**6.** All of the following statements about $Rh_o$(D) immune globulin are accurate EXCEPT:
**(A)** It provides Rh isoimmunization from fetal-maternal transfusion
**(B)** It is ineffective if administered more than 48 hours after exposure
**(C)** It is used for nonimmune females only
**(D)** It is categorized as passive immunization

## ANSWERS

**1.** Antibodies derived from human serum not only diminish the risk of hypersensitivity, but also have a much longer half-life than those from animal sources. For example, human IgG antibodies have a half-life of 23 days, compared with 5–7 days for the antibodies derived from animals. Smaller doses of human antibodies can be administered to provide therapeutic levels for several weeks. The answer is **(D)**.

**2.** Active immunization does not a priori result in permanent protection. Primary immunization against measles, mumps, poliomyelitis, and rubella appears to be permanent, and in each case live viruses are used. However, the duration of effect of active immunization with killed virus products ranges from 6 months for case of cholera, through 1–3 years for influenza, to 3+ years for tetanus. The answer is **(C)**.

**3.** Rabies immune globulin should be given as soon as possible after exposure and must be combined with immunization with human diploid cell-derived rabies vaccine. Passive immunization is not recommended for individuals with demonstrated antibody response to preexposure prophylaxis with rabies vaccine. The answer is **(B)**.

**4.** DTP contains diphtheria and tetanus toxoids and pertussis antigen. The answer is **(C)**.

**5.** The pertussis and antilymphocyte preparations are used in passive immunization. Both the mumps vaccine and BCG (used for tuberculosis) are used in active immunization, but they are live viruses. Pneumococcal vaccine is a polysaccharide recommended for individuals at high risk for pneumococcal disease. The answer is **(D).**

**6.** Ideally, $Rh_o(D)$ should be administered to a $Rh_o(D)$-negative woman within 72 hours of abortion, amniocentesis, obstetric delivery of an Rh-positive child, or transfusion of Rh-positive blood. However, it may be effective at much greater postexposure intervals and should be given even if more than 72 hours has elapsed. The answer is **(B).**

# Appendix I.

# Examination I

## General Principles, Autonomic Drugs, Cardiovascular Drugs, Renal Drugs, Autacoids, Drugs Used in Asthma*

**DIRECTIONS (items 1–52):** Each numbered item or incomplete statement in this section is followed by answers or by completions of the statement. Select the ONE lettered answer or completion that is BEST in each case.

**1.** Common effects of muscarinic stimulant drugs include all of the following EXCEPT
**(A)** tachycardia
**(B)** increased peristalsis
**(C)** mydriasis
**(D)** stimulation of sweat glands
**(E)** increased secretion by salivary glands

**2.** A patient is admitted to the emergency department for treatment of an overdose of a drug. The identity of the drug is unknown, but it is observed that when the urine pH is acidic, the renal clearance of the drug is less than the glomerular filtration rate, and that when the urine pH is alkaline, the clearance is greater than the glomerular filtration rate. The drug is probably a
**(A)** strong base
**(B)** weak base
**(C)** nonelectrolyte
**(D)** weak acid
**(E)** strong acid

**3.** Drugs that block the alpha receptor on effector cells at adrenergic synapses cause
**(A)** reversal of the effects of norepinephrine on the blood pressure
**(B)** reversal of the effects of epinephrine on the blood pressure
**(C)** reversal of the effects of epinephrine on adenylyl cyclase
**(D)** an increase in blood glucose levels
**(E)** mydriasis

**4.** Aminophylline, dobutamine, and digoxin can each
**(A)** increase the amount of cAMP
**(B)** increase cardiac contractile force
**(C)** decrease conduction velocity in the atrioventricular node
**(D)** increase peripheral vascular resistance
**(E)** decrease venous return

**5.** The polypeptide agent with the strongest vasodilator properties is
**(A)** bradykinin
**(B)** glucagon
**(C)** methysergide
**(D)** prostacyclin
**(E)** angiotensin II

*Examination I covers Chapters 1–20 of this review.

**6.** Common adverse effects of cimetidine include
**(A)** agranulocytosis
**(B)** systemic lupus erythematosus
**(C)** inhibition of hepatic metabolism of other drugs
**(D)** antiestrogenic effects
**(E)** hypertension

**7.** One property of quinidine that is not associated with procainamide is its
**(A)** ability to control atrial arrhythmias
**(B)** tendency to produce cinchonism
**(C)** activity by the oral route
**(D)** prolongation of the PR interval
**(E)** prolongation of the QRS interval

**8.** A patient discharged from the hospital after a myocardial infarction is receiving small doses of quinidine to suppress a ventricular tachycardia. One month later, his local physician prescribes high-dose hydrochlorothiazide therapy for the treatment of ankle edema, which he ascribes to congestive heart failure. Three weeks after beginning thiazide therapy, the patient is readmitted to the hospital with a rapid multifocal ventricular tachycardia. The most probable cause of this arrhythmia is
**(A)** quinidine toxicity caused by inhibition of quinidine metabolism by the thiazide
**(B)** direct effects of hydrochlorothiazide on the pacemaker of the heart
**(C)** thiazide toxicity caused by the effects of quinidine on the kidneys
**(D)** reduction of serum sodium caused by the diuretic action of hydrochlorothiazide
**(E)** reduction of serum potassium caused by the diuretic action of hydrochlorothiazide

**9.** Important therapeutic or toxic effects of loop diuretics when used in the treatment of hypertension include
**(A)** decreased heart rate
**(B)** decreased blood volume
**(C)** increased total body potassium
**(D)** metabolic acidosis
**(E)** increased serum sodium

**10.** Contraindications to the use of oral propranolol include
**(A)** glaucoma
**(B)** migraine
**(C)** benign prostatic hypertrophy
**(D)** asthma
**(E)** hypertension

**11.** Soon after being put to bed for a nap, a 4-year-old child is found convulsing. Diarrhea and a warm, moist skin are apparent. The heart rate is 70/min, and the pupils are markedly constricted. Drug intoxication is suspected. The most probable cause is
**(A)** an organophosphate-containing insecticide
**(B)** a nicotine-containing insecticide
**(C)** amphetamine-containing diet pills
**(D)** phenylephrine-containing eye drops
**(E)** an atropine-containing medication

**12.** A patient is admitted to the emergency room 2 hours after taking an overdose of phenobarbital. The plasma level of the drug at time of admission is 100 mg/L, and the apparent volume of distribution, half-life, and clearance of phenobarbital are 35 L, 4 days, and 6.1 L/d, respectively. The ingested dose was
**(A)** approximately 1 g
**(B)** approximately 3.5 g
**(C)** approximately 6.1 g
**(D)** approximately 40 g
**(E)** approximately 70 g

**13.** Most weak-acid drugs as well as weak-base drugs are absorbed primarily from the small intestine after oral administration, because
**(A)** both types are more ionized in the small intestine
**(B)** both types are less ionized in the small intestine
**(C)** the blood flow is greater in the small intestine than in other parts of the gut
**(D)** the surface area of the small intestine is greater than most other parts of the gut
**(E)** the small intestine has nonspecific carriers for most drugs

**14.** The primary site of action of tyramine is
**(A)** preganglionic sympathetic nerve terminals
**(B)** ganglionic receptors
**(C)** postganglionic sympathetic nerve terminals
**(D)** vascular smooth muscle cell receptors
**(E)** gut and liver catechol-O-methyltransferase

**15.** A drug suitable for producing a brief (5- to 15-minute) increase in cardiac vagal tone is
**(A)** pyridostigmine
**(B)** pralidoxime
**(C)** digoxin
**(D)** edrophonium
**(E)** ergotamine

**16.** A drug suitable for producing mydriasis and cycloplegia lasting more than 24 hours is
**(A)** atropine
**(B)** tropicamide
**(C)** echothiophate
**(D)** edrophonium
**(E)** ephedrine

**17.** Neostigmine and physostigmine differ in that
**(A)** neostigmine is inactive when given orally
**(B)** physostigmine is inactive when given orally
**(C)** the effects of neostigmine are irreversible
**(D)** physostigmine has more effect on the central nervous system
**(E)** neostigmine has less effect on skeletal muscle

**18.** Which of the following is useful for rapidly reducing serum calcium in hypercalcemia?
**(A)** furosemide
**(B)** spironolactone
**(C)** hydrochlorothiazide
**(D)** mannitol
**(E)** acetazolamide

**19.** A drug that decreases blood pressure by a CNS action is
**(A)** guanethidine
**(B)** trimethaphan
**(C)** nitroprusside
**(D)** prazosin
**(E)** clonidine

**20.** When treating hypertension, orthostatic hypotension is greatest with
**(A)** hydralazine
**(B)** guanethidine
**(C)** propranolol
**(D)** clonidine
**(E)** methyldopa

**21.** The antihypertensive drug most likely to aggravate angina pectoris is
(A) hydralazine
(B) guanethidine
(C) propranolol
(D) clonidine
(E) methyldopa

**22.** A drug lacking vasodilator properties that is useful in angina is
(A) nitroglycerin
(B) nifedipine
(C) metoprolol
(D) isosorbide dinitrate
(E) verapamil

**23.** An arachidonic acid derivative that reduces arterial clotting of blood (thrombi) is
(A) prostaglandin $E_2$
(B) prostaglandin $F_2$
(C) prostacyclin
(D) thromboxane $A_2$
(E) leukotriene $B_4$

**24.** A potent facilitator of platelet aggregation is
(A) prostaglandin $E_2$
(B) prostaglandin $F_2$
(C) prostacyclin
(D) thromboxane $A_2$
(E) leukotriene $B_4$

**25.** A drug useful in the treatment of asthma, although it lacks bronchodilator action, is
(A) aminophylline
(B) isoproterenol
(C) ephedrine
(D) metaproterenol
(E) cromolyn

**26.** The most common route of drug entry into cells is
(A) uptake by special carrier
(B) diffusion through the lipid phase
(C) endocytosis after combining with coated pits
(D) aqueous diffusion
(E) transport by amino acid carriers

**27.** Epinephrine reverses many effects of histamine, although it does not act at the histamine receptor. Epinephrine is a
(A) competitive inhibitor of histamine
(B) noncompetitive antagonist of histamine
(C) physiologic antagonist of histamine
(D) chemical antagonist of histamine
(E) metabolic inhibitor of histamine

**28.** Most drug receptors are
(A) small molecules with a molecular weight between 100 and 1000
(B) lipids arranged in a bilayer configuration
(C) proteins located on cell membranes or in the cytosol
(D) DNAs
(E) RNAs

**29.** After intravenous bolus administration of a drug, the major factors determining the initial plasma concentration are
(A) dose and clearance
(B) dose and apparent volume of distribution
(C) apparent volume of distribution and clearance
(D) clearance and half-life
(E) half-life and dose

**30.** Propranolol and hydralazine have which of the following effects in common?
(A) tachycardia
(B) bradycardia
(C) increased vascular resistance
(D) decreased mean arterial blood pressure
(E) decreased cardiac output

**31.** Intravenous administration of norepinephrine in a patient already taking an effective dose of atropine will often
(A) increase heart rate
(B) decrease total peripheral resistance
(C) decrease blood sugar
(D) increase skin temperature
(E) reduce pupil size

**32.** A drug that will produce mydriasis without cycloplegia is
(A) tropicamide
(B) phenylephrine
(C) isoproterenol
(D) atropine
(E) cyclopentolate

**33.** Which of the following statements is correct?
(A) "Maximum efficacy" of a drug is directly correlated with its potency
(B) The "therapeutic index" is the LD50 (or TD50) divided by the ED50
(C) A "partial agonist" has no effect on its receptors unless another drug is present
(D) Graded dose-response data provide information about the standard deviation of sensitivity to the drug in the population studied

**34.** The heart rate response to the infusion of a moderate dose of phenylephrine in conscious patients is NOT blocked by
(A) hexamethonium
(B) atropine
(C) phenoxybenzamine
(D) reserpine

**35.** All of the following statements about scopolamine are correct EXCEPT:
(A) It has depressant actions on the CNS
(B) It may cause hallucinations
(C) It is poorly distributed across the placenta to the fetus
(D) It may prevent motion sickness when applied as a patch to the skin
(E) It is similar to atropine in reducing gastrointestinal motility

**36.** All of the following statements about propranolol and timolol are correct EXCEPT:
(A) Timolol is a nonselective $\beta_1$- and $\beta_2$-blocker
(B) Propranolol cannot be given orally
(C) Timolol has useful cardiac effects after myocardial infarction
(D) Propranolol has more local anesthetic action than timolol

**37.** Correct differences between hydralazine and nitroglycerin include which of the following?
(A) Nitroglycerin cannot be given orally
(B) Hydralazine has a much longer half-life than nitroglycerin
(C) Hydralazine induces methemoglobinemia
(D) Hydralazine causes primarily venous vasodilation; nitroglycerin dilates both arteries and veins

**38.** The increase in heart rate and force of cardiac contraction normally induced by electrical stimulation of sympathetic nerves can be blocked by which of the following?
(A) Hydralazine
(B) Atropine
(C) Clonidine
(D) Neostigmine
(E) Propranolol

**39.** Treatments of angina that consistently increase the exercise time in a treadmill test and increase the product of heart rate and blood pressure at which anginal symptoms occur include
(A) nitroglycerin
(B) propranolol
(C) nifedipine
(D) coronary bypass surgery
(E) verapamil

**40.** Verapamil and diltiazem may diminish the symptoms of angina pectoris by causing all of the following EXCEPT
(A) reduction in blood pressure
(B) reduction in heart rate
(C) reduction in cardiac contractile force
(D) increase in heart size
(E) increase in diastolic interval

**41.** Which of the following has a self-limited diuretic action even when hypovolemia is prevented?
(A) Hydrochlorothiazide
(B) Triamterene
(C) Acetazolamide
(D) Furosemide
(E) Mannitol

**42.** Diuretics that increase the delivery of poorly absorbed solute to the thick ascending limb of the nephron include
(A) spironolactone
(B) mannitol
(C) indapamide
(D) furosemide
(E) all of the above

**43.** In a patient receiving digoxin for congestive heart failure, conditions that may facilitate the appearance of toxicity include
(A) hypocalcemia
(B) hypomagnesemia
(C) hyperkalemia
(D) hypernatremia
(E) all of the above

**44.** Causes of digitalis toxicity include
(A) intracellular calcium overload
(B) intracellular potassium overload
(C) increased parasympathetic activity
(D) increased adrenocorticosteroid levels
(E) all of the above

**45.** Methylxanthine drugs such as aminophylline cause all of the following EXCEPT
(A) vasodilation in many vascular beds
(B) increase in the amount of cAMP in mast cells
(C) bronchodilation
(D) activation of the enzyme phosphodiesterase

**46.** Drugs used in asthma that often cause tachycardia and tremor include
(A) isoproterenol
(B) cromolyn sodium
(C) ipratropium
(D) beclomethasone

**47.** Drugs with potentially useful effects in the treatment of inoperable metastatic pheochromocytoma include all of the following EXCEPT
(A) phenoxybenzamine
(B) reserpine
(C) phentolamine
(D) metyrosine
(E) propranolol

**48.** Agents that can readily cause edema if released near capillaries include
(A) norepinephrine
(B) serotonin
(C) histamine
(D) angiotensin II

**49.** Typical results of beta-receptor activation include all of the following EXCEPT
(A) hyperglycemia
(B) lipolysis
(C) glycogenolysis
(D) decreased skeletal muscle tremor
(E) increased renin secretion

**50.** Drugs that may be useful in the treatment of atrial fibrillation include
(A) quinidine
(B) mexiletine
(C) bretylium
(D) lidocaine
(E) all of the above

**51.** Atropine and similar drugs can
(A) block the cardiac acceleration induced by preganglionic sympathetic nerve stimulation
(B) block the cardiac deceleration induced by intravenous infusion of phenylephrine
(C) block the vasoconstriction induced by intravenous administration of nicotine
(D) block the vasodilation induced by the intravenous infusion of nitroglycerin

**52.** Drugs that readily enter the CNS when given intravenously include
(A) amphetamine
(B) dopamine
(C) guanethidine
(D) bethanechol

**DIRECTIONS (items 53–70):** Each group of items in this section consists of lettered headings followed by a set of numbered phrases. For each numbered phrase, select the ONE lettered heading that is most closely associated with it. Each lettered heading may be selected once, more than once, or not at all.

Items 53–55:
- **(A)** Diphenhydramine
- **(B)** Ergotamine tartrate
- **(C)** Terfenadine
- **(D)** Cimetidine
- **(E)** Ranitidine

**53.** A drug that is claimed to have significant action against motion sickness

**54.** A drug that decreases gastric acid secretion and has antiandrogenic effects

**55.** A drug with partial agonist effects at serotonin receptors and alpha receptors

Items 56–59:
- **(A)** Prazosin
- **(B)** Guanethidine
- **(C)** Reserpine
- **(D)** Methyldopa
- **(E)** Captopril

**56.** A drug that appears to block postsynaptic receptors more effectively than presynaptic receptors

**57.** A drug that blocks a carrier mechanism located in the membrane of synaptic transmitter storage vesicles

**58.** A drug that inhibits a peptidase enzyme in the blood

**59.** A drug that is converted into the active form in the brain

Items 60–63:
- **(A)** Quinidine
- **(B)** Digoxin
- **(C)** Verapamil
- **(D)** Lidocaine
- **(E)** Propranolol

**60.** A drug that predictably prolongs the PR interval and increases cardiac contractility

**61.** A drug that is useful in supraventricular tachycardias and angina pectoris and is not contraindicated in asthma

**62.** A drug that is useful in ventricular and atrial arrhythmias but may cause tinnitus

**63.** A drug that is very useful in early post-myocardial infarction ventricular arrhythmias but not very effective in atrial arrhythmias

Items 64–67:
- **(A)** Botulinus toxin
- **(B)** Tetrodotoxin
- **(C)** Saxitoxin
- **(D)** Cocaine
- **(E)** 3-Methoxy-4-hydroxy mandelic acid

**64.** A substance that inhibits reuptake of norepinephrine into sympathetic nerve terminals

**65.** A toxic substance that is synthesized in protozoans and concentrated in shellfish

**66.** A substance that prevents release of transmitter from cholinergic nerve endings

**67.** A substance that is excreted in large amounts by patients with increased catecholamine synthesis

Items 68–70:
- **(A)** Neostigmine
- **(B)** Nicotine
- **(C)** Bethanechol
- **(D)** Acetylcholine
- **(E)** Malathion

**68.** Converted to the active form by substitution of oxygen for sulfur; rapidly detoxified in mammals

**69.** Direct-acting muscarinic agonist with minimal susceptibility to cholinesterase

**70.** Cholinoceptor agonist that causes vasoconstriction

**DIRECTIONS* (items 71–90):** For each item in this section, ONE or MORE of the numbered options are correct. Select
- **(A)** if only **(1), (2), and** (3) are correct;
- **(B)** if only **(1) and** (3) are correct;
- **(C)** if only **(2) and** (4) are correct;
- **(D)** if only **(4)** is correct;
- **(E)** if all are correct.

**71.** Which of the following statements is (are) correct?
- **(1)** "Maximum efficacy" of a drug is directly correlated with its potency
- **(2)** The "therapeutic index" is the LD50 (or TD50) divided by the ED50
- **(3)** A "partial agonist" has no effect on its receptors unless another drug is present
- **(4)** Quantal dose-response data provide information about the standard deviation of sensitivity to the drug in the population studied

**72.** The heart rate response to the infusion of a moderate dose of phenylephrine in conscious patients can be blocked by
- **(1)** hexamethonium
- **(2)** atropine
- **(3)** phenoxybenzamine
- **(4)** neostigmine

**73.** Scopolamine
- **(1)** has depressant actions on the CNS
- **(2)** may cause hallucinations
- **(3)** is similar to atropine in reducing gastrointestinal motility
- **(4)** may prevent motion sickness when applied as a patch to the skin

**74.** Differences between propranolol and timolol include which of the following?
- **(1)** Timolol is a selective $\beta_1$-blocker
- **(2)** Propranolol cannot be given orally
- **(3)** Timolol has no cardiac effects
- **(4)** Propranolol has more local anesthetic action

*Questions 71–90 are "K-type" (multiple true/false) versions of questions 33–52. This format is no longer used in National Board examinations (see Preface); it is included here for review of the material and for course examinations in which this type of question is still used. See Appendix IV for strategies in dealing with this type of question.

**75.** Differences between hydralazine and nitroglycerin include which of the following?
(1) Nitroglycerin cannot be given orally
(2) Hydralazine has a much longer half-life
(3) Hydralazine induces methemoglobinemia
(4) Hydralazine causes primarily arterial vasodilatation

**76.** The increase in heart rate and force of cardiac contraction normally induced by sympathetic nerve discharge can be blocked by
(1) propranolol
(2) pindolol
(3) nadolol
(4) metoprolol

**77.** Treatments of angina that consistently increase the exercise time in a treadmill test without increasing the product of heart rate and blood pressure at which anginal symptoms occur include
(1) nitroglycerin
(2) propranolol
(3) nifedipine
(4) coronary bypass surgery

**78.** Verapamil and diltiazem may diminish the symptoms of angina pectoris by
(1) reducing blood pressure
(2) reducing heart rate
(3) reducing cardiac contractile force
(4) increasing heart size

**79.** Which of the following has (have) a self-limited diuretic action even when volume contraction is prevented?
(1) Hydrochlorothiazide
(2) Triamterene
(3) Furosemide
(4) Acetazolamide

**80.** Diuretics that increase the delivery of poorly absorbed solute to the thick ascending limb of the nephron include
(1) acetazolamide
(2) spironolactone
(3) mannitol
(4) indapamide

**81.** In a patient receiving digoxin for congestive heart failure, conditions that may facilitate the appearance of toxicity include
(1) hypercalcemia
(2) hypomagnesemia
(3) hypokalemia
(4) hypernatremia

**82.** Common forms of digitalis toxicity include
(1) nausea and vomiting
(2) junctional tachycardia arrhythmia
(3) atrial fibrillation arrhythmia
(4) ventricular extrasystoles and tachycardia

**83.** Methylxanthine drugs such as aminophylline
(1) cause vasodilatation in many vascular beds
(2) increase the amount of cAMP in mast cells
(3) cause bronchodilatation
(4) inhibit the enzyme phosphodiesterase

**84.** Drugs used in asthma that often cause tachycardia and tremor include
(1) isoproterenol
(2) cromolyn sodium
(3) aminophylline
(4) beclomethasone

**85.** Drugs with potentially useful effects in the treatment of inoperable metastatic pheochromocytoma include
(1) phenoxybenzamine
(2) propranolol
(3) phentolamine
(4) metyrosine

**86.** Agents that can readily cause edema if released near capillaries include
(1) histamine
(2) serotonin
(3) bradykinin
(4) angiotensin II

**87.** Typical results of beta-receptor activation include
(1) hyperglycemia
(2) lipolysis
(3) glycogenolysis
(4) increased renin secretion

**88.** Drugs that may be useful in the treatment of atrial fibrillation include
(1) quinidine
(2) digoxin
(3) procainamide
(4) lidocaine

**89.** Hexamethonium and similar ganglion blockers can
(1) block the cardiac acceleration induced by preganglionic sympathetic nerve stimulation
(2) block the cardiac acceleration induced by intravenous infusion of nitroglycerin
(3) block the vasoconstriction induced by intravenous administration of nicotine
(4) block the vasoconstriction induced by the intravenous infusion of tyramine

**90.** Drugs that readily enter the CNS when given intravenously include
(1) amphetamine
(2) dopamine
(3) methyldopa
(4) bethanechol

## Answer Key for Examination I*

**1.** C (6, 7)
**2.** D (1)
**3.** B (10)
**4.** B (9, 13, 19)
**5.** A (17)
**6.** C (16)
**7.** B (14)
**8.** E (14, 15)

*Numbers in parentheses indicate chapters in which answers may be found.

**9.** B (11, 15)
**10.** D (10)
**11.** A (9)
**12.** B (3)
**13.** D (1)
**14.** C (6, 9)
**15.** D (7)
**16.** A (8)
**17.** D (7)
**18.** A (15)
**19.** E (11)
**20.** B (11)
**21.** A (11)
**22.** C (12)
**23.** C (18)
**24.** D (18)
**25.** E (19)
**26.** B (1)
**27.** C (2)
**28.** C (2)
**29.** B (3)
**30.** D (11)
**31.** A (6, 8, 9)
**32.** B (8, 9)
**33.** B (16)
**34.** D (16)
**35.** C (16)
**36.** B (10, 11)
**37.** B (11)
**38.** E (11)
**39.** D (11)
**40.** D (13)
**41.** C (12)
**42.** B (14)
**43.** B (14)
**44.** A (6)
**45.** D (6)
**46.** A (6)
**47.** B (6)
**48.** C (7)
**49.** D (7)
**50.** A (7)
**51.** B (2)
**52.** A (6, 8, 9, 10)
**53.** A (8)
**54.** D (10)
**55.** B (11, 12)
**56.** A (10)
**57.** C (12)
**58.** E (12)
**59.** D (15)
**60.** B (15)
**61.** C (13)
**62.** A (13)
**63.** D (19)
**64.** D (19)
**65.** C (6, 10)
**66.** A (16, 17)
**67.** E (9)

**68.** E (13, 14)
**69.** C (6, 8)
**70.** B (7, 9, 11)
**71.** C (2)
**72.** A (6, 7, 8, 9, 10)
**73.** E (8)
**74.** D (10)
**75.** C (11, 12)
**76.** E (10)
**77.** A (12)
**78.** A (12)
**79.** D (15)
**80.** B (15)
**81.** A (13)
**82.** E (13)
**83.** E (19)
**84.** B (19)
**85.** E (6, 10)
**86.** B (16, 17)
**87.** E (9)
**88.** A (14)
**89.** A (6)
**90.** B (9, 11)

# Appendix II.

# Examination II

## CNS Drugs; Drugs Used for Diseases of the Blood, Inflammation, and Gout; Endocrine Drugs; Drugs Used for Infections and Cancer; Toxicology*

**DIRECTIONS (items 1–40):** Each numbered item or incomplete statement in this section is followed by answers or by completions of the statement. Select the ONE lettered answer or completion that is BEST in each case.

**1.** In the treatment of severe alcohol withdrawal syndrome,
**(A)** symptoms disappear after approximately 48 hours
**(B)** convulsions are best managed with diazepam or phenytoin
**(C)** if confusion and amnesia are prominent, the patient should be given chlorpromazine
**(D)** because of the short half-life of alcohol, sedative-hypnotics with similarly short half-lives should be used to reduce acute symptoms
**(E)** nausea and vomiting should be managed by giving marihuana derivatives

**2.** All of the following statements about ethanol are true EXCEPT:
**(A)** It is metabolized by alcohol dehydrogenase
**(B)** It is metabolized by a microsomal ethanol-oxidizing system
**(C)** Its rate of metabolism is relatively independent of its blood level over most of the pharmacologic range
**(D)** An important aspect of chronic use is the absence of any physical tolerance
**(E)** Psychic dependence is an important component of abuse

**3.** In the use of most modern general anesthetics,
**(A)** the state of surgical anesthesia is associated with complete muscle paralysis
**(B)** anesthetic potency is quantitated by the minimum alveolar concentration (MAC) that causes 50% of subjects to lose reflex response to a painful stimulus
**(C)** anesthesia is associated with increased blood pressure and total peripheral resistance
**(D)** gaseous agents are used for long procedures because intravenous anesthetics are too toxic to use for more than a few minutes
**(E)** agents that are very insoluble in the blood have a relatively slow onset of anesthetic action

**4.** Concerning the local anesthetics,
**(A)** ester-type drugs block large myelinated fibers first
**(B)** local anesthetics are structurally similar to antimuscarinic agents
**(C)** amides must be metabolized to terminate their anesthetic effect
**(D)** they block slowly firing fibers before rapidly firing fibers
**(E)** their actions on excitable cells are use-dependent

**5.** Neuromuscular blocking drugs
**(A)** may act by mimicking or blocking the action of acetylcholine at the neuromuscular endplate
**(B)** must be given by continuous intravenous infusion
**(C)** are excreted unchanged in the urine
**(D)** have adrenoceptor blockade as an important side effect
**(E)** are useful in the treatment of spastic conditions such as cerebral palsy

*Examination II covers Chapters 20–60 of this review.

**6.** In the treatment of chronic cancer pain,
**(A)** narcotics should be given only when requested in order to delay the development of addiction
**(B)** non-narcotic analgesics may control symptoms during a significant portion of the course of the disease
**(C)** the placebo effect is absent; thus, powerful analgesics are needed
**(D)** addiction occurs universally in the later stages of the disease because of the very large narcotic doses required
**(E)** heroin is documentably more effective than morphine

**7.** Effects of the narcotic analgesics include all of the following EXCEPT
**(A)** anticonvulsant action
**(B)** antitussive (cough suppressant) action
**(C)** constipation
**(D)** sedation
**(E)** reduction of heart rate

**8.** Which of the following drugs has the lowest addiction liability?
**(A)** Amphetamine
**(B)** Codeine
**(C)** Cocaine
**(D)** Nicotine
**(E)** LSD

**9.** Which of the following is an important factor regarding the use of anticoagulant drugs?
**(A)** Heparin is contraindicated in pregnancy
**(B)** Warfarin has a long onset of action that is related to the half-lives of blood clotting components
**(C)** Heparin is activated in the liver to an active agent
**(D)** The effect of warfarin is monitored by measuring the bleeding time
**(E)** Heparin is inactive in vitro

**10.** In the treatment of thromboembolic disorders,
**(A)** aspirin is contraindicated
**(B)** urokinase, especially when readministered in a patient, carries a major risk of an allergic reaction
**(C)** antiplatelet drugs may act through the inhibition of platelet thromboxane synthesis
**(D)** aminocaproic acid may be a useful antithrombotic agent
**(E)** patient intake of vitamin K should be reduced

**11.** Plasmid-mediated bacterial resistance to this drug group involves the synthesis of transferase enzymes that inactivate by addition of acetyl or other groups.
**(A)** Macrolides
**(B)** Tetracyclines
**(C)** Aminoglycosides
**(D)** Penicillins
**(E)** Erythromycin

**12.** All of the following antimicrobials inhibit bacterial protein synthesis EXCEPT
**(A)** erythromycin
**(B)** ciprofloxacin
**(C)** amikacin
**(D)** tetracycline
**(E)** clindamycin

**13.** Which of the following adverse effects is associated with the use of methicillin?
(A) Phototoxicity
(B) Maculopapular skin rashes
(C) Interstitial nephritis
(D) Agranulocytosis
(E) Acute hemolytic anemia

**14.** Of the following penicillins, which is most suitable for oral use in an oropharyngeal infection proved by culture to be due to a beta-hemolytic streptococcus?
(A) Procaine penicillin G
(B) Penicillin V
(C) Indanyl carbenicillin
(D) Nafcillin
(E) Ticarcillin

**15.** In addition to its effectiveness in infections caused by penicillinase-producing staphylococci, cefazolin has useful activity against
(A) *Pseudomonas* spp
(B) *Treponema pallidum*
(C) *Mycoplasma pneumoniae*
(D) *Bacteroides fragilis*
(E) *Klebsiella* spp

**16.** All of the following statements about tetracyclines are accurate EXCEPT:
(A) They bind to 30S ribosomal subunits of bacteria
(B) They are active against *Chlamydia*
(C) They may cause candidal superinfections
(D) They are usually active against methicillin-resistant staphylococci
(E) Oral absorption may be decreased by multivalent cations

**17.** A valid clinical use of chloramphenicol is
(A) chlamydial infections of the urinary tract
(B) viral infections of the upper respiratory tract
(C) treatment of syphilis in penicillin allergy
(D) empiric treatment of neonatal sepsis
(E) ampicillin-resistant *Haemophilus influenzae* infections

**18.** The drug most likely to be effective in a serious hospital-acquired infection due to *Serratia marcescens* is
(A) ampicillin
(B) netilmicin
(C) tetracycline
(D) cefazolin
(E) erythromycin

**19.** A drug active against methicillin-resistant staphylococcal strains is
(A) gentamicin
(B) cephalothin
(C) erythromycin
(D) vancomycin
(E) ampicillin

**20.** An inhibitor of DNA-dependent RNA polymerase, useful in tuberculosis, is
(A) isoniazid
(B) streptomycin
(C) rifampin
(D) ethambutol
(E) pyrazinamide

**21.** All of the following statements about aminoglycosides are accurate EXCEPT:
**(A)** They may cause dose-dependent vestibular dysfunction
**(B)** They are bactericidal inhibitors of protein synthesis
**(C)** They are primary drugs for gram-negative bacterial infections
**(D)** They are effective against anaerobes, including *Bacteroides* spp
**(E)** They are polar compounds eliminated mainly by renal glomerular filtration

**22.** The mechanism of antibacterial action of sulfonamides is to
**(A)** inhibit dihydrofolate reductase
**(B)** competitively inhibit thymidylate synthase
**(C)** block cell uptake of PABA
**(D)** inhibit glucose-6-phosphate dehydrogenase
**(E)** inhibit dihydropteroate synthetase

**23.** All of the following drugs have clinically useful activity against *Candida albicans* EXCEPT
**(A)** nystatin
**(B)** ketoconazole
**(C)** griseofulvin
**(D)** amphotericin B
**(E)** flucytosine

**24.** A drug that is phosphorylated rapidly by herpesvirus-specific thymidine kinase, eventually forming a compound that inhibits viral DNA polymerase, is
**(A)** amantadine
**(B)** azidothymidine
**(C)** idoxuridine
**(D)** acyclovir
**(E)** methisazone

**25.** Resistance to this drug involves methylation of the 23S rRNA receptor and block of drug binding.
**(A)** Streptomycin
**(B)** Tetracycline
**(C)** Chloramphenicol
**(D)** Sulfamethoxazole
**(E)** Erythromycin

**26.** A valid clinical use of clindamycin is
**(A)** treatment of gonorrhea
**(B)** severe infection due to *Bacteroides* spp
**(C)** respiratory infection due to *Mycoplasma* spp
**(D)** *Clostridium difficile* gastrointestinal infection
**(E)** rickettsial infections

**27.** This antiparasitic drug is bioactivated to toxic intermediates by the enzyme system pyruvate:ferredoxin oxidoreductase present in anaerobes.
**(A)** Metronidazole
**(B)** Pyrimethamine
**(C)** Chloroquine
**(D)** Emetine
**(E)** Quinine

**28.** This antimalarial is a blood schizonticide active against all 4 types of malaria, but resistant strains of *Plasmodium falciparum* occur. The drug may cause dose-dependent retinal damage.
**(A)** Chloroquine
**(B)** Quinine
**(C)** Primaquine
**(D)** Pyrimethamine
**(E)** Amodiaquin

**29.** Praziquantel is the drug of choice for *Schistosoma* infection. Its mechanism of action involves
(A) inhibition of microtubule synthesis
(B) muscle contraction and paralysis via increased $Ca^{2+}$ entry
(C) stimulation of the inhibitory effects of GABA
(D) inhibition of thiamine uptake
(E) activation of nicotinic receptors

**30.** All of the following statements about mebendazole are accurate EXCEPT:
(A) It is the drug of choice for hookworm and pinworm infections
(B) It causes the Mazzotti reaction, which is due to toxic products from dying worms
(C) Its absorption from the gut is increased by fatty foods
(D) It inhibits microtubule aggregation
(E) It has a high therapeutic index

**31.** This anticancer drug with specificity for the S phase of the cell cycle is activated by kinases to form an inhibitor of DNA polymerase.
(A) Etoposide
(B) Cyclophosphamide
(C) Methotrexate
(D) Procarbazine
(E) Cytarabine

**32.** The cardiotoxicity of doxorubicin involves
(A) inhibition of folate reductase
(B) intercalation between the base pairs of DNA
(C) generation of free radicals
(D) interaction with tubulin to block mitosis
(E) inhibition of thymidylate synthase

**33.** This anticancer drug is a component of regimens effective in testicular carcinoma. Its distinctive toxicity includes hyperkeratosis, fever with dehydration, pulmonary dysfunction, and anaphylactoid reactions.
(A) Dactinomycin
(B) Vinblastine
(C) Cyclophosphamide
(D) Bleomycin
(E) Mercaptopurine

**34.** Characteristic toxic effects of the anticancer plant alkaloid vincristine include
(A) cardiac abnormalities and tachycardia
(B) pulmonary infiltrates
(C) areflexia, peripheral neuritis, and paralytic ileus
(D) adrenal suppression
(E) renal dysfunction

**35.** This immunosuppressive agent causes selective destruction of T lymphoid cells, resulting in decreased cellular immunity with minor effects on humoral antibody formation.
(A) Prednisone
(B) Azathioprine
(C) Cyclophosphamide
(D) Antilymphocytic globulin
(E) $Rh_o$(D) immune globulin

**36.** All of the following statements about the urinary antiseptic nitrofurantoin are accurate EXCEPT:
(A) It may cause pulmonary infiltrates
(B) It has minimal systemic antimicrobial activity
(C) Its activity is increased by alkalization of urine
(D) It commonly causes gastrointestinal side effects
(E) It has no cross-resistance with other urinary antiseptics

**37.** The repeated application of this agent to the skin of neonates to protect against staphylococcal infections has resulted in cases of CNS white matter degeneration.
- **(A)** Hexachlorophene
- **(B)** Benzalkonium chloride
- **(C)** Undecylenic acid
- **(D)** Chlorhexidine
- **(E)** Nitrofurazone

**38.** This agent is used commonly for passive immunization (eg, in hepatitis A, hypogammaglobulinemia, and measles).
- **(A)** Antilymphocytic globulin
- **(B)** BCG vaccine
- **(C)** $Rh_o(D)$ immune globulin
- **(D)** Interferon
- **(E)** Human immune globulin

**39.** All of the following statements about cyclosporine are accurate EXCEPT:
- **(A)** It is an effective immunosuppressant in organ and bone marrow transplantations
- **(B)** It inhibits proliferation and early differentiation of lymphoid T cells
- **(C)** It causes marked bone marrow toxicity
- **(D)** It is a lipophilic peptide antibiotic
- **(E)** Its toxicity may be reduced by mannitol diuresis

**40.** Antimicrobial drug treatment of meningitis of suspected bacterial origin should not be started before
- **(A)** the patient has been hospitalized for at least 24 hours
- **(B)** the microbiologic laboratory has reported on the sensitivity of the pathogen
- **(C)** the organism is isolated by the microbiologic laboratory
- **(D)** specimens have been obtained for laboratory tests and cultures
- **(E)** intradermal penicillin is injected to check for hypersensitivity

**DIRECTIONS (items 41–76):** Each group of items in this section consists of lettered headings followed by a set of numbered phrases or statements. For each numbered phrase or statement, select the ONE lettered heading that is most closely associated with it. Each lettered heading may be selected once, more than once, or not at all.

Items 41–44:
- **(A)** Oral tolbutamide
- **(B)** Subcutaneous ultralente insulin
- **(C)** Intravenous crystalline insulin
- **(D)** Intramuscular glucagon
- **(E)** Intravenous hypertonic (50%) glucose

**41.** Most appropriate initial therapy for severe diabetic ketoacidosis

**42.** Most appropriate initial emergency room therapy for a comatose patient with known insulin-dependent diabetes

**43.** Most appropriate outpatient therapy for a patient with non-insulin-dependent diabetes

**44.** Most appropriate self-medication during early symptoms of hypoglycemia in a patient with insulin-dependent diabetes

Items 45–48:
- **(A)** Bromocriptine
- **(B)** Human growth hormone
- **(C)** Dexamethasone
- **(D)** Estradiol
- **(E)** Thyroid-stimulating hormone

**45.** Production increased by follicle-stimulating hormone

**46.** Inhibits the release of prolactin

**47.** Stimulates the formation of cAMP

**48.** A synthetic steroid hormone

Items 49–52:

**(A)** Propylthiouracil
**(B)** Fludrocortisone
**(C)** Spironolactone
**(D)** Methylprednisolone
**(E)** Corticotropin

**49.** Steroid useful in the management of inflammatory disease

**50.** Orally active agent useful in the treatment of thyrotoxicosis

**51.** Corticosteroid with high ratio of mineralocorticoid to glucocorticoid activity

**52.** Competitive inhibitor of aldosterone

Items 53–56:

**(A)** Ethinyl estradiol
**(B)** Chlorotrianisene
**(C)** Norethindrone
**(D)** Tamoxifen
**(E)** Clomiphene

**53.** Competitive estrogen inhibitor widely used for breast cancer

**54.** Partial estrogenic agonist used in the treatment of infertility

**55.** Progestational drug used in oral contraceptives

**56.** Estrogenic compound suitable for use in postmenopausal supplementation

Items 57–59:

**(A)** Dimercaprol (BAL)
**(B)** Penicillamine
**(C)** Edetate calcium disodium
**(D)** Deferoxamine
**(E)** Levamisole

**57.** Bidentate, oily, broad-spectrum chelating agent that must be given intramuscularly

**58.** Bacterial product that competes effectively for iron with ferritin but not with cytochrome or hemoglobin

**59.** Potentially nephrotoxic agent capable of displacing lead from the body

Items 60–61:

**(A)** Ethanol abstinence syndrome
**(B)** Ethylene glycol intoxication
**(C)** Acetaminophen overdose
**(D)** Parathion poisoning
**(E)** Heroin overdose

**60.** Best treated with diazepam and conservative management

**61.** Best treated with acetylcysteine

Items 62–64:
- **(A)** Amoxicillin
- **(B)** Cefazolin
- **(C)** Erythromycin
- **(D)** Chloramphenicol
- **(E)** Streptomycin

**62.** Effective against *Mycoplasma pneumoniae* and penicillinase-producing staphylococci

**63.** Detoxification normally is carried out with hepatic glucuronyl transferases, which may be deficient in neonates

**64.** Antibacterial activity may be enhanced by administration with penicillinase inhibitors

Items 65–67:
- **(A)** Tetracycline
- **(B)** Griseofulvin
- **(C)** Nystatin
- **(D)** Isoniazid
- **(E)** Amphotericin B

**65.** This polyene antibiotic is given intravenously and causes "shake and bake" chills and fever, electrolyte imbalance, cardiac irregularities, and nephrotoxicity.

**66.** This antifungal drug interferes with microtubule function. Its adverse effects include headaches, confusion, gastrointestinal upsets, and changes in liver function. It may be teratogenic.

**67.** The neurotoxic adverse effects of this antimicrobial drug can be alleviated by administration of pyridoxine.

Items 68–70:
- **(A)** Sulfisoxazole
- **(B)** Nafcillin
- **(C)** Methenamine
- **(D)** Vancomycin
- **(E)** Trimethoprim

**68.** This drug is an appropriate choice for treatment of hospital-acquired staphylococcal infections, including those caused by methicillin-resistant strains

**69.** Bacterial dihydrofolate reductases may be as much as $10^4$ times more sensitive than mammalian forms of the enzyme to inhibition by this drug.

**70.** Alkalization helps to avoid urinary crystallization of this drug and does not reduce its antibacterial activity

Items 71–73:
- **(A)** Chloroquine
- **(B)** Allopurinol
- **(C)** Stibocaptate
- **(D)** Praziquantel
- **(E)** Quinine

**71.** This drug is a good substrate for hypoxanthine-guanine phosphoribosyltransferase in parasites. It is incorporated into RNA, which loses its normal functions.

**72.** This antimonial compound is used in schistosomiasis. It inhibits glycolysis in these parasites, possibly by inhibiting phosphofructokinase.

**73.** Adverse effects of this drug include flushed, sweaty skin, tinnitus, impaired vision and hearing, gastrointestinal upset, and disturbances in cardiac rhythm and conduction.

Items 74–76:

**(A)** Procarbazine
**(B)** Mechlorethamine
**(C)** Cytarabine
**(D)** Vincristine
**(E)** Cyclophosphamide

**74.** This drug is a component of the "MOPP" regimen effective in Hodgkin's disease. It causes arrest of cancer cells in the M phase of the cell cycle.

**75.** This S-phase-specific antimetabolite is used primarily in the treatment of acute myelogenous leukemia.

**76.** This useful anticancer drug is biotransformed to a metabolite that inhibits MAO and can cause drug interactions. Unfortunately, the drug is leukemogenic and has teratogenic and mutagenic effects.

**DIRECTIONS (items 77–100):** Each numbered item or incomplete statement in this section is followed by answers or by completions of the statement. Select the ONE lettered answer or completion that is BEST in each case.

**77.** All of the following agents may be used to control status epilepticus seizures EXCEPT
**(A)** phenytoin
**(B)** diazepam
**(C)** chlorpromazine
**(D)** thiopental

**78.** Which of the following statements about local anesthetics is most accurate?
**(A)** They are more effective when used in infected tissues, because of the increased blood flow through such areas
**(B)** They are less toxic if combined with a vasoconstrictor agent
**(C)** They must be given locally because they are too toxic to be administered systemically
**(D)** They have a high affinity for sodium channels in the rested state

**79.** Drugs that are useful in the treatment of Parkinson's disease include all of the following EXCEPT
**(A)** pergolide
**(B)** trihexyphenidyl
**(C)** fluoxetine
**(D)** amantadine
**(E)** selegiline

**80.** Which of the following is a common adverse effect of the tricyclic antidepressants amitriptyline and doxepin?
**(A)** Sedation
**(B)** Cardiac arrhythmias
**(C)** Akinesia
**(D)** Hypertension

**81.** Phenothiazine effects result from blockade of all the following receptors EXCEPT
**(A)** peripheral alpha adrenoceptors
**(B)** central dopamine receptors
**(C)** nicotinic receptors
**(D)** muscarinic receptors

**82.** Which of the following is characteristic of narcotic analgesics?
**(A)** The ratio of maximal efficacy to addiction liability is a constant
**(B)** Tolerance to ocular and gastrointestinal effects develops during chronic use
**(C)** Mixed agonist-antagonists are less effective analgesics than the pure agonist agents in this group
**(D)** They have many effects in common with a group of endogenous polypeptides

**83.** Concerning the treatment of arthritis, which of the following is accurate?
**(A)** Aspirin (daily dose 4000 mg) is less effective than piroxicam (daily dose 20 mg)
**(B)** Gastrointestinal toxicity does not occur with the use of ibuprofen
**(C)** Phenylbutazone is associated with an increased incidence of thromboembolism
**(D)** Renal toxicity is an important toxic effect of long-term therapy with nonsteroidal anti-inflammatory drugs

**84.** All of the following statements about therapy of inflammatory joint disease are accurate EXCEPT:
**(A)** Gold salts are claimed to be able to halt the destruction of joint cartilage and bone
**(B)** The anti-inflammatory action of penicillamine is due to its ability to chelate heavy metals
**(C)** Antimalarial drugs are useful in some patients who are unresponsive to nonsteroidal anti-inflammatory agents
**(D)** Corticosteroids are effective in reducing symptoms temporarily but have major toxicity when used chronically

**85.** Naloxone is LEAST likely to be effective in reversing
**(A)** heroin overdose in an addict
**(B)** analgesia induced by meperidine in a cancer patient
**(C)** respiratory depression caused by nalbuphine overdose
**(D)** miosis that occurs during treatment with morphine

**86.** All of the following statements about the penicillins are accurate EXCEPT:
**(A)** Nafcillin is active against penicillinase-producing staphylococci
**(B)** Clavulanic acid with amoxicillin increases antibacterial activity
**(C)** Aminoglycosides antagonize the action of penicillin G against enterococci
**(D)** Renal elimination is decreased by probenecid

**87.** Appropriate clinical uses of tetracycline include treatment of all of the following EXCEPT
**(A)** staphylococcal osteomyelitis acquired in hospital
**(B)** upper respiratory tract infections due to *Mycoplasma pneumoniae*
**(C)** gonorrhea
**(D)** chlamydial infections of the urogenital system

**88.** Aminoglycoside antibiotics
**(A)** inhibit phosphoryl-group transferases
**(B)** intercalate between base pairs of DNA
**(C)** bind to the 30S ribosomal subunit to block initiation of peptide formation
**(D)** inhibit DNA gyrase

**89.** All of the following statements about the chemotherapy of tuberculosis are accurate EXCEPT:
**(A)** Combination drug therapy is desirable to delay the emergence of resistance
**(B)** Isoniazid affects liver function by increasing the activity of microsomal cytochrome P-450
**(C)** Adverse effects of rifampin include hepatotoxicity, decreased antibody responses, and a "flu" syndrome
**(D)** Ethambutol may cause optic neuritis when used at high doses

**90.** Characteristics of the cephalosporin drug group include all of the following EXCEPT:
**(A)** They are beta-lactam inhibitors of cell wall synthesis
**(B)** Cefazolin is appropriate for the treatment of pneumococcal meningitis
**(C)** Cephalothin is active against staphylococci, *Escherichia coli,* and *Klebsiella* spp
**(D)** Third-generation drugs may cause bleeding through impairment of vitamin K availability

**91.** Characteristics of chloramphenicol include all of the following EXCEPT:
**(A)** It blocks peptidyltransferase by binding to the 50S ribosomal subunit
**(B)** It causes dose-dependent, reversible bone marrow depression
**(C)** Resistance to the drug may involve plasmid-mediated induction of inactivating acetyltransferases
**(D)** It binds to cations in bone to delay long-bone growth

**92.** Which of the following statements about trimethoprim-sulfamethoxazole is accurate?
**(A)** Trimethoprim inhibits the synthesis of dihydropteroic acid
**(B)** The effects of sulfamethoxazole may be enhanced by PABA
**(C)** Sulfamethoxazole stimulates the formation of glucose-6-phosphate dehydrogenase
**(D)** The drugs cause a sequential blockade of folic acid synthesis

**93.** Gentamicin is a commonly used antibiotic, especially in hospitals. Its adverse effects include all of the following EXCEPT
**(A)** tinnitus and loss of perception of high-frequency sounds
**(B)** elevation of serum iron
**(C)** acute tubular necrosis
**(D)** respiratory impairment

**94.** Characteristics of ketoconazole include all of the following EXCEPT:
**(A)** It inhibits 14α-demethylation of lanosterol
**(B)** It is active against *Candida albicans*
**(C)** It inhibits glucocorticoid synthesis
**(D)** It is more effective than amphotericin B in the treatment of most systemic mycoses

**95.** Mechanisms of action of antiviral drugs include all of the following EXCEPT:
**(A)** Disoxaril prevents viral genome entry into host cells
**(B)** Azidothymidine is an inhibitor of reverse transcriptase
**(C)** Acyclovir is bioactivated to a toxic compound by hypoxanthine-guanine phosphoribosyltransferase
**(D)** Vidarabine is phosphorylated by cell kinases to form a compound that inhibits viral DNA polymerase

**96.** Valid clinical uses of metronidazole include all of the following EXCEPT
**(A)** bacterial infections due to aerobic gram-negative strains
**(B)** urogenital trichomoniasis
**(C)** intestinal giardiasis
**(D)** eradication of amebic tissue infections

**97.** Erythromycin
**(A)** is bactericidal
**(B)** may cause a hypersensitivity-based nephritis
**(C)** is a useful alternative to penicillins for coccal infections in allergic patients
**(D)** is associated with a high incidence of pseudomembranous colitis

**98.** All of the following are characteristics of the anthelmintic drugs EXCEPT:
**(A)** Niclosamide is the drug of first choice in most tapeworm infections
**(B)** Hematotoxicity a major problem during use of the antischistosomal agent niridazole
**(C)** The antiparasitic activity of metrifonate is due to formation of dichlorvos, a cholinesterase inhibitor
**(D)** Levamisole stimulates cell-mediated immune responses

**99.** Which of the following is an anticancer drug that is cytotoxic through the formation of reactive intermediates that alkylate nucleophilic groups on DNA bases?
**(A)** Dactinomycin
**(B)** Cisplatin
**(C)** Methotrexate
**(D)** Cyclophosphamide

**100.** Characteristics of azathioprine include all of the following EXCEPT:
**(A)** It is cytotoxic to both B and T lymphoid cells
**(B)** It selectively inhibits cellular immunity, sparing antibody formation
**(C)** Allopurinol increases its toxicity
**(D)** It is metabolized to 6-mercaptopurine

## Answer Key for Examination II*

**1.** B (21, 22)
**2.** D (22)
**3.** B (24)
**4.** E (25)
**5.** A (26)
**6.** B (30)
**7.** A (30)
**8.** E (30, 31)
**9.** B (33)
**10.** C (33)
**11.** C (42, 45)
**12.** B (42)
**13.** C (43)
**14.** B (43)
**15.** E (43)
**16.** D (44)
**17.** E (44)
**18.** B (45)
**19.** D (50, 52)
**20.** C (46)
**21.** D (45)
**22.** E (47)
**23.** C (48)
**24.** D (49)
**25.** E (50)
**26.** B (50)
**27.** A (54)
**28.** A (54)
**29.** B (55)
**30.** B (55)
**31.** E (56)
**32.** C (56)
**33.** D (56)
**34.** C (56)
**35.** D (57)
**36.** C (50)
**37.** A (51)
**38.** E (57)
**39.** C (57)
**40.** D (52)
**41.** C (40)
**42.** E (40)
**43.** A (40)
**44.** D (40)
**45.** D (36, 39)
**46.** A (36)

*Numbers in parentheses are chapters in which answers may be found.

**47.** E (36)
**48.** C (38)
**49.** D (38)
**50.** A (37)
**51.** B (38)
**52.** C (38)
**53.** D (39)
**54.** E (39)
**55.** C (39)
**56.** A (39)
**57.** A (59)
**58.** D (59)
**59.** C (59)
**60.** A (22, 60)
**61.** C (35, 60)
**62.** C (50)
**63.** D (44)
**64.** A (43)
**65.** E (48)
**66.** B (48)
**67.** D (46)
**68.** D (50)
**69.** E (47)
**70.** A (47)
**71.** B (53, 54)
**72.** C (55)
**73.** E (54)
**74.** D (56)
**75.** C (56)
**76.** A (56)
**77.** C (23)
**78.** B (25)
**79.** C (27)
**80.** A (29)
**81.** C (28)
**82.** D (30)
**83.** D (35)
**84.** B (35)
**85.** C (30)
**86.** C (43)
**87.** A (44)
**88.** C (45)
**89.** B (46)
**90.** B (43)
**91.** D (44)
**92.** D (47)
**93.** B (45)
**94.** D (48)
**95.** C (49)
**96.** A (50, 54)
**97.** C (50)
**98.** B (55)
**99.** D (56)
**100.** B (57)

# Appendix III.

# Case Histories

This Appendix contains a series of case histories that illustrate some aspects of pharmacologic management of clinical problems. Each case is followed by a series of general self-evaluation questions. Answers are found at the end of the Appendix.

***Note:*** Ranges of numbers without units in parentheses or brackets are the ranges of normal at the institution where the patient was studied.

## CASE 1. THE GARDENER*

A 55-year-old man was found unconscious by his wife in the greenhouse behind their home. During the past week, he had been complaining of abdominal discomfort and frequent stools. His history was restricted to mild hypertension controlled by salt restriction (about 5 years) and non insulin-dependent diabetes mellitus controlled by diet (about 10 years). He had no history of mental illness or of alcohol or tobacco use, and he was not taking any medication. His last trip outside the country had been to Mexico 5 years earlier. He and his wife operated a small flower shop, and he was an enthusiastic home gardener.

Upon arrival at the emergency room, the patient was unconscious, salivating profusely, and breathing shallowly. His skin was warm and moist. Blood pressure was 140/90 mm Hg, pulse 72/min and regular, respirations 30/min, and temperature normal. There was no evidence of trauma. Both pupils were constricted and did not respond to light. Auscultation of the chest revealed moderate wheezing and numerous rhonchi. The heart was normal. Examination of the abdomen revealed no abnormalities other than hyperactive bowel sounds. The rectal examination was unremarkable, and the occult blood test of the stool was negative. The extremities showed subcutaneous muscle fasciculations at the time of admission. These disappeared during the course of the examination, but muscle tone decreased and breathing became shallower during this time. The neurologic examination revealed coma with no response to painful stimuli, no localizing signs, and no abnormal reflexes.

### Questions, Case 1

1. What are the possible toxicologic causes of the patient's signs and symptoms?
2. What immediate steps must be taken?
3. What drugs may be considered for the treatment of this patient? What are the risks and benefits of their use?

## CASE 2. THE SUICIDAL CARDIAC PATIENT†

A 39-year-old man had ingested 90 digoxin tablets (0.25 mg each) in a suicide attempt approximately 2 hours before admission. His medical history included rheumatic fever at age 10 and subsequent mitral stenosis with mild congestive failure after age 30. There was a history of mental depression during the past 2 years.

Upon admission, the patient was ethanol-intoxicated, lethargic, uncooperative, and vomiting frequently. The blood pressure was 110/70 mm Hg, pulse 40–60/min and irregular, and temperature

*Modified and reproduced, with permission, from Goldfrank L, Kirstein R: SLUD. *Hosp Physician* (Nov) 1976;**12:**20.
†Modified and reproduced, with permission, from Smith TW et al: Reversal of advanced digoxin intoxication with Fab fragments of digoxin-specific antibodies. *N Engl J Med* 1976;**294:**797.

normal. The lungs were clear and the abdomen unremarkable. Examination of the heart revealed a murmur at the apex and the left sternal border.

Initial laboratory data included a blood ethanol of 190 mg/dL, urea nitrogen 9 mg/dL (8–29), and serum creatinine 1.3 mg/dL (0.7–1.5). Electrolytes 2 hours after admission were sodium 141 meq/L (136–145), potassium 4.6 (3.5–5), chloride 101 (96–106), and bicarbonate 29 (24–28). An electrocardiogram revealed atrial fibrillation with a high degree of atrioventricular block and periods of atrioventricular junctional and atrial tachycardias. Ventricular rate did not exceed 50/min. Atropine, 3 mg, was given intravenously without producing any increase in ventricular rate. A transvenous pacing catheter was placed and ventricular pacing instituted at 60/min.

During the next 8 hours, the spontaneous ventricular rate, determined by briefly interrupting pacing and measuring the escape interval, progressively decreased to 33 and then to 13/min. No atrial activity could be detected on the ECG. The QRS duration reached a maximum of 0.33 s (normal: 0.1 s). Serum potassium increased to 8.7 meq/L despite intravenous infusion of glucose plus insulin and a retention enema containing polystyrene sulfonate, a potassium exchange resin.

Treatment with digoxin antibodies was begun 12 hours after ingestion of the digoxin. Fab fragments were administered intravenously over 2 hours. One hour after the start of Fab fragment administration, the spontaneous ventricular rate had risen to 30/min, and at 90 minutes atrial fibrillation with a ventricular rate of 40–50/min was observed. Two hours after the start of Fab administration, sinus rhythm with a rate of 75/min was present and the PR interval was 0.24 s (normal: less than 0.2 s). The serum potassium had fallen to 7.4 meq/L and continued to fall, eventually reaching 3.4 meq/L, a level that required administration of additional potassium.

The patient made a complete recovery from this episode of poisoning.

### Questions, Case 2

1. What was the cause and the primary source of the elevated serum potassium?
2. Describe the probable basis for the cardiac rhythm and electrocardiographic abnormalities.
3. Outline the conventional therapy for less severe digitalis intoxication and explain why it was not used in this case.
4. What treatment is available for severe intoxication with digitoxin?

## CASE 3. A SEED EATER*

A 15-year-old boy was brought to the emergency room by the police because he "had a flushed face and was acting crazy." He had been found nude, incoherent, and wandering about aimlessly.

Physical examination showed blood pressure 170/100 mm Hg, respirations 44/min, pulse 144/min, and temperature 38 °C. He was comatose, unresponsive to verbal stimuli, and minimally responsive to deep painful stimuli. Occasional decerebrate posturing was noted. The skin was flushed, dry and hot to the touch. The pupils were widely dilated and equal, with a minimal response to light.

Within 1 hour after admission, the vital signs were blood pressure 140/50 mm Hg, respirations 60/min, pulse 160/min, and rectal temperature 39.8 °C. The patient's coma had deepened.

At this time, physostigmine salicylate, 2 mg, was given intravenously under electrocardiographic, electroencephalographic, and temperature monitoring. Within 15 minutes, the rectal temperature had fallen to 38.8 °C, while blood pressure, respirations, and pulse were 160/68 mm Hg, 40/min, and 112/min, respectively. The patient became more alert and responsive to verbal commands but remained agitated. When questioned about ingestion of a toxic agent, the patient said that he had eaten "loco seeds," small black seeds of a weed that grew freely in the area. Remote memory was intact, but recent memory was grossly impaired.

Six hours later, the rectal temperature was 37 °C and other vital signs were stable. The patient was talking spontaneously in a rapid and garbled manner. Although completely oriented, he continued to speak of imaginary objects and voices.

The patient's condition rapidly improved, and he was discharged on the eighth hospital day without neurologic deficit.

---

*Modified and reproduced, with permission, from Mikolich JR, Paulson GW, Cross CJ: Acute anticholinergic syndrome due to Jimson seed ingestion: Clinical and laboratory observation in six cases. *Ann Intern Med* 1975;**83**:231.

## Questions, Case 3

1. What is the probable drug or drug group contained in "loco seeds"?
2. What is the most life-threatening effect of the intoxicant in this case?
3. What other treatments, pharmacologic or nonpharmacologic, might have been used in this case?
4. What are the dangers of physostigmine therapy? What are the risks of the other treatments you have suggested in answer to question 3?
5. What is the correlation of age with mortality rate in this type of poisoning?

## CASE 4. THE HYPERTENSIVE*

A 43-year-old man was found to be hypertensive in 1970 during a routine physical examination. He recounted a history of attacks of flushing, headache, palpitations, and excessive sweating, but the condition was diagnosed as essential hypertension. His blood pressure was controlled with difficulty by using a combination of hydrochlorothiazide, hydralazine, and propranolol. In 1977, during surgery for repair of an inguinal hernia, the patient had a sudden increase in blood pressure to 240/140 mm Hg, with tachycardia and ventricular premature beats. This paroxysm was controlled with sodium nitroprusside.

Postoperatively, the possibility of pheochromocytoma was raised. He was found to have high concentrations of 24-hour urinary catecholamines, "vanillylmandelic acid" (3-methoxy-4-hydroxymandelic acid), and metanephrines. Intravenous urography and adrenal angiography revealed no abnormality. Catheterization of the inferior vena cava and venous sampling for catecholamines showed a higher level of norepinephrine in the left adrenal vein. Exploratory laparotomy was performed, but no tumor could be found. Postoperatively, the patient remained hypertensive and received phenoxybenzamine, 10 mg twice a day, and propranolol, 20 mg 3 times a day.

The patient was referred to University Hospital for further evaluation and management. At that time he had no specific complaints. His blood pressure was 130/80 mm Hg, and the rest of the physical examination revealed no abnormality. The 24-hour levels of urinary catecholamines, 3-methoxy-4-hydroxymandelic acid, and metanephrines were, respectively, 3455 μg (0–280), 22 mg (2–10), and 3 μg (0–1). Chest roentgenography gave normal results. Computed tomography of the abdomen, pelvis, and chest gave normal results except for a faint, questionable lesion in the right thoracic paravertebral region.

In October 1982, the patient underwent midline sternotomy. A 3 × 2-cm mass was found at the root of the aorta, firmly adherent to the walls of both atria. It was removed with some difficulty.

After 4 days in the surgical intensive care unit under close monitoring, the patient was transferred to a hospital room in satisfactory condition. His blood pressure remained within the normal range, although all antihypertensive medication had been withdrawn. Twelve days after surgery, 24-hour levels of urinary catecholamines, 3-methoxy-4-hydroxymandelic acid, and metanephrines were 408 μg, 10 mg, and 1.4 μg, respectively. On the 14th postoperative day, the patient was discharged in good condition, receiving no medications.

## Questions, Case 4

1. Why is phenoxybenzamine preferred over the competitive alpha-receptor-blocking agents in the treatment of pheochromocytoma? What other groups of drugs may be useful?
2. Had the physicians suspected pheochromocytoma during the inguinal hernia surgery, how should the patient's paroxysm of hypertension have been managed?
3. Why did the surgeon performing exploratory surgery for the tumor look only in the abdomen when it ultimately was found in the chest?
4. What hemodynamic hazards are associated with surgery for pheochromocytoma?
5. In cases involving metastatic or inaccessible pheochromocytoma, what therapy can be used?

*Modified and reproduced, with permission, from Saad MF et al: Intrapericardial pheochromocytoma. *Am J Med* 1983;**75**:371.

## CASE 5. VASOCONSTRICTION & SYNCOPE*

The patient, a 55-year-old woman, was noted to be hypertensive upon physical examination in 1975. Because she weighed 114 kg, she was instructed to lose weight. Shortly after she began her weight reduction regimen, she began to notice symptoms typical of Raynaud's phenomenon involving all 5 fingers of both hands, more severe on the left than on the right. A typical episode began as blanching, coldness, and discomfort and then progressed to cyanosis followed by reddening. This occurred at any time and did not require cold induction, although her symptoms were more severe in cold weather.

In 1976, she was evaluated by being given a series of sympathetic ganglion blocks in the pain therapy clinic at the County General Hospital. Subsequently, she began receiving phenoxybenzamine. After a few months of improvement, her symptoms began to recur. At that time, because of the good response to the ganglion blocks, cervicodorsal sympathectomy on the left was performed through the transaxillary transthoracic route. Six months later, because of the good results on the left and with persistent symptoms on the right, right cervicodorsal sympathectomy was performed in a similar fashion. This also produced considerable improvement.

In the meantime, Raynaud symptoms had developed in both feet. Bilateral lumbar sympathectomy led to improvement in her feet. However, a few months later, the symptoms in her hands began to recur. Severe symptomatic postural hypotension also developed and was only partially relieved by use of Jobst elastic stockings. She also received fludrocortisone, ephedrine, and 12 g of sodium chloride daily. For treatment of Raynaud symptoms, she was initially given reserpine, but this drug caused behavioral depression and was discontinued. Papaverine tablets were also tried, with little benefit. Repeated workups at 2 medical centers failed to identify any underlying collagen disease responsible for Raynaud's phenomenon. Her postural symptoms consisted of dizziness upon sitting up from a supine position and upon standing from a sitting position. On several occasions, she had episodes of syncope in which she completely lost consciousness while walking.

She was hospitalized at the Clinical Research Center in 1979 for further evaluation of her orthostatic hypotension. Physical examination showed her weight to be 62 kg and height to be 152 cm. Her blood pressure (mm Hg) was 150/94 supine, 132/84 sitting, and 100/68 standing. Pulse was 88/min and regular and did not change with posture. Findings on examination of the head, eyes, ears, throat, and neck were essentially normal. She had normal carotid pulses with no bruit. Examination of the chest, heart, and abdomen revealed well-healed surgical scars but no other abnormalities. Her brachial, radial, femoral, popliteal, and pedal pulses were normal. The hands and feet were noted to be dry, but there were no ulcerations of fingers or toes or skin changes suggestive of scleroderma.

Laboratory evaluation of blood and urine gave normal results, as did measurements of plasma renin activity, catecholamines, and aldosterone levels. Responses to a cold pressor test were blunted but not abolished.

Since that study, she has been maintained on a high-salt diet, and various combinations of drugs have been tried for the simultaneous treatment of orthostatic hypotension and Raynaud's phenomenon. The agents used include fludrocortisone, vasoconstrictors, prostaglandin inhibitors, alpha-adrenoceptor blockers, vasodilators, angiotensin-converting enzyme inhibitor, and calcium channel blockers.

### Questions, Case 5

1. What is the purpose of the high-salt intake and administration of fludrocortisone?
2. What is the importance of arteriolar versus venous vasoconstrictors and vasodilators in this case?
3. In retrospect, what treatment should have been offered the patient instead of surgical sympathetic ganglionectomy?

## CASE 6. IATROGENIC SHOCK†

A 61-year-old patient had suffered from severe chronic asthmatic bronchitis with episodes of respira-

*Modified and reproduced, with permission, from Kochar MS: Simultaneous treatment of Raynaud's phenomenon and orthostatic hypotension. *Am J Med* 1983;**75**:537.

†Modified and reproduced, with permission, from Spoerel WE, Seleny FL, Williamson RD: Shock caused by continuous infusion of metaraminol bitartrate (Aramine). *Can Med Assoc J* 1964;**90**:349.

tory failure in the past and was admitted on this occasion with bronchopneumonia. Despite therapy with antibiotics and bronchodilators, his condition deteriorated and he became confused.

His arterial blood pH was 7.29 (7.35–7.45), $PCO_2$ 73 mm Hg (35–45), and hemoglobin 15.7 g/dL (14–18). A tracheostomy was performed under general anesthesia, and he was admitted to the intensive care unit.

Thirty minutes later, his pH was 7.41 and his $PCO_2$ 59 mm Hg, but his $O_2$ saturation remained very low (64% [94–100]). Intermittent positive-pressure breathing was begun, and his condition improved.

Two hours later, however, his blood pressure had fallen to 60 mm Hg systolic, and an infusion of the vasoconstrictor metaraminol (a sympathomimetic drug) was started. His heart rate promptly decreased from 120 to 75/min. During the next 36 hours, he received an average of 7 mg of metaraminol per hour, but he steadily developed the picture of shock, with a falling urine output. His heart rate gradually increased to 90/min. An attempt to overcome these changes by increasing the dosage of metaraminol (up to 50 mg/h) did not influence the progressive deterioration. He had cold extremities and peripheral cyanosis despite adequate respiratory exchange on 100% oxygen from the respirator. At this time, his arterial hematocrit was 70 (40–52), hemoglobin 20 g/dL, pH 7.52, and $PCO_2$ 25 mm Hg.

In an attempt to correct the severe hemoconcentration, the patient was given 1500 mL of dextran solution over the next 18 hours, and the blood pressure was maintained with norepinephrine infusion. With this treatment, his urine output rose, his extremities became warmer, and his color improved. His blood pressure was stable for about 48 hours, requiring only occasional support with norepinephrine in small doses. Two days after initiation of this treatment, his blood volume was measured at 5.5 L (4.6–6.8), with a hematocrit of 47%.

### Questions, Case 6

1. What is the mechanism by which metaraminol reduced the heart rate?
2. Why did the patient's hemoglobin and hematocrit rise?
3. What was the cause of the patient's deteriorating renal function, cold extremities, and cyanosis?
4. What were the effects of the dextran infusion and of the norepinephrine infusion in improving the patient's condition?

## CASE 7. AN ASTHMATIC BUSINESSWOMAN*

A businesswoman with a history of mild asthmatic attacks had onset of symptoms of bronchoconstriction in a restaurant during a business luncheon. Self-administration of 2 doses of a drug from an inhaler did not provide relief, and symptoms progressed until she became cyanotic. Paramedics were called and administered a subcutaneous drug upon arrival. She was admitted to the hospital emergency room in severe respiratory distress. Her pulse was 100/min, respiratory rate 32/min, and blood pressure 140/90 mm Hg. There was severe wheezing. Measurements of pulmonary function showed a $FEV_1$ (forced expiratory volume in 1 second) of 1.3 L (predicted 3.2 L). Blood gases were $PO_2$ of 60 and $PCO_2$ of 28 mm Hg (80–100 and 35–45 respectively).

The medical history revealed intolerance to foods containing metabisulfite (a preservative) and possibly to aspirin. There was no evidence of exposure to other possible allergens, but she had taken aspirin several hours before the luncheon. She had previously eaten the foods contained in her meal without reaction. There was no history of recent illness.

After this evaluation, she was given another dose of the subcutaneous medication that had been previously administered by the paramedics. Fifteen minutes later, her symptoms had decreased markedly but she still had respiratory wheezing. Use of a bronchodilator administered by hand-held nebulizer abolished the wheezing, and she was discharged 3 hours later.

### Questions, Case 7

1. What are the probable mediators of the bronchoconstriction evidenced in this woman's asthmatic attack?

---

*Modified and reproduced, with permission, from Simon RA: Management of severe asthma in relapse: Case discussion. Chap 28, page 241, in: *The Practical Management of Asthma.* Dawson A, Simon RA (editors). Grune & Stratton, 1984.

2. What medications are commonly used for the outpatient treatment of mild and moderate asthma? What are their mechanisms of action?
3. Which drug did she probably take by inhaler in the restaurant?
4. What drug was administered subcutaneously by the paramedics and later in the emergency room? What agent would be suitable for nebulizer use?

## CASE 8. ERGOTAMINE TOXICITY*

A 44-year-old woman with a history of moderate intake of ergotamine for migraine was admitted to hospital because of 3 days of increasingly cold and painful legs. Upon examination, the legs were found to be cyanotic and cold, with no detectable pulses distal to the femoral arteries. Transfemoral aortography showed normal aortic and pelvic vessels. However, the external iliac and femoral arteries were severely constricted, as were the smaller arteries of both legs.

A continuous epidural blockade, using bupivacaine, was established with complete bilateral anesthesia from the sixth thoracic to the fifth sacral segment. No vasodilatation was observed during the next 3 hours. A continuous infusion of nitroprusside was then begun, starting at 25 μg/min and increasing by 25 μg/min every 15 minutes. When the infusion rate reached 100 μg/min, the skin temperature of the great toe suddenly rose from 21.8 to 31.0 °C, the cyanosis cleared, and a normal pulse was felt in the peripheral vessels. A fall in arterial and central venous blood pressures was corrected by intravenous infusion of saline. The skin temperature of the toe rose to 36 °C. Despite brief interruption of the nitroprusside infusion after 4 hours, the vasodilatation continued.

Eleven hours after the infusion was started, nitroprusside infusion was discontinued, while the epidural anesthetic was continued. Signs of intense vasospasm occurred 90 minutes later. Infusion of nitroprusside at 25 μg/min rapidly increased the skin temperature and reestablished normal color and pulses in the legs. The epidural blockade was discontinued, and the patient was maintained on nitroprusside infusion alone. Thirty-six hours after admission, the infusion could be withdrawn without recurrence of vasoconstriction.

### Questions, Case 8

1. What is the mechanism of ergot-induced vasospasm?
2. What is the safe limit of ergot consumption?
3. What is the mechanism of vasodilatation induced by epidural blockade? Why was it ineffective in this case?
4. What is the mechanism of action of nitroprusside?
5. What medications should this patient receive to reduce her dependence on ergotamine for migraine relief?

## CASE 9. ABSENCE SEIZURES†

An 18-year-old woman was admitted for evaluation of therapy for frequent epileptic absence attacks associated with minor automatisms. The patient had a history of unsuccessful treatment with ethosuximide. The electroencephalograph showed generalized 3/s spike-and-wave complexes and intermittent left temporal discharges.

Therapy was restarted with sodium valproate, carbamazepine, and primidone. A 24-hour electroencephalographic study revealed 71 absence attacks. Increasing the valproate dosage from 1200 to 2400 mg/d was associated with a significant but transient decline in absence frequency. Serum levels of valproic acid at this time were 81 mg/L mean, 109 mg/L maximum, and 36 mg/L minimum on a twice-daily dosage regimen. Carbamazepine and primidone were slowly withdrawn, with no change in the number of clinical or electroencephalographic attacks. Addition of ethosuximide, 1000 mg/d, resulted in disappearance of all seizure activity. The mean serum ethosuximide level was 70 mg/L.

Six months later, an attempt was made to reduce the dosage of valproate. On a twice-daily dose of 300 mg (600 mg/d total), serum levels dropped to 34 mg/L mean, 57 mg/L maximum, and 23 mg/L minimum. There was a prompt recurrence of seizures, but they declined again when the valproate

---

*Modified and reproduced, with permission, from Christensen KN et al: Sodium nitroprusside and epidural blockade in the treatment of ergotism. *N Engl J Med* 1977;**296:**1271.

†Modified and reproduced, with permission, from Rowan AJ et al: Valproate-ethosuximide combination therapy for refractory absence seizures. *Arch Neurol* 1983;**40:**797.

dosage was returned to 2400 mg/d. A follow-up study 8 months later demonstrated a continuing favorable response.

## Questions, Case 9

1. Why were carbamazepine and primidone used at the beginning of the study?
2. Why were blood levels of the drugs measured several times during the day?
3. What interactions are of importance in regulating antiepileptic drug dosage?
4. What are the hazards of therapy with ethosuximide? With sodium valproate?

## CASE 10. THE TIRED (DEPRESSED) PATIENT*

A 37-year-old man visited the outpatient clinic with a chief complaint of chronic tiredness. He reported that over the past 6 months he had experienced frequent bouts of stomach upset, a weight loss of 5 kg, and occasional headaches.

Physical examination was within normal limits. Laboratory studies, including blood count and blood chemistry panel, urinalysis, thyroid function tests, and upper gastrointestinal tract x-ray series, were all normal.

When the patient returned to the clinic for a follow-up visit 1 week later, a more complete history was taken. He had come to the clinic at the request of his wife. He reported having early morning insomnia, loss of appetite, loss of interest in his work, and difficulty in remembering details related to his job. He also admitted a loss of interest in sex.

A diagnosis of major depression was made. Amitriptyline, 50 mg, was prescribed, to be taken at bedtime daily for 3 nights, followed by 100 mg daily thereafter, also taken at bedtime.

Two weeks later, a blood sample was taken to determine the plasma amitriptyline level. An interview at this time indicated that the patient was sleeping better but that his memory and appetite remained poor. The blood level was reported to be 100 ng/mL. The dose of drug was increased to 150 mg/d.

Five weeks after the initial visit, the patient was feeling much better, with improved interest in his job, family life, and food. He had regained most of his lost weight and no longer had insomnia.

## Questions, Case 10

1. What are the major drug groups used in the treatment of endogenous depression?
2. What mechanisms have been proposed for their actions?
3. What are the adverse effects associated with each group?
4. What factors must be considered when evaluating the dosage regimen and plasma drug levels?
5. Should fluoxetine have been substituted for amitriptyline after 2 weeks?

## CASE 11. THYROTOXICOSIS†

A 27-year-old woman was referred for evaluation of thyroid disease. She had a 3-month history of intermittent heat intolerance, sweats, tremor, tachycardia, and muscle weakness. She had lost weight despite a marked increase in appetite. She denied taking any medications before seeing her family physician. She had been taking iodide drops since seeing her doctor and initially noted a decrease in symptoms. For the past month, however, they had worsened. Physical examination revealed blood pressure 180/90 mm Hg, heart rate 110/min, minimal proptosis, and an enlarged thyroid gland. Laboratory tests showed elevated thyroxine, resin T3 uptake, radioactive iodine uptake, and antimicrosomal antibodies. A diagnosis of hyperimmune hyperthyroidism (Graves' disease) was made.

## Questions, Case 11

1. What therapeutic measures should be considered in this case? Why did the iodide drops the patient was taking reduce symptoms at first and then lose their effectiveness?

---

*Modified and reproduced, with permission, from Coleman JH, Johnston JA: Affective disorders. Page 1021 in: *Applied Therapeutics,* 3rd ed. Katcher BS, Young LY, Koda-Kimble MA (editors). Applied Therapeutics, Inc., 1983.

†Modified and reproduced, with permission, from Dong BJ: Thyroid diseases. Page 1313 in: *Applied Therapeutics,* 3rd ed. Katcher BS, Young LY, Koda-Kimble MA (editors). Applied Therapeutics, Inc., 1983.

2. What are the benefits and hazards of pharmacologic therapy in hyperthyroidism?
3. What are the mechanisms of action of antithyroid drugs?
4. What therapy should be considered if thyrotoxic crisis (thyroid storm) occurs?

## CASE 12. A DIABETIC STUDENT*

An 18-year-old woman was referred to the endocrine clinic at her student health service because a routine physical examination urinalysis revealed glycosuria and a random plasma glucose measured subsequently was 250 mg/dL.

The history disclosed that this was the student's first time away from home and that she had had a number of symptoms she attributed to anxiety associated with the move to college. These symptoms included weight loss (5 kg), polydipsia, nocturia, fatigue, and 3 episodes of vaginal yeast infections in the past 3 months. Before moving, she had a long series of recurrent upper respiratory infections.

The family history was negative for diabetes, and she was taking no medications. The physical examination was within normal limits. Her weight was 50 kg, which is in the 20th percentile for her height.

The laboratory results were as follows: fasting plasma glucose 280 mg/dL (<115 ), urine glucose and ketones strongly positive. On the basis of these and other findings, a diagnosis of type I diabetes was made.

### Questions, Case 12

1. What are the primary therapeutic strategies available in this case?
2. What are the complications and hazards of the major therapies for diabetes?
3. What methods of monitoring and adjusting therapy are available to the patient?

## CASE 13. SEVERE RHEUMATOID ARTHRITIS†

A 60-year-old woman was referred for management of severe rheumatoid arthritis. She had had the disease for 15 years and had been managed until age 55 with aspirin. She was then switched to ibuprofen, which diminished the gastrointestinal adverse effects she had developed from aspirin. One year before referral she had started to complain of increased joint pain and stiffness, and laboratory studies confirmed that the disease had become more active. Several attempts to control her symptoms with an increased dosage of ibuprofen and with a trial of another NSAID had not been effective, and the decision was made to add corticosteroids to the regimen.

Prednisone was started in a dose of 5 mg daily, given in the morning. After a period of evaluation, the dose was increased to 10 mg and then to 15 mg daily. At this dose, the patient's symptoms were reduced to a degree that permitted normal activity.

### Questions, Case 13

1. What are the relative advantages and disadvantages of corticosteroids versus corticotropin in the treatment of inflammatory disease?
2. Why was prednisone given to this patient in the morning?
3. What is the advantage of alternate-day therapy with corticosteroids? Which steroids are unsuitable for alternate-day therapy?
4. What are the hazards of long-term glucocorticoid therapy in chronic disease?

## CASE 14. AN INFANT WITH FEVER‡

A 19-month-old girl was hospitalized with fever and signs indicative of bacterial meningitis. She was

*Modified and reproduced, with permission, from Koda-Kimble MA, Rotblatt MD: Diabetes mellitus. Page 1357 in: *Applied Therapeutics,* 3rd ed. Katcher BS, Young LY, Koda-Kimble MA (editors). Applied Therapeutics, Inc., 1983.

†Modified and reproduced, with permission, from Kishi DT: Disorders of the adrenals. Page 1279 in: *Applied Therapeutics,* 3rd ed. Katcher BS, Young LY, Koda-Kimble MA (editors). Applied Therapeutics, Inc., 1983.

‡Adapted from Centers for Disease Control: Ampicillin and chloramphenicol resistance in systemic Haemophilus influenzae disease. *MMWR* (Jan 27) 1984;**33:**35.

treated with ampicillin and chloramphenicol for 72 hours and then placed on chloramphenicol alone on the basis of the results of microbiologic laboratory examinations.

After 12 days of antibiotic treatment, the patient was afebrile and cerebrospinal fluid was sterile, with normal protein and glucose levels. Drug treatment was discontinued, but after 3 days she developed vomiting and fever to 40.5 °C, and cerebrospinal fluid examination showed a white cell count of 300/μL (0–20), glucose 50 mg/dL (50–85), and protein 52 mg/dL (20–45). Cerebrospinal fluid culture was sterile, but counterimmunoelectrophoresis was positive for *Haemophilus influenzae*, type b polyribosylribitol phosphate antigen.

The patient was treated for 12 days with moxalactam and remained afebrile after the second day. At completion of therapy, cerebrospinal fluid was sterile, counterimmunoelectrophoresis was negative, and the white cell count and protein levels were returning toward the normal range.

### Questions, Case 14

1. Why was antibiotic treatment started before microbiologic laboratory examinations were completed?
2. What was the basis for the initial choice of ampicillin and chloramphenicol?
3. Why was ampicillin therapy stopped after 3 days?
4. What is the most likely cause of the apparent relapse after discontinuance of chloramphenicol?
5. What was the basis for the choice of moxalactam?
6. What are the possible adverse effects of chloramphenicol in this patient?

## CASE 15. A DRUG REACTION*

A 64-year-old man was hospitalized for evaluation and treatment of carcinoma of the tongue. Following a course of chemotherapy, the patient was brought to the operating room for radical neck dissection. He was intubated and given 2 g of cefoxitin intravenously. Ten minutes later, he had developed severe hypotension with a systolic blood pressure of 40–50 mm Hg, wheezing over both lung fields, and urticaria.

The operation was postponed, and the patient was given intravenous epinephrine, dexamethasone, diphenhydramine, and fluids over the next 2 hours. Blood pressure was restored and maintained by intravenous infusion of dopamine. In the intensive care unit, electrocardiography suggested acute cardiac injury; the patient had no history of angina pectoris or heart disease. Subsequent chest x-ray revealed a normal heart size with bilateral pulmonary edema. The latter responded to supportive care over the ensuing 5 days.

### Questions, Case 15

1. Why was an antimicrobial drug given at the time of surgery?
2. What was the basis for the choice of cefoxitin?
3. What type of drug allergy did the patient experience?
4. What are the mechanisms underlying this type of immunologic reaction?
5. Why were epinephrine, diphenhydramine, and a corticosteroid administered?
6. Can you offer any explanation for the cardiovascular changes?

## CASE 16. DIARRHEA FOLLOWING ANTIBIOTICS†

A 10-year-old girl received erythromycin for a prolonged respiratory tract infection. She continued to have headaches and stuffy nose, and a facial x-ray suggested maxillary sinusitis, which could not be confirmed following sinus puncture. She was then given amoxicillin (250 mg 3 times a day) for 10 days.

On the last day of amoxicillin treatment, she developed diarrhea, with some abdominal pain but no vomiting. Initially the stools were alternately watery and solid, but later they became mucoid, with

*Adapted and reproduced, with permission, from Austin SM, Barooah B, Chung SK: Reversible acute cardiac injury during cefoxitin-induced anaphylaxis in a patient with normal coronary arteries. *Am J Med* 1984;**77**:729.

†Adapted and reproduced, with permission, from Vesikari T et al: Pseudomembranous colitis with recurring diarrhea and prolonged persistence of *Clostridium difficile* in a 10-year-old girl. *Acta Paediatr Scand* 1984;**73**:135.

some blood. After 11 days of these symptoms, she was given loperamide for her diarrhea, and a stool culture was positive for *Clostridium difficile*.

She was hospitalized, and sigmoidoscopy revealed colitis with pseudomembranes, confirmed histologically. Stool culture was positive for *C difficile* and negative for *Salmonella, Shigella, Yersinia,* and *Campylobacter;* no rotavirus antigen was detectable by immunoassay. The girl was treated with oral vancomycin, 250 mg 4 times daily for 7 days, and was discharged following rectoscopic examination that proved normal and a negative *C difficile* stool culture.

### Questions, Case 16

1. What is the rationale for treatment of upper respiratory tract infections with erythromycin?
2. Why was amoxicillin used to treat the suspected sinusitis?
3. What was the most likely cause of the diarrhea and the presence of large numbers of *C difficile* in the gastrointestinal tract?
4. What was the cause of the pseudomembranous colitis?
5. Why was oral vancomycin used in this case? What other clinical uses of vancomycin are accepted?

## CASE 17. DIARRHEA FOLLOWING A TRIP*

After returning from a trip to Mexico, a 41-year-old woman had a week-long bout of diarrhea that resolved spontaneously. She did not feel well for the succeeding 4 months, and then abdominal discomfort became severe and fever (but no bowel symptoms) occurred. There was no history of jaundice, gallstones, or hepatitis, but acute cholecystitis was suspected, and the patient was admitted to hospital for what proved to be an unrewarding oral cholecystogram.

Following the x-ray studies, diarrhea reappeared. She was treated with penicillin and ampicillin for her fever. She was referred to another institution and was initially treated with metronidazole, ampicillin, and gentamicin for presumed amebic liver abscesses or acute cholecystitis with liver abscesses. At that time, laboratory values were hemoglobin 13 g/dL (12–16), hematocrit 37.3 (37–47), white blood cell count 19,800/μL (4300–10,000), sedimentation rate 120 (0–20), and a differential of 75% segs (25–62), 7% bands (0–21), and 10% lymphs (20–53). Alkaline phosphatase was 1315 (21–91); SGOT, bilirubin, and total protein were normal. Further examinations were negative for ova and parasites in the stool, but a serologic test for amebic infection was positive. Liver and spleen scans confirmed the presence of abscesses, and on the basis of this and the positive amebic serologic test, gentamicin and ampicillin were discontinued.

The patient's symptoms improved with a 10-day course of oral metronidazole and tetracycline. She became afebrile, and amebic serologic tests reverted to negative. Oral iodoquinol was given for 3 weeks, and follow-up examinations showed resolution of the abscess cavities and no recurrence of symptoms.

### Questions, Case 17

1. What are the most likely causes of diarrhea in a tourist following a trip to Mexico? Should such cases of "traveler's diarrhea" be routinely treated with antibiotics?
2. What activity is anticipated for ampicillin and gentamicin used in this case?
3. Why was metronidazole added to the regimen after discontinuance of the above antibiotics? What does tetracycline add to the therapeutic regimen?
4. What are the possible adverse effects of oral treatment with metronidazole and tetracycline?
5. What was the rationale for the 3 weeks of oral treatment with iodoquinol?

## CASE 18. THE AFRICAN TRAVELER†

A 20-year-old woman in good health was one of a party of American students visiting Kenya in a travel and study program. She was immunized against tetanus, typhoid, cholera, and yellow fever,

*Modified and reproduced, with permission, from Strum WB: Persistent pain, fever after a trip to Mexico. *Hosp Pract* (Oct) 1984;**19:**86.

†Adapted from Centers for Disease Control: Acute schistosomiasis with transverse myelitis in American students returning from Kenya. *MMWR* (Aug 10) 1984;**33:**445.

received human immune globulin, and in Kenya took chloroquine and Fansidar (pyrimethamine-sulfadoxine) for malarial prophylaxis. After 10 weeks, she was one of 15 (of 18) students to become ill, with fever, abdominal pain, and nonbloody diarrhea. Five days later, she developed severe back pain and then rapidly lost ambulatory ability. Stool examination showed ova of *Schistosoma mansoni,* and she was diagnosed as having schistosomiasis with transverse myelitis.

She was treated with oxamniquine and transported to the USA, where evaluation showed flaccid paralysis and decreased sensation of touch and temperature in the legs. The spinal lesion was localized at L1–2. Cerebrospinal fluid examination showed pleocytosis and protein elevation. Serologic tests for *Mycoplasma* and viral agents were negative. A myelogram showed no masses amenable to surgical removal.

The patient was treated with praziquantel and large doses of dexamethasone. The patient's motor function and sensation improved with treatment, and within a month she was ambulating with assistance in a rehabilitation center.

### Questions, Case 18

1. What are the mechanisms of action of chloroquine and the combination of pyrimethamine-sulfadoxine against plasmodia?
2. Why was oxamniquine used for the initial treatment of schistosomiasis in this case? What other drugs could have been used?
3. How does praziquantel differ from other drugs used in schistosomiasis? What is known about its mechanism of action?
4. What are the anticipated adverse effects of oxamniquine and praziquantel?
5. Is there any reason to believe that oxamniquine or praziquantel might have been contraindicated in this patient?
6. Why was dexamethasone administered?

## ANSWERS: CASE HISTORIES

### Answers, Case 1

1. The most probable chemical intoxicants in the case of the 55-year-old gardener are insecticides. The most common constituents of currently available insecticides that produce acute poisoning are the cholinesterase inhibitors and nicotine. The signs of muscarinic excess that this patient shows developed over a period of a week (abdominal discomfort and diarrhea), suggesting that a long-acting drug was gradually accumulating to a toxic level. The symptoms of cholinergic toxicity can be remembered by the use of the mnemonic DUMBELS—for diarrhea, urination, miosis, bronchospasm, excitability (of the neuromuscular end-plate or central nervous system), lacrimation, and salivation. Another mnemonic, SLUD, signifies salivation, lacrimation, urination, and defecation. Miosis and perspiration are common signs of cholinesterase inhibition. Nicotine rarely produces this pattern of slow onset and usually induces signs of sympathetic as well as parasympathetic discharge. The diagnosis can be confirmed by measuring the patient's blood cholinesterase level and by identifying a carbamate or organophosphate-containing insecticide among the patient's stock of garden supplies.
2. Immediate measures must be taken to maintain vital signs and to ensure that exposure to the intoxicant has ceased. Because the patient is unconscious, induction of emesis is contraindicated, and gastric lavage should not be attempted unless a cuffed endotracheal tube is in place. Since the patient's symptoms developed over a 1-week period, it is unlikely that the present stomach contents are contributing much to his intoxication. Since the organophosphates can be absorbed across the skin, the clothing should be removed and the skin cleansed (with care to avoid contamination of medical personnel). With the endotracheal tube in place, mechanical respiratory assistance can be applied as required to maintain normal blood gases, and gastric lavage may be done if there is any chance that the intoxicant was ingested. An intravenous line should be placed for the administration of drugs and for the maintenance of good hydration.
3. Drugs to be considered for this patient include atropine, for control of muscarinic effects; pralidoxime, for regeneration of cholinesterase, especially at the neuromuscular junction; and cardiovascular stimulants, but only if required to maintain a normal tissue perfusion. (They

are rarely required.) The use of atropine is likely to be beneficial in this case. Reduction of excess airway secretion and bronchoconstriction should reduce the risk of pulmonary complications, and decreased cholinergic activity in the gastrointestinal tract will decrease the likelihood of emesis or ulceration. Although pralidoxime is much less effective when administered late after the onset of poisoning, it is almost always used if the poisoning is associated with serious muscle weakness. With some organophosphates, the aging of the enzyme-inhibitor complex makes the inhibition irreversible. Mechanical ventilation may be necessary.

## Answers, Case 2

1. The cause of the dramatic rise in serum potassium was the poisoning of membrane $Na^+,K^+$-ATPase (the sodium pump) in the entire body. The serum potassium concentration can be used as an index of the severity of poisoning and may be more accurate as a prognostic tool than the blood level of digoxin. The source of the ion is the intracellular space, particularly that of skeletal muscle (because of the large mass of this tissue). Because the flux of potassium out of cells is significant, inhibition of the pump will result in depletion of intracellular $K^+$ early in an intoxication. However, the extracellular $K^+$ concentration does not rise unless the kidneys are unable to handle the amounts presented to them. In the present case, the amount of $K^+$ appearing in the serum was far in excess of the excretory ability of the kidneys (which was probably depressed under these conditions).
2. Digitalis has the reputation of causing any and all types of cardiac arrhythmias. The most common are junctional tachycardia (originating in the atrioventricular node) and ventricular tachycardia. The patient's atrial fibrillation detected on admission was probably a chronic condition related to mitral stenosis. The high degree of atrioventricular block, with the low ventricular rate, could reflect the strong vagal effects of the cardiac glycoside, but in view of the resistance to atropine in this case it probably represents direct depression by the drug. The widened QRS complex and the prolonged escape interval when pacing was interrupted reflect severe depression of Purkinje and ventricular cell automaticity and excitability. Such depression could have been caused by depolarization by the high extracellular potassium level. Under these circumstances, administration of antiarrhythmic agents, which are also cardiac depressants, was clearly contraindicated. The effects noted in this patient are unusually severe. At the more common levels of toxicity observed in nonsuicidal patients, automaticity is usually increased, not decreased. In such patients, depressant interventions such as administration of potassium or antiarrhythmic drugs are often successful in controlling arrhythmias.
3. Conventional therapy of mild to moderate cardiac glycoside intoxication consists of the following: (a) Normalization of low serum $K^+$. In the present case—and in most cases of gross overdosage—the serum $K^+$ is high. However, in many cases of mild to moderate toxicity, the serum $K^+$ is low or normal. In some cases (usually involving vomiting or diarrhea), low serum magnesium is found and correction of this deficiency corrects the arrhythmia. (b) Use of antiarrhythmic drugs. (Lidocaine is usually tried first.) (c) Avoidance of DC cardioversion unless ventricular fibrillation occurs. The first 2 of these approaches were clearly not suitable for this much more severely intoxicated patient.
4. Fortunately, severe intoxication is less common with digitoxin than with digoxin. Anti-digoxin Fab fragments cross-react sufficiently to be useful in reversing digitoxin effects. Trapping of drug in the small intestine with steroid-binding resins (eg, cholestyramine) has been of value in some cases. The success of such treatment reflects the importance of enterohepatic circulation of digitoxin.

## Answers, Case 3

1. The case description is typical of antimuscarinic drug poisoning. A common source of such agents in nature is Jimson weed *(Datura stramonium)*. The patient had ingested several of the 2- to 3-mm round black seeds from the pods of this plant.
2. The most life-threatening effect of the antimuscarinic agents in many patients is hyperthermia. This is particularly true of small children and infants, who are very dependent on sweating as a means for dissipating body heat. Unsupervised hallucinating patients may try to fly in the conviction that this is now possible, so they may fall from heights and injure themselves. Convulsions may occur. Other effects of these drugs, although uncomfortable, are not life-threatening.
3. Other treatments include temperature control blankets and sponge baths to prevent dangerous

hyperthermia and neostigmine for peripheral cholinesterase inhibition. Direct-acting cholinergic stimulants such as bethanechol and carbachol are never indicated.

4. The chief danger of physostigmine is its central stimulant effect, which may lead to convulsions. Most emergency departments now prefer to treat antimuscarinic poisoning symptomatically because of this hazard. Other anticholinesterase drugs, such as neostigmine, do not enter the CNS as readily as physostigmine; they are less dangerous but also less effective in reversing the central effects of the intoxicant.
5. As noted above, children are particularly at risk of dangerous hyperthermia from the atropinelike drugs. In general, patients with a strong dependence on sweating as a major means of temperature control (as in a very hot environment) are more susceptible. In the absence of hyperthermia, deaths are surprisingly rare.

## Answers, Case 4

1. A noncompetitive blocker such as phenoxybenzamine is preferred over agents such as phentolamine or prazosin, because the irreversible agent decreases the maximum or ceiling effect of the agonist (norepinephrine). Competitive drugs only shift the dose-response curve to higher dose levels, and in the presence of these agents a sufficiently large release of catecholamines can still cause dangerously high spikes of blood pressure.

   Other drugs of potential value include the beta-adrenoceptor-blocking agents. These drugs are especially important if an arrhythmia is present or if the tumor releases catecholamines with a high epinephrine:norepinephrine ratio.
2. During surgery, a rapidly acting and reversible alpha-blocking drug is preferred. Phentolamine is suitable.
3. The surgeon looked in the usual place for pheochromocytomas, the adrenal glands. The tumor is most commonly derived from adrenal medullary cells but can develop in any structure with similar embryonic origins, such as the sympathetic ganglia.
4. The major hazards are hypertensive crises before the tumor is removed, as demonstrated in this patient's history, and hypotensive events immediately after removing the tumor. In some cases, hypertension results from direct handling of the tumor by the surgeon; in others, from reflex discharge of catecholamines. Hypotension following removal of the tumor is the result of marked reduction of blood volume and normal adrenergic tone. Before removal of the tumor, an untreated patient has a greatly increased vasomotor tone, and therefore the blood volume is reduced by salt and water excretion—a compensatory mechanism for maintaining a normal blood pressure. When the source of the excessive catecholamines is removed, the heart may not be able to maintain normal pressure. This potential complication is usually prevented (as in the present case) by pretreatment with alpha-adrenoceptor-blocking drugs until the blood volume is normal.
5. Nonresectable pheochromocytoma can be treated with receptor antagonists, preferably phenoxybenzamine and, if needed, propranolol. In addition, synthesis of catecholamines can be reduced by use of metyrosine, which inhibits tyrosine hydroxylase.

## Answers, Case 5

1. The chief symptoms of orthostatic hypotension are the result of inadequate blood flow to the brain. The immediate cause is usually a decrease in venous vascular tone and venous return. These lead to a fall in cardiac output, aortic blood pressure, and cerebral perfusion. Since cerebral vascular resistance is not readily modified by vasoactive drugs, perfusion of the cerebral vascular bed is best maintained by supporting venous return and, indirectly, cardiac output. These goals can sometimes be accomplished by increasing blood volume. Thus, a high salt intake and administration of a salt-retaining hormone can improve the blood flow response to postural stress.
2. Because the patient has Raynaud's phenomenon, it would be very undesirable to cause constriction of the arteries, especially in the limbs. Furthermore, venoconstrictors are much more effective in reversing orthostatic symptoms. Unfortunately, there are no selective venoconstrictor drugs. On the other hand, some vasodilators are relatively selective: nitrates for veins, hydralazine and minoxidil for arteries. Thus, the dilator of choice for the patient's Raynaud's phenomenon would be an arterial vasodilator such as hydralazine.
3. It is obvious, from the unobstructed vantage point of hindsight, that this patient should have been treated with vasoactive drugs such as alpha-adrenoceptor blockers and direct-acting vasodilators rather than by an irreversible surgical procedure. If ganglionectomy was believed to

be especially effective in this patient, pharmacologic ganglionectomy with a drug such as mecamylamine should have been tried.

## Answers, Case 6

1. Because metaraminol is an alpha-receptor agonist, it causes marked vasoconstriction, which can be accompanied by reflex bradycardia. This patient rapidly became dependent on the exogenous stimulant for maintenance of cardiac output, and attempts to stop the infusion resulted in hypotension.
2. The hemoglobin and hematocrit increased because of hemoconcentration. Marked vasoconstriction results in increased Starling forces outward across the capillary wall and increased capillary permeability, caused by local ischemia; both of these facilitate the movement of plasma water out of the vascular compartment and into the tissues and the urine.
3. The patient went into shock because of the loss of blood volume described in answer 2 and because the increased cardiac work was causing heart failure. The result was a form of hypotension that responds well to volume replacement and renal vasodilators.
4. As noted in answer 3, volume replacement (eg, with dextran solution) is the most important aspect of therapy in this situation. Because the patient's cardiovascular system had become dependent on exogenous sympathomimetics, norepinephrine was necessary for a short time. However, rapid removal of this stimulus was indicated and was successfully accomplished in this case.

## Answers, Case 7

1. The mediators probably most important in causing asthmatic bronchoconstriction are leukotrienes $LTC_4$ and $LTD_4$. Another leukotriene ($LTB_4$), prostaglandins, and histamine probably also play a role.
2. The most important bronchodilators are the beta-adrenoceptor agonists and the methylxanthines. In some patients, muscarinic blocking drugs have a useful bronchodilating effect. Cromolyn inhibits the degranulation of mast cells and is useful as a prophylactic agent in some patients. Corticosteroids are given to patients with asthma who do not respond adequately to other agents.
3. The drugs most commonly used by the inhalation route are the $\beta_2$ stimulants. These agents have a reduced ratio of cardiac to bronchiolar effects compared with nonselective agents such as isoproterenol. Metaproterenol, albuterol, and terbutaline are $\beta_2$-selective agents currently available in aerosol form. Nonselective beta-stimulant agents available in inhalers include epinephrine and isoproterenol.
4. The drug administered by the paramedics and personnel in the emergency room was epinephrine. This agent is extremely effective and has a rapid onset of action. However, it is probably no more effective than inhaled $\beta_2$-selective agonists. The drugs commonly used in nebulizers include epinephrine, isoproterenol, and the $\beta_2$-selective agonists listed above.

## Answers, Case 8

1. Ergot causes vasoconstriction through the activation of several receptors, including alpha adrenoceptors and serotonin receptors. Additional receptors may be involved, since blockade of both adrenoceptors and serotonin receptors is often ineffective in reversing ergot-induced vasospasm.
2. The recommended limits of ergotamine consumption are 2–6 mg of ergotamine tartrate per episode of migraine and not more than 10 tablets (10 mg) per week. For severe migraine, intravenous administration of dihydroergotamine mesylate is sometimes effective. A maximum of 2 mg per dose of this drug is recommended, with a limit of 6 mg per week.
3. Epidural blockade interrupts preganglionic sympathetic outflow and thereby eliminates sympathetic vasoconstriction. In the present case, release of catecholamines from sympathetic nerves was not the cause of the severe vasoconstriction; therefore, little improvement could be expected.
4. The mechanism of action of nitroprusside is not fully understood. It is active in vivo and in vitro. It probably breaks down spontaneously to release nitric oxide in vascular smooth muscle. (NO is also released in vascular endothelium by muscarinic agonists.) Nitric oxide increases the conversion of GTP to cGMP, which causes smooth muscle relaxation.
5. If the patient has frequent attacks of migraine, prophylactic medication is indicated. Ergono-

vine and methysergide, a semisynthetic ergot derivative, have been used successfully in some patients. Propranolol, amitriptyline, and cyproheptadine have also been effective.

## Answers, Case 9

1. Carbamazepine and primidone were probably used at the start of the study to prevent the automatisms (complex partial seizures) that were reportedly part of the patient's seizure repertoire. Carbamazepine is considered the drug of choice for this seizure type. When it became apparent that such seizures were actually infrequent in this patient, the drugs were withdrawn.
2. Monitoring of blood levels is very important in the management of epilepsy. Effective, highly effective, and toxic plasma levels are listed in several textbooks. The effective levels listed for valproate and ethosuximide are 50–100 mg/L. Thus, the levels measured in this patient while receiving the high dose of valproate were within the effective range for both agents. When the dose of valproate was reduced to 600 mg/d, the mean and minimum plasma levels dropped below the effective range and seizures recurred.
3. Pharmacokinetic drug interactions are very important in the treatment of epilepsy. Many antiseizure drugs, eg, phenytoin, barbiturates, and carbamazepine, are capable of inducing production of hepatic microsomal enzymes. Valproate inhibits the metabolism of some drugs, including phenobarbital, phenytoin, and carbamazepine. Some anticonvulsants displace other drugs from plasma protein-binding sites; eg, valproate displaces phenytoin.
4. Ethosuximide is associated with a very low incidence of serious adverse effects. Gastric irritation, lethargy, fatigue, and other CNS effects are reported. In contrast, valproate has a low but significant risk of serious hepatic injury. It is contraindicated in pregnant women because it has been shown to cause spina bifida in infants born to mothers taking the drug.

## Answers, Case 10

1. Three drug groups are available for the treatment of major or endogenous depression. The traditional drug groups used are the tricyclic agents and the monoamine oxidase (MAO) inhibitors. Another group of drugs has recently been released that resembles the tricyclic drugs in many ways but may differ in terms of adverse effects. Typical members of the tricyclic group are imipramine, amitriptyline, desipramine, doxepin, and others. Members of the MAO inhibitor group include phenelzine, tranylcypromine, and isocarboxazid. Members of the new "second-generation" antidepressant subgroup include amoxapine, fluoxetine, maprotiline, and trazodone.
2. The mechanisms of action of the antidepressants are still poorly understood. The leading hypothesis is that some change in amine metabolism in the central neurons is involved. This concept is supported by the fact that the tricyclic agents inhibit reuptake of catecholamines into adrenergic nerve endings and the MAO inhibitors increase the concentration of catecholamines in these nerve terminals. However, the second-generation agents do not fully conform with this pattern. For example, fluoxetine is a selective blocker of serotonin reuptake.
3. The toxicity of antidepressant drugs is very important, because these drugs are often taken for long periods and because depressed patients often use medications close at hand in attempting suicide. The tricyclic drugs have autonomic effects much like those of the phenothiazine antipsychotic agents, which are chemically similar to tricyclic drugs. In addition, they can cause serious cardiac arrhythmias that are very difficult to treat. The MAO inhibitors cause serious interactions with catecholamine-releasing agents such as vasoconstrictor drugs (eg, ephedrine) and food constituents (eg, tyramine in fermented foods).
4. Factors that should be considered when interpreting blood levels of any drug include patient compliance and patient variations in pharmacokinetics. These factors are particularly important in the use of tricyclic antidepressants, since depressed patients may be very noncompliant. Furthermore, there is a large natural variation in the bioavailability and clearance of these drugs, and this variation must be accounted for in adjusting dosage with this group of drugs.
5. Antidepressant drugs have a slow onset of therapeutic action, and it may take several weeks of drug therapy before symptoms of depression are reversed. You would not consider an alternative drug after just 2 weeks of treatment. Although fluoxetine appears to be effective in some patients who fail to respond to tricyclic antidepressants, there is some concern that it may promote suicidal ideation in a few individuals.

## Answers, Case 11

1. The major therapies available for Graves' disease are surgery, thyroid-suppressant drugs, and

radioactive iodine in sufficient dosage to destroy the gland. Iodide therapy (usually a saturated solution of potassium iodide) is useful in reducing thyroid hormone release and in decreasing the vascularity of the gland prior to surgery. However, escape from the inhibitory effect of iodide often occurs in Graves' disease, and the increased iodine substrate made available by the therapy may actually accentuate the disease.

2. Radioactive iodine is often the treatment of choice for young adult patients. This treatment provides a permanent cure (in fact, hypothyroidism is common after treatment and is managed with levothyroxine replacement therapy). There is no evidence that the exposure to radioactivity causes increased incidence of disease, even after 35 years of follow-up. However, radioactive iodine should not be used in pregnant women, because it crosses the placenta and will damage the fetal thyroid as well as the maternal thyroid.

   Antithyroid drugs include iodide (discussed above) and the thionamides. The principal thionamides are propylthiouracil and methimazole. Almost all patients respond promptly to these agents. However, immunologic complications are not rare. Skin rashes are the most common. Agranulocytosis, cholestatic jaundice, hepatocellular damage, and exfoliative dermatitis are uncommon. Surgical thyroidectomy is the treatment of choice for patients with very large or multinodular glands. Patients must be treated preoperatively with antithyroid drugs until they are euthyroid, and they receive iodine for 2 weeks prior to surgery to reduce vascularity of the gland.

3. Radioactive iodine is therapeutically effective by virtue of the radiation damage caused by the beta rays emitted by the isotope. The damage is limited to the thyroid because the element is so avidly concentrated by the gland.

   Antithyroid thionamides appear to act through several mechanisms. The most important is inhibition of incorporation of iodine into protein tyrosine residues by peroxidase. A second effect is inhibition of the coupling of diiodotyrosines to form thyroxine. In addition, the drugs may have an immunosuppressive effect. Propylthiouracil also inhibits the conversion of thyroxine to triiodothyronine.

   The actions of nonradioactive iodide have been mentioned above. The primary mechanism of action is the inhibition of hormone release. The mechanism for the reduced glandular vascularity caused by iodide is not known.

4. Patients in a thyrotoxic crisis usually have multiple system involvement. The cardiovascular system is particularly susceptible, and severe tachycardia, arrhythmias, and heart failure are common. The sympathetic nervous system is hyperactive, and this is one of the major causes of the cardiovascular effects. The CNS is also affected, and signs may include severe agitation, delirium, and coma.

   Sympathoplegic drugs are very useful in thyrotoxicosis. Propranolol is the most commonly used. Further release of hormone from the gland is blocked by intravenous administration of sodium iodide, supplemented with oral potassium iodide. Synthesis is inhibited by oral or, if necessary, parenteral antithyroid drugs. Corticosteroids are sometimes used.

## Answers, Case 12

1. In a young diabetic of normal weight with a history of viral infections preceding the onset of hyperglycemia, it is likely that the disease is due to loss of functioning pancreatic islet B cells. The diagnosis of insulin-dependent (type I) diabetes mellitus was made in this case. The oral hypoglycemic agents are not useful in type I diabetes. Therefore, the strategies available are dietary management and insulin.

2. The most important acute complication of insulin therapy is hypoglycemia. This is an emergency that the patient and his or her family must be prepared to deal with, since it may occur suddenly or insidiously and can result in death or brain damage if not treated promptly and effectively. Treatment is by administration of glucose or glucagon.

   The long-term complications of insulin therapy include immunologic problems such as insulin allergy and insulin resistance caused by formation of antibodies to the insulin used. These effects can be minimized by the use of purified preparations, which contain lower concentrations of noninsulin protein, or by the use of human insulin preparations.

   Another complication of insulin therapy is lipodystrophy at the site of injection. This consists of atrophy of the subcutaneous lipid tissue. It has become much less common since the advent of improved methods of purifying insulin, and even the standard preparations are relatively free of the effect. In fact, lipid hypertrophy may occur.

   The complications of the oral hypoglycemic drugs are more varied than those of insulin therapy. Tolbutamide is associated with a low incidence of skin rashes and interactions with other drugs that result in prolonged hypoglycemia. Chlorpropamide causes prolonged hypoglycemia more often than tolbutamide, as well as jaundice and an antidiuretic effect. The latter action may cause dilutional hyponatremia. The "second-generation" agents (glipizide, glyburide) are so much more potent than the older sulfonylureas that care must be exercised to avoid significant hypoglycemia.

3. Most patients should monitor their blood or urine glucose as an aid to adjustment of insulin dosage. The major reason for daily adjustment of dosage is that insulin requirement is altered by many factors—diet, exercise, disease, etc.

   The major adjustments made by most patients are the total number of units of insulin injected and the proportions of rapid-acting and intermediate- or long-acting preparations used.

## Answers, Case 13

1. The only significant advantage of adrenocorticotropin (ACTH) over corticosteroids is the prevention of adrenal suppression. There may be less suppression of growth in children when ACTH is used. However, it must be given parenterally and it causes increased mineralocorticoid as well as glucocorticoid secretion. Therefore, glucocorticoids are almost always selected for the treatment of chronic inflammatory disease.
2. The normal diurnal variation of glucocorticoid release includes a peak in the morning hours and a trough late at night. Therefore, a single dose of a long-acting (12–24 hours) agent such as prednisone mimics the normal variation and reduces the degree of suppression of the pituitary.
3. Alternate-day therapy permits a greater degree of pituitary-adrenal interaction to be maintained and also allows temporary recovery of peripheral tissues from stimulation by high levels of glucocorticoid. This is particularly valuable in growing children.

   The longest-acting corticosteroids are not suitable for alternate-day regimens, because the duration of pituitary suppression is over 48 hours and so nothing is gained. These agents include paramethasone, dexamethasone, and betamethasone.
4. The toxic effects of corticosteroids include adrenocortical suppression, iatrogenic Cushing's syndrome (weight gain, buffalo hump, striae, osteoporosis, diabetes), peptic ulcers, cataracts, glaucoma, and psychoses. Because of the serious nature of these adverse effects, strenuous attempts should be made to switch this patient to another form of therapy. Alternative drugs include the gold compounds, hydroxychloroquine, and penicillamine.

## Answers, Case 14

1. The principal justification for empiric, presumptive antimicrobial therapy is that the infection is best treated early to avoid serious morbidity or death. Suspected bacterial meningitis is a classic example of the need to initiate therapy immediately on the basis of the clinical diagnosis and the initial microbiologic diagnosis. The latter should include history, physical signs, and Gram stain.
2. *Haemophilus influenzae* type b is a common cause of bacterial meningitis in patients of this age group. Ampicillin is effective against many strains of this organism and will also cover for infections caused by pneumococci, meningococci, and *Escherichia coli*. However, *H influenzae* resistance to ampicillin is increasing, and it is not uncommon to use chloramphenicol (in combination with ampicillin) until microbiologic laboratory results identify the infecting organism and document its susceptibility to antimicrobial drugs.
3. The microbiologic laboratory confirmed *H influenzae* type b and demonstrated that the isolate was beta-lactamase-positive. Remember that ampicillin and amoxicillin are inactivated by penicillinases and that production of such enzymes by gram-negative bacilli (and staphylococci) is a mechanism of bacterial resistance to these drugs.
4. Although the cerebrospinal fluid was apparently sterile, the counterimmunoelectrophoresis analysis suggests a relapse due to *H influenzae* type b, because either of inadequate treatment with chloramphenicol or development of resistance. Further microbiologic laboratory examinations revealed that the isolate was relatively insensitive to chloramphenicol (ie, high minimum bactericidal concentration and minimum inhibitory concentration) and also produced acetyltransferases that could inactivate the drug. The production of this drug-inactivating enzyme is a mechanism of plasmid-mediated resistance.
5. Resistance of *H influenzae* isolates to both ampicillin and chloramphenicol is rare. The treatment of infections due to such organisms may be difficult. In this case, certain third-generation cephalosporins such as moxalactam and ceftriaxone may be effective in meningi-

tis and presently have activity against several important gram-negative pathogens. Moxalactam is more toxic than ceftriaxone and is now rarely used. ***Note:*** Resistance has occurred to the newer cephalosporins, and they should therefore be used judiciously.

6. This patient was not a neonate; therefore, her liver glucuronyltransferase activity would probably be adequate to prevent accumulation of chloramphenicol leading to the "gray baby" syndrome. Gastrointestinal irritation, a problem in adults, is rare in children. The most likely toxicity in this case is dose-dependent reversible arrest of red cell maturation, leading to anemia and reticulocytopenia. Remember that aplastic anemia, although rare, is a potential toxic effect of chloramphenicol.

## Answers, Case 15

1. Chemoprophylaxis is indicated when the wound infection rate for surgical procedures, under optimal conditions, is 5% or more. This patient had been treated for cancer, possibly with immunosuppressive agents, and may have been at particular risk for infection.
2. The cephalosporins are the most commonly used antimicrobial agents for surgical prophylaxis because they have activity against gram-positive cocci and selected gram-negative bacilli that are likely pathogens. Frequently, a first-generation drug (cephalothin or cefazolin) is used, but under certain circumstances a second-generation cephalosporin, such as cefoxitin, may be given. Cefoxitin is somewhat less active against gram-positive organisms and more active against *Serratia marcescens,* indole-positive *Proteus,* and other beta-lactamase-producing gram-negative bacteria.
3. The patient experienced a classic type I (immediate) IgE-mediated allergic reaction, which often includes anaphylaxis, urticaria, and angioedema. Antimicrobial drugs, particularly members of the penicillin group, can cause type I reactions, and the cephalosporins also have this potential since they have some features of molecular structure in common with penicillins. The degree of cross-allergenicity between the 2 drug groups remains controversial, perhaps between 6 and 16%. Skin testing with a dilute solution of drug may reveal drug sensitivity but often gives false-negative results.
4. The afferent limb of this immune response involves the drug acting as a hapten (often via a carrier protein), proliferation of lymphoid B cells to produce IgE antibodies, and their fixation to blood basophils or tissue mast cells. Upon reexposure to the drug (efferent limb), the sensitized basophils or mast cells bind the antigens and are stimulated to release chemical mediators (histamine, leukotrienes, etc) that initiate tissue responses, which in turn cause tissue injury, inflammation, and, sometimes, lethal effects.
5. Epinephrine, isoproterenol, and theophylline block the release of mediators from mast cells and basophils (via cAMP mechanisms) and produce bronchodilation. Diphenhydramine competitively blocks histamine actions at $H_1$ receptors, actions that would otherwise cause bronchoconstriction and increased capillary permeability. Dexamethasone probably has multiple effects, including inhibition of IgE-producing clone proliferation, block of T helper cell function, and anti-inflammatory actions.
6. Cardiovascular changes during a type I drug allergic reaction could be secondary to hypoxia due to bronchoconstriction, especially in the presence of ischemic heart disease. Animal studies also show that the heart may be a target organ in systemic allergic reactions (Capurro N, Levi R: *Circ Res* 1975;**36:**520) and, as inferred by the reporters of this case, the acute cardiac injury that followed cefoxitin administration may reflect cardiac sensitization to IgE-mediated antigens.

## Answers, Case 16

1. There is no information in the history of the original upper respiratory tract infection regarding possible (or confirmed) pathogens or their susceptibility to antimicrobial drugs. Erythromycin has activity against common streptococci, staphylococci (including penicillinase-producing strains), and *Mycoplasma pneumoniae,* as well as other less commonly occurring respiratory tract bacterial pathogens. Such data presumably underlie the choice of the drug in this case. However, erythromycin has limited activity against most strains of *Haemophilus influenzae*. The drug has few adverse effects, although some gastrointestinal irritation and occasional liver dysfunction may occur. There is no cross-allergenicity with the penicillin group, which is another reason some physicians prefer erythromycin.
2. The suspected sinusitis had not responded to erythromycin. Since attempts to positively confirm bacterial infection had failed, amoxicillin therapy was started on empiric grounds. Re-

sembling ampicillin but better absorbed orally, amoxicillin has activity against many streptococci and *H influenzae* strains as well as selected gram-negative rods. It is not resistant to penicillinase, including that produced by *Staphylococcus aureus,* and it has no activity against *M pneumoniae*. However, these organisms should have been eradicated by the prior treatment with erythromycin. Allergic reactions to amoxicillin can occur if a patient is sensitive to any penicillin.

3. Ampicillin is more likely to cause diarrhea than other penicillins, partly by causing direct gastrointestinal irritant effects and partly by disturbing the normal gut flora. In this case, its close congener, amoxicillin, resulted in diarrhea that persisted for over a week after drug discontinuance, suggesting the possibility of microbial overgrowth. This was confirmed by culture revealing colonization by *Clostridium difficile*. This organism has been identified more commonly in recent years as an opportunistic pathogen of the gastrointestinal tract following antimicrobial drug treatment. It causes colitis following therapy with various antibiotics, including clindamycin, the tetracyclines, and beta-lactam agents.
4. Pseudomembranous colitis is a superinfection associated with the elaboration of toxins by *C difficile*. The toxins are cytotoxic to mucosal cells, causing ulceration and "pseudomembrane" formation revealed by sigmoidoscopy. Diarrhea may be severe (with abdominal pain), with stools containing mucous membrane shreds, blood, and many neutrophils. Fever is usually present. The syndrome may be lethal.
5. When given orally, vancomycin has been effective in the treatment of colitis caused by toxin-producing bacteria, including *C difficile*. It is also a first-choice drug in the treatment of gastrointestinal superinfections due to staphylococci, including penicillinase-producing and methicillin-resistant strains. Vancomycin is poorly absorbed after oral administration, and there is a low risk of causing the ototoxicity and nephrotoxicity that occur with intravenous administration.

## Answers, Case 17

1. The most common causes of traveler's diarrhea are infections due to coliform bacteria and viruses. Although antibiotics, including doxycycline, may be used for prophylaxis against bacterial dysentery, antimicrobial therapy should not be used for routine treatment for several reasons. Most such infections are self-limiting, and fluid and electrolyte replacement is usually adequate treatment. The antibiotics are not effective in gastrointestinal infections due to viruses and have minimal activity against intestinal protozoan parasites, including amebas.
2. Ampicillin and gentamicin were included in the drug regimen on the basis of a possible bacterial involvement in acute cholecystitis, a component of the initial clinical diagnosis. Ampicillin would give coverage for streptococci (including enterococci) and selected gram-negative enteric organisms, including *Escherichia coli, Shigella,* and *Salmonella* strains. Gentamicin is active against gram-negative rods, including *E coli, Enterobacter, Klebsiella,* and *Pseudomonas* strains. Neither drug has good activity against gram-negative anaerobes, and anaerobic bacteria are a major cause of bacterial liver abscess.
3. The confirmed diagnosis of amebic disease justified empiric therapy with metronidazole, which is the drug of choice in most cases of extraluminal amebiasis, although it is not a luminal amebicide. Metronidazole also has antibacterial actions, including activity against gram-negative anaerobes. Chloroquine is sometimes added, since it is a hepatic amebicide. Oral tetracycline is an inhibitor of bacteria that associate with *Entamoeba histolytica* in the gut, and it may indirectly affect luminal amebas by such an action. Diloxanide furoate and iodoquinol are more effective as luminal amebicides.
4. Common adverse effects of metronidazole include metallic taste, glossitis, gastrointestinal irritation, and headache. Rarely, the drug causes leukopenia, dizziness, and ataxia. It can also cause disulfiramlike reactions to ethanol. Tetracyclines cause gastrointestinal irritation, superinfections due to *Candida albicans* or bacteria, renal dysfunction, skin reactions, and, rarely, hepatotoxicity.
5. The halogenated hydroxyquinolines such as iodoquinol are not effective in severe intestinal disease due to *E histolytica* or in amebic hepatic abscess. They are used to treat concurrent intestinal infection and to totally eradicate the protozoan, preventing treatment failures and recurrence of symptoms of disease.

## Answers, Case 18

1. Chloroquine and its 4-aminoquinoline congeners complex with DNA by insertion between

base pairs and prevent its replication or transcription to RNA. A chloroquine-concentrating mechanism in parasitized cells accounts for the selective toxicity of the drug. The pyrimethamine-sulfadoxine combination inhibits the synthesis of folic acid via sequential blockade of dihydropteroate synthase and dihydrofolate reductase.

2. Oxamniquine is active against mature and immature forms of *Schistosoma mansoni* (but not other *Schistosoma* spp), although resistance can occur. Its choice was presumably based on identification of the parasite ova in stools, its ease of administration (it is orally effective), and its low incidence of adverse effects. Praziquantel is equivalent as the drug of choice in this case and also has activity against all *Schistosoma* spp. Other possible drugs for schistosomiasis include niridazole (which has adverse effects, including psychiatric symptoms), metrifonate (active only against *Schistosoma haematobium* and therefore not applicable in this case), and antimony compounds (which have more serious toxic potential).
3. Praziquantel is effective in infections with all species of schistosomes. It increases the permeability of the parasite cell membrane to calcium, causing initial contraction and then paralysis of its musculature. The tegmen becomes vacuolized and disintegrates, causing parasite death.
4. Adverse effects of oxamniquine include dizziness, headache, drowsiness, gastrointestinal irritation, and pruritus. Effects probably due to dying parasites include eosinophilia, pulmonary infiltrates, and urticaria. Stimulation of the CNS may occur, resulting in hallucinations and seizures. The most common toxic effects of praziquantel are malaise, headache, dizziness, gastrointestinal irritation, urticaria, and fever. Some of these effects may be caused by dying parasites.
5. Praziquantel is contraindicated in pregnancy, since animal studies show that it increases the abortion rate. The drug may act as a comutagen in test systems. Oxamniquine is also mutagenic and is embryocidal in animal test systems.
6. Corticosteroids are used to suppress host immune responses and inflammation, including reactions to eggs deposited in the venules in and around the spinal cord.

# Appendix IV.

# Strategies for Improving Test Performance

There are many "strategies" for studying and exam taking, and decisions about which ones to use are partly a function of individual habit and preference.

## FIVE BASIC STUDY RULES

1. Never read more than a few pages of dense textual material without stopping to write out the gist of it from memory. This is a universal rule for effective study. Refer to the material just read as required. After finishing a chapter, make up tables of the major drugs, receptor types, mechanisms, etc, and fill in as many of the blanks as you can. This is active learning; just reading is passive and far less effective unless you happen to have a photographic memory. Notes should be legible and saved for ready access in reviewing before exams.
2. Experiment with other study methods until you find out what works for you. This may involve solo study or group study, flash cards, or text reading. You won't know how effective these techniques are until you have tried them.
3. Don't scorn "cramming," but don't rely on it either. Some steady, day-by-day reading and digestion of conceptual material is usually needed to avoid last-minute indigestion.
4. When taking "objective" examinations such as the National Boards, don't change your first "guess" unless you find a convincing reason for doing so.
5. If you are taking a lecture course, make every effort to attend *all* of the lectures. The lecturer's view of what is important may be very different from that of the author of the textbook, and the chances are good that exam questions will be based on the instructor's own lecture notes.

## STRATEGIES FOR SPECIFIC QUESTION FORMATS

A certain group of students—often characterized as "good test-takers"—may not know every detail about the subject matter being tested but seem to perform extremely well most of the time. The strategy used by these people is not a secret, although few instructors seem to realize how easy it is to break down their questions into much simpler ones. Lists of these strategies are widely available, eg, in the descriptive material distributed by the National Board of Medical Examiners to its candidates. A paraphrased compendium of this advice is presented below.

### A. Strategies for the "Choose the one best answer" (of 5 choices) Type Question:

1. If 2 statements are contradictory (ie, only one can be correct), chances are better than 50% that one is the correct answer; ie, the other 3 choices are distractors. For example, consider the following:

In treating quinidine overdose, the best strategy would be to

(A) Alkalize the urine
(B) Acidify the urine
(C) Give procainamide
(D) Give potassium chloride
(E) Administer a calcium chelator such as EDTA

The correct answer is **(B)**, acidify the urine. The instructor revealed what was being tested for in the first pair of choices and used the last 3 as "filler." Therefore, *if you don't know the answer,* you are better off guessing **(A)** or **(B)** (a 50% success rate) than **(A)** or **(B)** or **(C)** or **(D)** or **(E)** (a 20% success rate).

2. A statement is not false just because changing a few words will make it somewhat more true than you think it is now. "Choose the one best answer" does not mean "Choose the only correct statement."
3. Statements that contain the words "always," "must," etc, are usually false. For example,

   Acetylcholine always increases the heart rate when given intravenously because it lowers blood pressure and evokes a strong baroreceptor-mediated reflex tachycardia.

   The statement is false, because although acetylcholine often increases the heart rate by the reflex mechanism mentioned in the question, it can also cause bradycardia. (When given as a bolus, it may reach the sinus node in high enough concentration to cause initial bradycardia.) The use of "trigger" words such as "always" and "must" suggests that the instructor had some exception in mind.

## B. Strategies for the "Answer A if 1, 2, and 3 are correct" Type Question:*

For this type of question, one rarely must know the truth about all 4 statements to arrive at the correct answer. The instructions are to select

(A) if only **(1)**, **(2)**, and **(3)** are correct;
(B) if only **(1)** and **(3)** are correct;
(C) if only **(2)** and **(4)** are correct;
(D) if only **(4)** is correct;
(E) if all are correct.

Useful strategies include the following:

1. If choice **(1)** is right and **(2)** is wrong, the answer must be **(B)**, ie, **(1)** and **(3)** are correct. You don't need to know anything about **(3)** or **(4)**.
2. If statement **(1)** is wrong, then statement **(3)** must also be wrong and answers **(A)**, **(B)**, and **(E)** are automatically excluded. Concentrate on statements **(2)** and **(4)**.
3. The converse of 1 above: If choice **(1)** is wrong and **(2)** is right, the answer must be **(C)**, ie, **(2)** and **(4)** are correct.
4. If statement **(2)** is correct and **(4)** is wrong, the answer is **(A)**, ie, **(1)** and **(3)** must be correct and you need not even look at them. (See example below.)
5. If statements **(1)**, **(2)**, and **(4)** are correct, the answer must be **(E)**. You need not know anything about **(3)**.
6. Similarly, if statements **(2)** and **(3)** are right and **(4)** is wrong, the answer must be **(A)**, and statement **(1)** must be correct.
7. If statements **(2)**, **(3)**, and **(4)** are correct, then the answer must be **(E)**, and statement **(1)** must be correct.

No doubt more of these rules exist. In general, if you "know" whether 2 or 3 of the 4 statements in each question are right or wrong (ie, 50–75% the material), you should achieve a perfect score on this kind of question. The best way to learn these rules is to apply them to practice questions until the principles are firmly ingrained.

*This question type ("K type") will no longer be used in the United Stated Medical Licensure Examination (USMLE) Step 1.

Consider the following question. Using the above rules, you should be able to answer it correctly even though there is no reason why you should know anything about the information contained in 2 of the 4 statements. The answer follows.

| A | B | C | D | E |
|---|---|---|---|---|
| 1, 2, 3 only | 1, 3 only | 2, 4 only | 4 only | All are correct |

**(1)** The "struck bushel" is equal to 2150.42 cubic inches
**(2)** Medicine is one of the health sciences
**(3)** The fresh meat of the Atlantic salmon contains 220 IU of vitamin A per 100-g edible portion
**(4)** Hippocrates was the founder of modern psychoanalysis

The answer is **(A).** Since statement **(2)** is clearly correct, and **(4)** is just as patently incorrect (let's give Freud the credit), the answer can only be **(A),** and statements **(1)** and **(3)** must be correct. (The data are from Lentner C [editor]: *Geigy Scientific Tables,* 8th ed. Vol. 1. Ciba-Geigy, 1981.)

# Index

Page numbers in **boldface** type indicate a major discussion. Page numbers followed by a t or an f indicate tables or figures, respectively.

## Basic Science Textbooks

*Jawetz, Melnick & Adelberg's*
**Medical Microbiology, 19/e**
*Brooks, Butel & Ornston*
1991, ISBN 0-8385-6241-8, A6241-2

**Concise Pathology**
*Chandrasoma & Taylor*
1991, ISBN 0-8385-1320-4, A1320-9

**Correlative Neuroanatomy, 21/e**
*deGroot & Chusid*
1991, ISBN 0-8385-1332-8, A1332-4

**Review of Medical Physiology, 15/e**
*Ganong*
1991, ISBN 0-8385-8418-7, A8418-4

**Physiology: A Study Guide, 3/e**
*Ganong*
1989, ISBN 0-8385-7875-6, A7875-6

**Basic Histology, 7/e**
*Junqueira, Carniero & Kelly*
1992, ISBN 0-8385-0576-7, A0576-7

**Basic & Clinical Pharmacology, 5/e**
*Katzung*
1992, ISBN 0-8385-0562-7, A0562-7

**Pharmacology: Examination & Review, 3/e**
*Katzung & Trevor*
1992, ISBN 0-8385-7807-1, A7807-9

**Medical Microbiology & Immunology**
***Examination & Board Review, 2/e***
*Levinson & Jawetz*
1991, ISBN 0-8385-6262-0, A6262-8

**Harper's Biochemistry, 22/e**
*Murray, et al.*
1991, ISBN 0-8385-3640-9, A3640-8

**Basic Histology**
***Examination & Board Review, 2/e***
*Paulsen*
1992, ISBN 0-8385-0569-4, A0569-2

**Basic & Clinical Immunology, 7/e**
*Stites & Terr*
1991, ISBN 0-8385-0544-9, A0544-5

**Basic Human Immunology**
*Stites & Terr*
1991, ISBN 0-8385-0543-0, A0543-7

## Clinical Science Textbooks

**Fluid & Electrolytes**
***Physiology & Pathophysiology***
*Cogan*
1991, ISBN 0-8385-2546-6, A2546-8

**Basic and Clinical Biostatistics**
*Dawson-Saunders & Trapp*
1990, ISBN 0-8385-6200-0, A6200-8

**Review of General Psychiatry, 3/e**
*Goldman*
1992, ISBN 0-8385-8428-4, A8428-3

**Principles of Clinical Electrocardiography, 13/e**
*Goldschlager & Goldman*
1989, ISBN 0-8385-7951-5, A7951-5

**Basic and Clinical Endocrinology, 3/e**
*Greenspan*
1990, ISBN 0-8385-0545-7, A0545-2

**Occupational Medicine**
*LaDou*
1990, ISBN 0-8385-7207-3, A7207-2

**Clinical Anatomy**
*Lindner*
1989, ISBN 0-8385-1259-3, A1259-9

**Clinical Anesthesiology**
*Morgan & Mikhail*
1992, ISBN 0-8385-1324-7, A1324-1

**Dermatology**
*Orkin, Maibach & Dahl*
1991, ISBN 0-8385-1288-7, A1288-8

**Clinical Neurology, 2/e**
*Simon, Aminoff & Greenberg*
1992, ISBN 0-8385-1311-5, A1311-8

**Clinical Cardiology, 5/e**
*Sokolow, McIlroy & Cheitlin*
1990, ISBN 0-8385-1266-6, A1266-4

**Clinical Thinking in Surgery**
*Sterns*
1988, ISBN 0-8385-5686-8, A5686-9

**Smith's General Urology, 13/e**
*Tanagho & McAninch*
1992, ISBN 0-8385-8600-2, A8608-0

**General Ophthalmology, 13/e**
*Vaughan, Asbury & Riordan-Eva*
1992, ISBN 0-8385-3115-6, A3115-1

## CURRENT Clinical References

**CURRENT Pediatric Diagnosis & Treatment, 11/e**
*Hathaway, et al.*
1992, ISBN 0-8385-1440-5, A1440-5

**CURRENT Obstetric & Gynecologic Diagnosis & Treatment, 7/e**
*Pernoll*
1991, ISBN 0-8385-1424-3, A1424-9

**CURRENT Emergency Diagnosis & Treatment, 4/e**
*Saunders & Ho*
1992, ISBN 0-8385-1347-6, A1347-2

**CURRENT Medical Diagnosis & Treatment 1992, 31/e**
*Schroeder, et al.*
1992, ISBN 0-8385-1438-3, A1438-9

**CURRENT Surgical Diagnosis & Treatment, 9/e**
*Way*
1991, ISBN 0-8385-1426-X, A1426-4

***Order information on reverse.***

## LANGE Clinical Manuals

**Dermatology**
***Diagnosis and Therapy***
*Bondi, Jegasothy & Lazarus*
1990, ISBN 0-8385-1274-7, A1274-8

**Office & Bedside Procedures**
*Chesnutt & Dewar*
1992, ISBN 0-8385-1095-7, A1095-7

**Psychiatry**
***Diagnosis & Treatment, 2/e***
*Flaherty, Davis & Janicak*
1992, ISBN 0-8385-1267-4, A1267-2

**Neonatology**
***Management, Procedures, On-Call Problems, Diseases, Drugs, 2/e***
*Gomella*
1992, ISBN 0-8385-1284-4, A1284-7

**Clinician's Pocket Reference, 6/e**
*Gomella*
1989, ISBN 0-8385-1212-7, A1212-8

**Drug Therapy, 2/e**
*Katzung*
1991, ISBN 0-8385-1312-3, A1312-6

**Poisoning and Drug Overdose**
*Olson*
1990, ISBN 0-8385-1297-6, A1297-9

**Ambulatory Medicine**
***Primary Care of Families***
*Schwiebert & Mengle*
1992, ISBN 0-8385-1294-1, A1294-6

**Internal Medicine**
***Diagnosis and Therapy, 2/e***
*Stein*
1991, ISBN 0-8385-1299-2, A1299-5

**Surgery**
***Diagnosis & Therapy***
*Stillman*
1989, ISBN 0-8385-1283-6, A1283-9

**Medical Perioperative Management**
*Wolfsthal*
1989, ISBN 0-8385-1298-4, A1298-7

## LANGE Handbooks

**Handbook of Gynecology & Obstetrics**
*Brown & Crombleholme*
1992, ISBN 0-8385-3608-5, A3608-5

**Handbook of Clinical Endocrinology, 2/e**
*Fitzgerald*
1991, ISBN 0-8385-3615-8, A3615-0

***Silver, Kempe, Bruyn & Fulginiti's***
**Handbook of Pediatrics, 16/e**
*Merenstein, Kaplan & Rosenberg*
1991, ISBN 0-8385-3639-5, A3639-0

**Pocket Guide to Commonly Prescribed Drugs**
*Levine*
1992, ISBN 0-8385-8023-8, A8023-2

**Pocket Guide to Diagnostic Tests**
*Detmer, et al.*
1992, ISBN 0-8385-8020-3, A8020-8